Infection Prevention in Athletes

EDITOR | Deverick J. Anderson | MD, MPH, FSHEA, FIDSA

Director, Duke Center for Antimicrobial Stewardship and Infection Prevention
Professor of Medicine
Division of Infectious Diseases
Duke University Medical Center
Durham, North Carolina

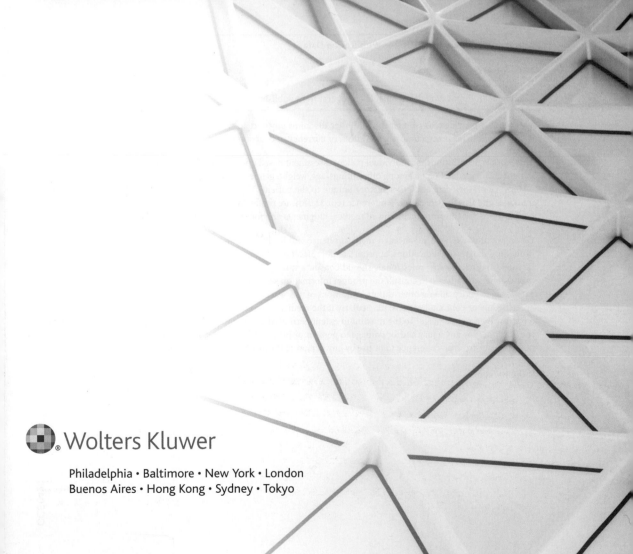

. Wolters Kluwer

Philadelphia • Baltimore • New York • London
Buenos Aires • Hong Kong • Sydney • Tokyo

D0713592

Executive Editor: Sharon Zinner
Development Editor: Thomas Celona
Editorial Coordinator: Julie Kostelnik
Marketing Manager: Phyllis Hitner
Production Project Manager: Kirstin Johnson
Design Coordinator: Holly McLaughlin
Manufacturing Coordinator: Karin Duffield
Illustrator: Holly R. Fischer
Prepress Vendor: TNQ Technologies

Copyright © 2021 Wolters Kluwer.

All rights reserved. This book is protected by copyright. No part of this book may be reproduced or transmitted in any form or by any means, including as photocopies or scanned-in or other electronic copies, or utilized by any information storage and retrieval system without written permission from the copyright owner, except for brief quotations embodied in critical articles and reviews. Materials appearing in this book prepared by individuals as part of their official duties as U.S. government employees are not covered by the above-mentioned copyright. To request permission, please contact Wolters Kluwer at Two Commerce Square, 2001 Market Street, Philadelphia, PA 19103, via email at permissions@lww.com, or via our website at shop.lww.com (products and services).

9 8 7 6 5 4 3 2 1

Printed in China

Library of Congress Cataloging-in-Publication Data

ISBN-13: 978-1-9751-3724-3

Cataloging in Publication data available on request from publisher.

This work is provided "as is," and the publisher disclaims any and all warranties, express or implied, including any warranties as to accuracy, comprehensiveness, or currency of the content of this work.

This work is no substitute for individual patient assessment based upon healthcare professionals' examination of each patient and consideration of, among other things, age, weight, gender, current or prior medical conditions, medication history, laboratory data and other factors unique to the patient. The publisher does not provide medical advice or guidance and this work is merely a reference tool. Healthcare professionals, and not the publisher, are solely responsible for the use of this work including all medical judgments and for any resulting diagnosis and treatments.

Given continuous, rapid advances in medical science and health information, independent professional verification of medical diagnoses, indications, appropriate pharmaceutical selections and dosages, and treatment options should be made and healthcare professionals should consult a variety of sources. When prescribing medication, healthcare professionals are advised to consult the product information sheet (the manufacturer's package insert) accompanying each drug to verify, among other things, conditions of use, warnings and side effects and identify any changes in dosage schedule or contraindications, particularly if the medication to be administered is new, infrequently used or has a narrow therapeutic range. To the maximum extent permitted under applicable law, no responsibility is assumed by the publisher for any injury and/or damage to persons or property, as a matter of products liability, negligence law or otherwise, or from any reference to or use by any person of this work.

shop.lww.com

CCS0420

Dedication

To Ann, Henry, William, and Charlie—whom I love and adore

Acknowledgments

The authors would like to acknowledge the numerous athletic trainers and team physicians who have provided input, feedback, and support for our program. In particular, we would like to thank Mr. Ronnie Barnes, Head Athletic Trainer of the New York Football Giants and long-term advocate for player safety. Our program and this text book would not be possible without his support.

Foreword

There are many reasons to participate in sports. Sports are part of our culture. They are part of our lives. And for good reason. Sports bring joy, excitement, discipline, and improved health. Sports teach many lessons that translate directly and indirectly to life in our complicated world. Among the many lessons learned through sports, athletes learn strategies to (1) optimize performance and health and (2) overcome adversity.

Of course, sports can lead to risks for athletes. Anyone who has participated in sports has likely suffered bumps, bruises, or in some cases, more serious injuries such as sprained ankles, concussions, or torn ACLs. In my job and for most of my career, I have tried to answer the question, "What can we do to improve the health of athletes and decrease risk of harm?"

One risk for athletes explored in detail in this textbook is the risk of infection. Many of us in the medical community have seen an athlete contract an infection. Most of the time, these infections are minor and do not cause long-lasting effects. Occasionally, infections in athletes can be devastating, leading to lost careers or, worst of all, loss of life.

The Duke Infection Control Outreach Network (DICON) Program for Infection Prevention in the NFL has been in place for 7 years. I have had the pleasure of working with Dr Anderson and his team during my tenure as the Chief Medical Officer for the NFL for the past 3 years. Dr Anderson's program is highly regarded among physicians and athletic trainers throughout all 32 NFL clubs. When an infection-related issue comes up in our league, the DICON team is the go-to group. As a direct result of this program, our clubs now systematically use standardized strategies to reduce the risk of infections in our athletes. I'm confident the materials and approach promoted by DICON and used in the NFL can be translated to other settings, sports, and levels of competition, where appropriate.

One critical component of the DICON Program in the NFL is the extensive data review and information that Dr Anderson and colleagues have gathered. Presented as best practices and recommendations, these authors do an excellent job of translating science, data, and expert guidance into practical advice for physicians, athletic trainers, and athletes. I have made it clear to Dr Anderson and others in our medical community that I want to promote, where relevant, the best practices used in the NFL to all other sports and at all other levels. So, I was thrilled when Dr Anderson began discussing the development of this textbook. I'm equally thrilled to write the foreword for this impressive work.

The authors have taken the material developed for the NFL and expanded it so it is relevant for all athletes. A key component of the presented material is the use of the "Framework" for infection prevention. Dr Anderson and his team provide crucial information about risks and strategies to mitigate those risks in four components of the framework: personal and social behaviors, medical care, interactions with other athletes, and shared equipment. Throughout the textbook, you'll receive practical tips and advice for strategies to move from a recommendation written on a piece of paper to effective action in the athletic training facility. Dr Anderson's team invokes important themes for prevention but most importantly *make it easy to do the right thing*.

I'd recommend this book, whether you are an athlete, an athlete's parent, or a member of team medical staff working with athletes. Material presented in this book can help to reduce risk and keep players safe. The approach taken by the authors should be familiar to most athletes and coaches—focus on the fundamentals, educate to develop a solid foundation of knowledge, and utilize strategies that are most likely to succeed.

In summary, Dr Anderson and the DICON team are leading experts on infection prevention in athletes. We must continue to pursue and implement the best strategies to improve athletes' health and reduce risks at every opportunity. I strongly encourage you to use the information provided in this book in that pursuit.

Dr Allen Sills
NFL Chief Medical Officer

Introduction

Risk of infection is an occupational hazard for athletes. In other words, infections among athletes will occur and should be expected. While infection risk for athletes will never be zero, the goal is to reduce this risk to the lowest level possible. In this book, we provide best practices, recommendations, strategies, and tips to achieve this goal. Through this content, we want to improve the quality and increase the safety of care provided to athletes in all settings.

The foundation for the recommendations included in this book is based on one major tenet: **athletic training facilities are medical facilities**. Many of the same infection prevention practices and recommendations related to medical care provided in hospitals and outpatient clinics are applicable guides for infection prevention in athletic training facilities. As a result, this book includes many of the guiding principles and basic practices used in these medical facilities to reduce the risk of infection.

Infection risks for athletes can be separated into four categories: personal and social behaviors, medical care, interactions with other athletes, and use of facilities and equipment (Figure 1). Transmission can be direct (eg, person to person from other athletes, training staff, or clinicians) or indirect (eg, via contamination of the environment or equipment). Transmission of pathogens among athletes is facilitated by frequent skin injuries, the close proximity of players in training facilities and team activities, and by the frequent administration of routine medical care. Implementation of and adherence to the best practices throughout this book are the best strategies to decrease these risks.

The basic principles to reduce the risk of infection can be summarized in a few simple statements and concepts that permeate the materials in this book:

- Develop a culture of safety
- Make it easy to do the right thing
- Use a systematic approach to implementation
- Hygiene
- Preferentially use single-use disposable medical equipment

We use the term "culture of safety" throughout this book. The sum of our proposed best practices and recommendations will augment this culture of safety, but this culture must ultimately be generated and fostered within each facility, training staff, and team. When a culture of safety is in place, all members of the athletic training staff and players are actively engaged in monitoring and improving safe practices. Pressure to improve comes from peers and, more importantly, leaders. According to the Institute for Healthcare Improvement, an organization can develop a "culture of safety" only when leaders are openly and visibly committed to change, improvement, and open sharing of information.

Knowledge of best practices is easier to achieve than rigorous implementation of best practices. Increasing knowledge is important but insufficient on its own. Additional effort is required within each facility to ensure action and adherence to best practices and recommendations. One basic approach to assist implementation is to ensure easy access to materials necessary to implement best practices. For example, all athletic trainers know hand hygiene is important, but washing hands is a more difficult task if the only available alcohol dispenser

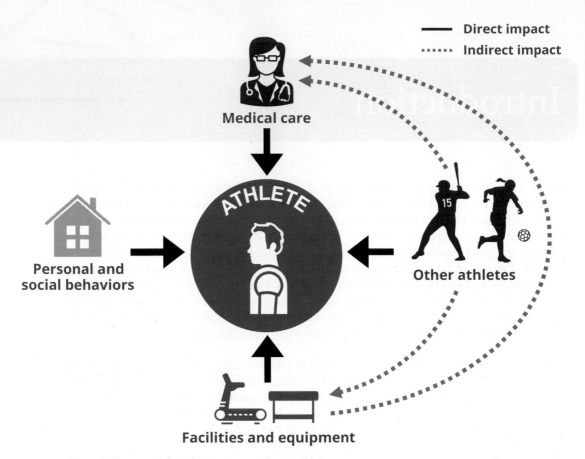

Figure 1 Framework for infection transmission in athletes.

or sink is located across the training room. Similarly, using a systematic approach improves implementation. For example, we recommend that facilities identify a single agent for disinfection and use it throughout the facility instead of using a unique disinfectant agent in every setting. Following a systematic approach improves understanding of why *and* how practices must be completed. Finally, while athletes inevitably will be exposed to potentially infectious organisms, exposure can be limited by strict adherence to (1) hand and body hygiene and (2) the use of single-use items. Hygiene breaks the transmission cycle, preventing exposure from turning into infection. Use of single-use items eliminates the risk of cross-transmission *and* simplifies processes (making it easier to do the right thing).

This book includes information for athletes and medical personnel. For each group, material is presented using the four components of the Framework for Prevention. Regardless of your role—athlete, athlete's parent, athletic trainer, team physician—we believe the material included in this book will help you practice, perform, and play in a safer environment.

Contributors

Christopher J. Hostler, MD

Assistant Professor of Medicine
Division of Infectious Diseases
Duke University School of Medicine
Durham, North Carolina
Staff physician and Associate Hospital
    Epidemiologist
Infectious Diseases Section
Durham VA Health Care System
Durham, North Carolina

Samuel Hume, MBBS (Hons), FRACP

Associate Professor
Department of Medicine
University of Melbourne (Royal Melbourne
    Hospital)
Victorian Infectious Diseases Service
Melbourne, Victoria, Australia

Tori Kinamon, BA

Medical Student, MD Candidate 2023
Duke University School of Medicine
Durham, North Carolina

Jessica Seidelman, MD, MPH

Medical Instructor
Division of Infectious Diseases
Duke University School of Medicine
Durham, North Carolina

Daniel J. Sexton, MD, FACP, FIDSA, FSHEA

Professor
Department of Medicine
Division of Infectious Diseases
Duke University School of Medicine
Durham, North Carolina

Nicholas A. Turner, MD, MHSc

Medical Instructor
Department of Medicine
Division of Infectious Diseases
Duke University School of Medicine
Durham, North Carolina

Contents

3A Cellulitis

3B MRSA

3C Abscess

3D Herpes Gladiatorum

3E Hand, Foot, and Mouth Disease

3F Tinea

3G Hepatitis A and B

3H Norovirus

3I The Flu

3J Mono

3K Whooping Cough

3L Tuberculosis

3M Chicken Pox

3N Measles

3O Mumps

3P HIV

1

Common Infections in Athletes—The Basics

Jessica Seidelman | Nicholas A. Turner

Introduction

Athletes are at increased risk for infections for several reasons. For example, athletes have frequent skin-to-skin contact and are often in crowded locker room environments. Infections can lead to adverse outcomes in athletes, including lost practice time and lost playing time. In extreme cases, infections can end athletic careers. While infections in athletes may not be entirely preventable, early recognition of infections can decrease the risk of adverse events.

This chapter summarizes common infections in athletes. We encourage athletes, parents, coaches, and team medical personnel to review the information herein. Essential information is included for each type of infection, including basic information and typical presentation. Infections highlighted in this chapter are presented because they are more common in athletes. In most instances, these infections are highlighted because they can be transmitted from athlete to athlete. As a result, this chapter also includes high-level information about strategies to prevent transmission in a locker room. Additional details on effective prevention strategies are provided throughout the remainder of the book.

Infections in this chapter are highlighted because (1) they are more common in athletes and/or (2) can be transmitted from athlete to athlete.

Localized Cutaneous Infections

Bacterial Skin Infections

DISEASE BASICS

Infections of the skin can be divided into two clinical categories: infections with pus (purulent) and infections without pus (nonpurulent).[1] Purulent skin infections are associated with drainage of pus and/or abscesses, whereas nonpurulent skin infections have inflamed skin without pus. These infections are typically caused by bacteria such as staphylococci or streptococci that are present on the skin. Infection occurs when there is a break in the skin that allows bacteria to enter.[2]

Streptococci are a group of gram-positive bacteria that cause several clinically important illnesses, including skin infections. They are broadly organized into two groups: pyogenic (beta-hemolytic) and alpha-hemolytic. For example, *Streptococcus pyogenes* (group A Strep) is a beta-hemolytic *Streptococcus* that commonly causes skin infections and can even cause necrotizing soft-tissue infection. In general, streptococci lead to cellulitis and nonpurulent skin infections.

Staphylococcus aureus is another gram-positive bacterium that commonly causes skin infections.[3] An estimated 30% of humans are colonized with *S. aureus* on their skin and in their nostrils.[3,4] However, when the skin or mucosal barriers are disrupted, *S. aureus* causes significant infections. Methicillin-resistant *Staphylococcus aureus* (MRSA) are strains of *S. aureus* that are resistant to β-lactam antibiotics and therefore can be more difficult to treat. In general, *S. aureus*—and particularly MRSA—leads to purulent skin infections.

Skin + Pus = MRSA until proven otherwise.

Risk factors for developing a bacterial skin infection include (1) a recent injury to the skin through shaving or a cut, abrasion, or scrape suffered during athletic activities; (2) the presence of a viral or fungal infection such as herpes or athlete's foot; or (3) chronic skin conditions such as eczema or psoriasis. Bacterial skin infections occur primarily in athletes with prolonged skin-to-skin contact, including wrestlers, rugby, judo, hockey, basketball, and football players. However, these infections can occur even in athletes with no risk factors and among athletes with little skin-to-skin contact.[5] Recurrence of skin infections is common: 22% to 49% of patients with a skin infection report at least one prior episode.[2]

Risk factors for skin infections? Anything that disrupts the skin barrier.

TYPICAL PRESENTATION

Bacterial skin infections can manifest in several clinical syndromes (**Figure 1.1**). One form of skin infection is called impetigo, which is characterized by well-defined, yellow crusted, scaling plaques. Erysipelas is a well-defined, erythematous plaque. Furunculosis occurs when multiple smaller boils (or pockets of pus) in the same area join together to form a large boil. Lastly, folliculitis presents as small pustules around hair follicles. *Pseudomonas* folliculitis or "hot tub folliculitis" can also occur in athletes who use hot tubs and whirlpools for rehabilitation.[6] This infection typically presents as pruritic pustules that emerge on the skin that was submerged in the whirlpool. More specifically, the affected area typically involves skin covered by the bathing suit.[6]

The most common symptom of a bacterial skin infection is a dull ache or pain at the area of involvement. Other symptoms include swelling, warmth, or redness. These symptoms typically worsen with the redness spreading over a period of hours to days. The onset of skin infections can be gradual or sudden. Itching is not a common symptom. Fever and chills can accompany bacterial skin infections but are not always present. That is, bacterial skin infections may occur in the absence of fever.

TRANSMISSION

S. aureus can spread through contact with pus or drainage from an infected wound, skin-to-skin contact with an infected person, or indirectly through a contaminated environment. These routes of transmission are common in the athletic setting due to the number of athletes

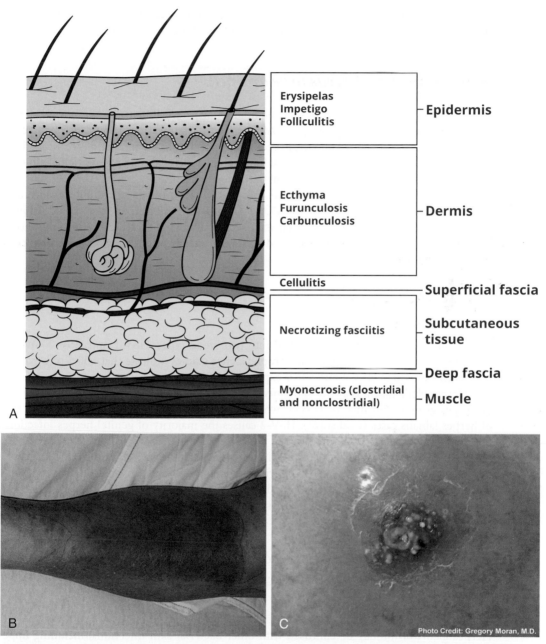

Figure 1.1 A, Skin infections and skin structures involved. B, Cellulitis. C, Abscess. (B, Reproduced with permission from: Berg D, Worzala K. *Atlas of Adult Physical Diagnosis*. Philadelphia: Lippincott Williams & Wilkins; 2006. Copyright © 2006 Lippincott Williams & Wilkins. C, Photo by Gregory Moran, MD.)

sharing the training facility and frequent, close interaction. Outbreaks of *S. aureus* skin infections have occurred in football, wresting, rugby, and basketball athletes, among others.[7-10] In one outbreak among fencers, sharing of equipment was linked to transmission of MRSA.[8]

PREVENTION MEASURES

Treatment typically includes antibiotic therapy and drainage of pus if present (typically via an incision and drainage or "I&D"). Skin lesions should be properly covered until they are healed.

Implementing therapy, covering the infection, and promptly removing infected athletes from contact with other athletes (ie, "isolation") can help decrease the number of missed practices and risk of transmission.[5]

If pus is present, it needs to be drained.

In general, athletes should not share equipment or personal items such as towels, razors, knee/elbow pads, or other athletic gear.[11] Athletes with skin infections should also avoid common areas (eg, weight rooms) and the hydrotherapy pools until the infection is controlled and can be covered. If the infected area cannot be covered, athletes should not participate in team activities such as practice and competition until the lesions heal.

For the prevention of *Pseudomonas* folliculitis, athletic trainers should ensure adequate chlorine levels and proper pH (7.0-7.4) in pools and whirlpools.[5] In addition, if trainers suspect that a pool has been exposed to an infected athlete, the pool should be drained and cleaned.[5] **See Chapter 4 for more details about routine maintenance of hydrotherapy pools.**

Herpes Gladiatorum

DISEASE BASICS

Herpes simplex virus (HSV) is classified into two broad types, HSV-1 and HSV-2. Overall, HSV infection is extremely common. Seroprevalence studies indicate that >50% of US adults have been exposed to HSV-1 and >15% exposed to HSV-2.[12]

Herpes gladiatorum is a viral skin infection caused by HSV. Nearly all reported outbreaks of herpes gladiatorum involve HSV-1, which is the same virus responsible for nearly 80% of herpes labialis cases (cold sores). HSV-2 causes the majority of genital herpes infections, but neither virus is strictly limited to one body site.[13] Since the virus gains entry to the body via small breaks in the skin, athletes involved in contact sports are at increased risk.[13] While the majority of outbreaks have been described among wrestlers, transmission between rugby players has also been described (informally called "scrum pox").[13-16] The same mechanisms of transmission—frequent abrasions and skin-to-skin contact between athletes—put athletes at risk.

HSV most commonly causes cold sores. Herpes gladiatorum occurs when HSV enters breaks in skin.

TYPICAL PRESENTATION

Herpes gladiatorum may be confused with other bacterial skin infections, including impetigo or folliculitis, leading to delayed diagnosis and ongoing transmission. The incubation period for herpes gladiatorum ranges from 4 to 11 days after exposure. Some people experience numbness at the site of inoculation prior to the development of skin lesions. Eventually a papulovesicular rash (small, fluid-filled spots) develops, usually in a localized distribution corresponding to areas of direct skin-to-skin contact (**Figure 1.2**).[17] The rash is often painful and may be accompanied by a low-grade fever and malaise. After 7 to 10 days, the lesions crust over and resolve. Rarely, scarring or postinflammatory hyperpigmentation persists at the site. After the initial infection resolves, the virus persists in a latent state within sensory neurons. As a result, herpes infections can recur. Recurrence may be triggered by stress, other illnesses, sun exposure, or trauma.

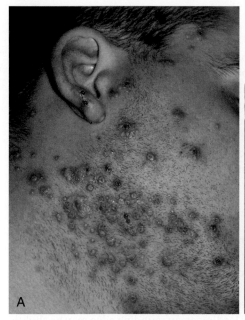
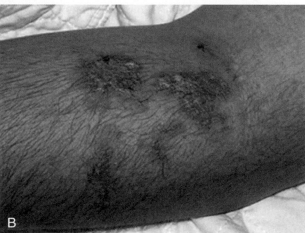

Figure 1.2 Herpes gladiatorum involving face (A) and more localized involvement of arm (B). (Part A, Reprinted with permission from Craft N, Fox LP, Goldsmith LA, et al. *VisualDx: Essential Adult Dermatology*. Philadelphia, PA: Wolters Kluwer Health; 2010. Part B, Reprinted with permission from McDonagh DO, Micheli LJ, Frontera WR, et al. *FIMS Sports Medicine Manual*. Philadelphia, PA: Wolters Kluwer Health; 2011.)

Ocular involvement is a rare but serious complication of herpetic skin infection. Herpes keratitis (infection of the cornea) can occasionally result in blindness. Prompt evaluation by an ophthalmologist is warranted for cases involving the eye.

TRANSMISSION

HSV is transmitted by direct physical contact and may enter the skin through small abrasions or breaks. Viral shedding is most active when lesions are present; however, shedding may also occur for a few days before any visible rash develops. Outbreaks related to contact sports such as rugby or wrestling are common.[13,14] Epidemiologic studies have yet to demonstrate a clear role for indirect transmission through contamination of training mats or shared gym equipment, but disinfection of equipment is still strongly recommended.[18]

PREVENTION MEASURES

Athletes with active herpes skin lesions should be excluded from competition until the skin lesions have dried and fully crusted over. Antiviral agents (acyclovir, valacyclovir, or famciclovir) inhibit replication of the herpes virus and may be prescribed to shorten the course of infection. For individuals with frequently recurrent herpes simplex outbreaks, the same antiviral agents may be prescribed for suppression. The determination of when an athlete is no longer contagious is best made by a physician after examining the lesions. In general, all lesions should be fully crusted over and no new lesions occurring before clearance to return to contact sports.

Although the role for indirect transmission of herpes simplex remains unclear, HSV can survive on various surfaces. Consequently, some facilities disinfect surfaces as a precaution, particularly in the setting of outbreaks.

Tinea

DISEASE BASICS

Tinea refers to superficial fungal skin infections caused by dermatophytes. The dermatophytes contain three genera of fungi: *Microsporum, Epidermophyton,* and *Trichophyton*.[19] Dermatophyte infections are common and can affect nearly any body site. In one recent US survey, tinea accounted for >25% of skin infections among athletes.[20] Athlete's foot refers to one of the most common sites of involvement. Warm, damp conditions produced by occlusive footwear place football and soccer players at particularly high risk.[21] Transmission via direct contact at other body sites has also been reported, mostly among contact sports participants such as wrestlers.[22] Compared to bacterial skin and soft-tissue infections, tinea infections are less invasive and severe but usually require longer courses of therapy.

TYPICAL PRESENTATION

As tinea can affect multiple body sites, specific names have been given to each site of infection: tinea capitis involves the scalp, tinea unguium: the nails (also called onychomycosis), tinea pedis: the feet, tinea corporis: the trunk, tinea faciei/barbae: the face/beard, and tinea cruris: the inguinal region (groin).[19]

While appearance may vary by site, most tinea infections present as a localized scaly, erythematous rash (**Figure 1.3**). Most are pruritic. The leading or surrounding edge may be slightly elevated, referred to by the common name "ringworm." Distribution often favors moist flexural regions (skin creases) of the body. Onychomycosis, or involvement of the nails, results in thickened, brittle, sometimes discolored nails.

The diagnosis of tinea is often made by appearance alone. In cases where uncertainty exists, a Wood lamp examination can confirm infection due to *Microsporum*, which fluoresces green.[19] A skin scraping can also be performed for KOH prep and dermatophyte culture. For onychomycosis, fungal culture of nail clippings can confirm the diagnosis.

Treatment varies by body site. Topical therapy is effective for tinea pedis, tinea cruris, and tinea corporis. Allylamines (eg, terbinafine) and azoles (eg, clotrimazole, econazole, miconazole) are first-line therapies and readily available over the counter.[23] Successful

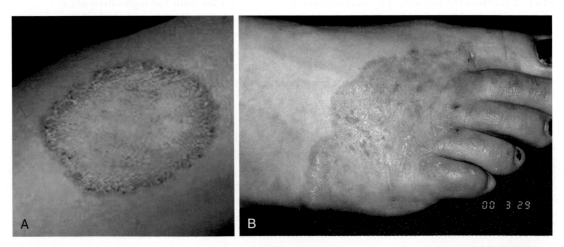

Figure 1.3 Tinea corporis (A) and tinea pedis (B). (Part A, Reprinted with permission from Gru AA, Wick M. *Pediatric Dermatopathology and Dermatology*. 1st ed. Philadelphia, PA: Wolters Kluwer Health; 2018. Part B, Reprinted with permission from Chung EK, Atkinson-McEvoy LR, Lai NL, Terry M. *Visual Diagnosis and Treatment in Pediatrics*. 3rd ed. Philadelphia, PA: Wolters Kluwer Health; 2014.)

treatment usually requires at least 2 to 6 weeks, with many providers recommending continuation for 1 to 2 weeks after visual resolution of the lesion to minimize risk of recurrence. Tinea capitis and onychomycosis respond poorly to topical therapies. Oral, systemic therapies such as griseofulvin or terbinafine are commonly used for tinea capitis. Treatment duration ranges from 6 to 12 weeks. Onychomycosis usually requires 3 to 6 months of oral terbinafine or occasionally itraconazole.

TRANSMISSION

Damp conditions produced by occlusive footwear likely account for the increased risk of tinea pedis seen among soccer and football players.[21] Tinea can also be spread by direct skin-to-skin contact, as outbreaks have been reported among athletes.[18] Finally, tinea pedis may be acquired or spread via shower floors in shared bathing facilities.[24]

Tinea pedis (athlete's foot) can be acquired from shower and locker room floors.

PREVENTION MEASURES

As tinea often favors moist body sites, removal of sweaty clothing, shoes, and socks promptly after activity may help reduce risk. Similarly, complete drying after showering may help to reduce susceptibility to tinea in flexural surfaces. Wearing sandals in the hydrotherapy and shower rooms can help athletes avoid exposure.

Central Nervous System Infections

Aseptic Meningitis

DISEASE BASICS

Aseptic meningitis refers to inflammation of the lining around the brain (meninges) without any bacterial growth on cerebrospinal fluid (CSF) culture. Because aseptic meningitis may closely resemble bacterial meningitis (see below), diagnosis is not always straightforward and often requires lumbar puncture (spinal tap) to rule out potentially life-threatening causes of meningitis. The majority of cases are caused by viral infection, particularly the enteroviruses. However, certain medications (especially nonsteroidal anti-inflammatory agents or NSAIDs) can cause aseptic meningitis as well.[25-27] For particular regions of the United States, tickborne diseases such as Rocky Mountain spotted fever (caused by *Rickettsia*) can also cause an aseptic meningitis (see **Table 1.1**). Fortunately, if other more serious causes can be ruled out, aseptic meningitis is generally self-resolving and requires only supportive care.

Diagnosis of meningitis typically requires a lumbar puncture ("spinal tap").

Outbreaks of aseptic meningitis have been reported among athletes.[28,29] Close contact among athletes and sharing of water bottles are presumed to put athletes at increased risk of enteroviral transmission.[30] The tendency for enteroviral transmission to peak in summer may also correspond with training camps and other preseason activities.[31]

Table 1.1 Causes of Aseptic Meningitis

Type of Aseptic Meningitis	Example Causes

Infectious causes	Common:
	    Enterovirus
	    Herpes simplex virus
	    Varicella zoster virus
	
	Less common/rare:
	    Arboviruses
	        St Louis encephalitis virus
	        Eastern equine encephalitis virus
	        West Nile virus
	    Coxsackievirus
	    Epstein-Barr virus
	    HSV
	    HIV
	    Measles
	    Mumps
	    Influenza
	    Rocky Mountain spotted fever (*Rickettsia*)
	    Ehrlichia
	    Leptospirosis
	    Syphilis
	    Tuberculosis
	    Mycoplasma
	    Neuroborreliosis

Medication-related	Nonsteroidal anti-inflammatories (NSAIDs) Azathioprine Carbamazepine IVIg (immune globulin)
Autoimmune	Sarcoidosis Lupus Behçet disease

Adapted from Hasbun R. The acute aseptic meningitis syndrome. *Curr Infect Dis Rep*. 2000;2(4):345-351 and Kupila L, Vuorinen T, Vainionpää R, Hukkanen V, Marttila R, Kotilainen P. Etiology of aseptic meningitis and encephalitis in an adult population. *Neurology*. 2006;66(1):75-80.

TYPICAL PRESENTATION

Aseptic meningitis can closely resemble bacterial meningitis. Headache, fever, neck stiffness, and photophobia are common. Presence of sore throat/pharyngitis or rash may hint at a viral cause, but the presence of these symptoms cannot reliably rule out other causes. Enterovirus has a strong seasonal trend, with the majority of cases occurring in summer.[26] Lumbar puncture is usually required to rule out bacterial meningitis. Care is supportive, and recovery is spontaneous once more serious causes (eg, bacterial meningitis) are ruled out.

TRANSMISSION

While medication-related aseptic meningitis is not communicable, enterovirus is transmissible through a variety of mechanisms. Enterovirus has been detected in respiratory secretions, blister fluids from rashes, and saliva. Enterovirus is also capable of survival on surfaces touched by infected individuals, so indirect transmission via touching contaminated surfaces can occur as well. Poor hand hygiene and sharing of water bottles have been implicated in some of the reported outbreaks among team athletes.[29]

Viruses that cause aseptic meningitis can be spread by sharing water bottles.

PREVENTION MEASURES

There are no specific vaccinations for enterovirus, the most common viral cause of aseptic meningitis. Based on modes of transmission and a high propensity for survival on surfaces, good hand hygiene and avoidance of sharing water bottles with infected individuals can reduce risk of infection.

Bacterial Meningitis

DISEASE BASICS

Bacterial meningitis is a serious infection that can be caused by a variety of pathogens. *Streptococcus pneumoniae*, *Haemophilus influenzae*, and *Neisseria meningitidis* are three of the most common causes in adults.[32] While any can be lethal, *N. meningitidis* is the most feared due to its particularly high mortality rate, extremely rapid progression, and tendency to occur in outbreaks among young adults. Risk for meningococcal meningitis occurs in two peaks: one in the first year of life and a second peak between the ages of 15 and 24 years. This second peak is the most likely to affect young athletes.

Bacterial meningitis is a medical emergency requiring rapid treatment with antibiotics. Although vaccination against *N. meningitidis* is now recommended for all adolescents and required by most colleges, awareness of the disease remains relevant for any sport involving young athletes staying in close quarters.

Bacterial meningitis is a medical emergency.

TYPICAL PRESENTATION

Meningitis classically presents with fever, headache, neck stiffness, and confusion—although fewer than half of patients will have all of these signs at the time of first presentation.[33] Some patients with *N. meningitidis* will develop a characteristic rash; in severe cases, it can lead to gangrene of the extremities as sepsis progresses (**Figure 1.4**). Lumbar puncture should be undertaken without delay in order to confirm the diagnosis, unless the patient has evidence of high intracranial pressure or a focal brain lesion. Final diagnosis is confirmed by culture, but polymerase chain reaction (PCR) testing is increasingly used to provide rapid preliminary identification of pathogens. Empiric antibiotics (vancomycin plus ceftriaxone for most otherwise healthy adults) should be started immediately, ideally after blood and CSF cultures are obtained, as mortality climbs by the hour without treatment.

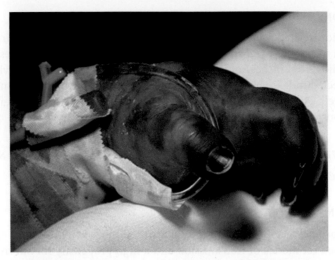

Figure 1.4 Gangrene of extremities in severe meningococcal sepsis. (Reprinted with permission from Kline-Tilford AM, Haut C. *Lippincott Certification Review: Pediatric Acute Care Nurse Practitioner*. 1st ed. Philadelphia, PA: Wolters Kluwer Health; 2015.)

TRANSMISSION

N. meningitidis may colonize the nose and upper throat of otherwise healthy individuals. Colonization converts to infection when these bacteria attach and invade through mucosal surfaces, leading to meningitis. Since *N. meningitidis* is found in saliva and respiratory secretions, it can be spread by kissing, coughing, or sharing of cups/eating utensils. Outbreaks are well reported in dense settings such as college dormitories.

PREVENTION MEASURES

Vaccination is highly effective, currently recommended for all adolescents, and generally required prior to attending college in the United States. There are several different vaccines available. The most widely used meningococcal conjugate vaccine (MCV4) protects against four common strains, but not meningitis B. MCV4 is recommended for all first-year college students residing on campus, all military recruits, individuals living with human immunodeficiency virus (HIV), those with asplenia or a complement deficiency, or those who may contract meningitis through travel or exposure to an outbreak. Because meningitis B is still a relatively common cause of outbreaks in the United States and abroad, separate vaccination with *N. meningitidis* group a polysaccharide antigen is recommended for individuals who have had their spleen removed, those with complement deficiency, or those with exposure to meningitis B through either occupation or an outbreak.

Antibiotic prophylaxis can be given to unvaccinated close contacts of patients with *N. meningitidis* to reduce risk of disease.

Gastrointestinal Infections

Hepatitis A

DISEASE BASICS

Hepatitis A is an acute, self-limiting viral infection involving the liver. Hepatitis A is typically acquired through contaminated food. Although overall incidence declined significantly following introduction of an effective vaccine in 1995, hepatitis A continues to occur in outbreaks spanning multiple US states.[34,35] Although several recent outbreaks predominantly occurred among urban homeless populations, transmission via infected food handlers or contaminated water is well-documented.[36] Consequently, transmission via contaminated foods at restaurants or banquets poses a potential threat to traveling sports teams.

Outbreaks of hepatitis A are increasingly common.

TYPICAL PRESENTATION

Disease severity varies with age. Childhood hepatitis A infection is usually asymptomatic. In contrast, adults are much more likely to experience fever, fatigue, jaundice (**Figure 1.5**), and right upper quadrant abdominal pain. Most adults recover spontaneously within 2 months, but some experience prolonged or waxing/waning disease occasionally lasting up to 6 months. Laboratory testing generally reveals significant elevations of the transaminases (aspartate aminotransferase [AST] and alanine aminotransferase [ALT], often in the thousands) and bilirubin. Diagnosis is confirmed by the presence of anti-HAV IgM antibodies.

There are no antiviral treatments for hepatitis A. Care is supportive and includes avoidance of alcohol or other hepatotoxins during convalescence.

TRANSMISSION

Transmission occurs via fecal-oral route (contaminated food/water), sexual contact, and illicit drug use. In developed countries with widespread access to safe drinking water, hepatitis A is most commonly acquired either through consumption of contaminated food or water during international travel or through consumption of contaminated foods. Virus may be shed for 1 to 2 weeks prior to symptomatic disease.

PREVENTION MEASURES

Receipt of hepatitis A vaccine leads to immunity. If exposure occurs prior to vaccination, the vaccine can still be given to reduce risk of disease if given within 2 weeks of exposure.

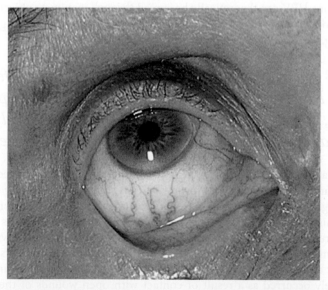

Figure 1.5 Scleral icterus/jaundice. (Used with permission from Bickley LS. *Bates' Guide to Physical Examination and History Taking.* 12th ed. Philadelphia, PA: Wolters Kluwer Health; 2016.)

Preexposure vaccination is recommended for adults traveling to certain regions with high rates of hepatitis A or for individuals with known liver disease. For the prevention of food-borne outbreaks, cooking to temperatures >185°F for >1 minute inactivates the virus.

Hepatitis B

DISEASE BASICS

Hepatitis B virus (HBV) causes an infection of the liver. HBV is a global health issue; more than 250 million people are infected with HBV in the world.[37] Approximately 80% of HBV infection in adults are clinically silent. While 20% of patients are symptomatic, fewer than 0.5% develop fulminant hepatitis. Almost 95% of adults with HBV infection achieve viral clearance, while the remaining 5% become chronic hepatitis B carriers.[38,39]

TYPICAL PRESENTATION

Symptoms from acute hepatitis B begin an average of 90 days after exposure (range 60-120 days).[40,41] Symptoms can include fever, abdominal pain, fatigue, dark urine, loss of appetite, clay-colored bowel movements, nausea, vomiting, joint pains, muscle aches, or jaundice (yellowing of the eyes).[42] Acute hepatitis B symptoms typically last for a few weeks but can persist up to 6 months.[40,41] In contrast, chronic hepatitis B infection is typically asymptomatic. Symptoms from chronic hepatitis B typically do not occur until a person has been infected with the virus for 10 to 30 years.[43]

TRANSMISSION

Hepatitis B is typically acquired as a result of exposure to blood or blood products, intravenous drug use, sexual transmission, tattooing, body piercing, acupuncture, and needlestick injuries.[44] During competition and training, athletes may be exposed to HBV through bleeding wounds and mucous membranes. The risk of transmission following high-risk exposures to blood infected with hepatitis B is approximately 33% (one in three). HBV is more likely to be transmitted than HIV because of its higher concentration in the blood and its stability in the environment.[45] In addition, HBV can remain stable in the environment for up to 7 days.[45] Therefore, HBV can theoretically be spread through inanimate objects contaminated with infected blood. However, HBV is not spread through food, water, sharing eating utensils, hugging, kissing, hand-holding, coughing, or sneezing.

Hepatitis B is highly contagious. Exposure to blood infected with hepatitis B leads to transmission in one out of three exposures. In contrast, hepatitis C is transmitted in approximately 1 of 30 exposures, and HIV is transmitted in 1 of 300 exposures.

Athletes may have a higher risk of hepatitis B due to injuries with bleeding and close contact with teammates. The estimates for risk of HBV transmission during athletic activity are wide ranging. The risk is estimated to be between one transmission in every 10,000 games and one transmission in every 4.25 million games.[46] An outbreak of hepatitis B among sumo wrestlers occurred in 1980.[47] This outbreak was caused by an asymptomatic wrestler. Another case series summarized an outbreak among 11 of 65 American football players who developed hepatitis B over a period of 19 months.[48] This outbreak was also caused by an asymptomatic carrier that likely occurred as a result of contact with open wounds of the carrier during sporting activity.

Why vaccinate against hepatitis B? Transmission of hepatitis B can happen during athletic activities.

PREVENTION MEASURES

Vaccination is highly effective in reducing the risk of acquiring HBV to near zero, is long lasting, and is safe.[49] Hepatitis B vaccination has been recommended by the ACIP for all children since 1991. The National Collegiate Athletic Association (NCAA) has recommended HBV vaccination for all student athletes since 1994.[50]

Theoretically, bloodborne infections may be transmitted through sharing a water container, as bleeding around the mouth is common in contact sport.[51] Therefore, ideally, athletes should use squeeze water bottles to reduce the risk of oral and blood contamination.

Any blood spills (including dried blood) can be infectious.[52] Therefore, blood on any surfaces or equipment should be cleaned with a blood spill kit while wearing gloves.

Norovirus

DISEASE BASICS

Norovirus is a leading cause of both sporadic and epidemic gastroenteritis. Norovirus is highly contagious; inoculation with fewer than 100 viral particles can lead to infection. Norovirus can spread through aerosols, direct contact, from person to person, or through contaminated foods. Outbreaks most often occur due to contaminated food. In fact, outbreaks associated with contaminated foods have been described on cruise ships, in schools, and among sports teams.[53-55] While infection usually begins with exposure to food contaminated by ill food handlers, norovirus can spread rapidly among members of a team traveling together.

TYPICAL PRESENTATION

Norovirus presents with sudden onset of nausea, vomiting, cramping abdominal pains, diarrhea, and sometimes fever. The incubation period is brief (<48 hours), and illness generally resolves in <72 hours.[56] Diagnosis is primarily clinical, though confirmatory stool tests do exist. There are no effective treatments specific to norovirus. Supportive care generally involves oral rehydration given in frequent small volumes. For more severe cases, antiemetics or even intravenous fluids are occasionally necessary.

TRANSMISSION

Transmission occurs mainly by the fecal-oral route. Norovirus can survive wide temperature ranges and as a result can also be transmitted through water sources, fomites, and environmental contamination. Foodborne outbreaks are typically associated with contamination of food by ill food handlers but have also been associated with raw oyster consumption.[56,57] In adults, children are often the cause of norovirus transmission in a household.

Because norovirus consists of many distinct and constantly evolving strains, prior infection does not confer immunity to future disease recurrence. A small subset of the population is impervious to norovirus infection.[56]

PREVENTION MEASURES

With its extremely low infectious dose and capability of surviving in the environment, preventing norovirus transmission is challenging. Most importantly, any player with diarrhea should be removed from the facility as soon as possible. Strict attention to hand hygiene, especially before eating or drinking, is essential, but alcohol-based hand cleaners are ineffective against norovirus. Individuals with norovirus should not be involved in any food preparation for at least 48 hours after full resolution of symptoms. Cooking temperatures higher than 145°F may be necessary to inactivate norovirus in potentially contaminated foods. Finally, *as outlined in Chapter 6*, norovirus is not eliminated with many disinfectant chemicals. As a result, if a diarrheal illness occurs in players, cleaning and disinfection in the facility must be performed with a bleach- or hydrogen peroxide–containing disinfectant.

Pharyngitis and Respiratory Tract Infections

Hand, Foot, and Mouth Disease

DISEASE BASICS

Hand, foot, and mouth disease (HFMD) is a typically mild viral infection that occurs in children in the summer and fall; it can be caused by several viruses but is typically caused by coxsackievirus or enterovirus.[58] The coxsackievirus A16 is the most common cause of HFMD in the United States.

TYPICAL PRESENTATION

HFMD typically leads to mouth or throat pain in children, often accompanied by low-grade fever. Rash on the hands (often vesicular on the palms or soles) and lesions in the mouth (mild ulcers) are often visible on physical examination.

In children, oral lesions (**Figure 1.6**) are often the first clinical sign of this infection (and sometimes the only sign). The oral lesions are vesicular in nature. Lesions on the extremities (**Figure 1.7**) typically occur after the oral ulcers. On the extremities, HFMD appears as a red rash, without itching but sometimes with blistering. The rash is typically on the palms, soles, and sometimes the buttocks.

Adults may not have the same type of rash or skin lesions seen on children with HFMD. Instead, HFMD in adults is typically a mild illness with widely varying presentations; most adult patients believe they have a "cold" when infected with HFMD. These nonspecific symptoms typically last about 2 to 7 days. Occasionally, the rash may be the only symptom present in adults.

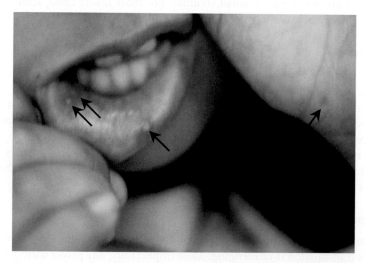

Figure 1.6 Vesicular oral lesions of hand, foot, and mouth disease. (Reprinted with permission from Salimpour RR, Salimpour P, Salimpour P. *Photographic Atlas of Pediatric Disorders and Diagnosis.* Philadelphia, PA: Wolters Kluwer; 2013.)

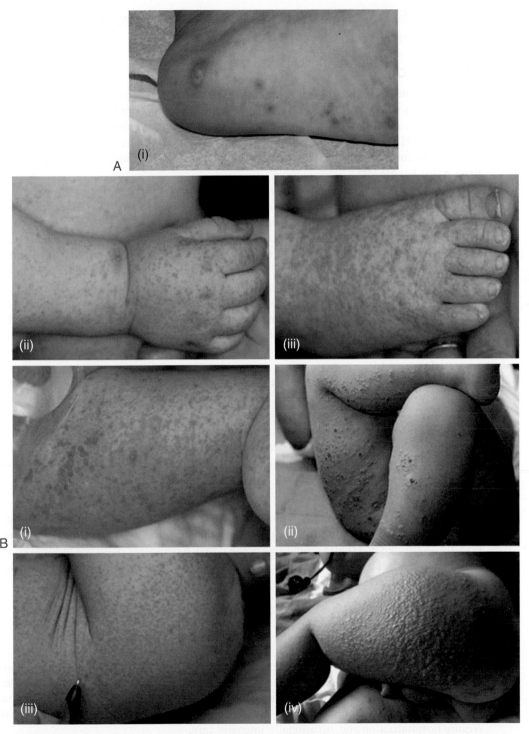

Figure 1.7 Erythematous rash of hand, foot, and mouth disease on the extremities. Top three panels: classic vesicular rash involving hands and feet. Bottom four panels: more extensive involvement of legs, thighs, and buttocks. (Part A (i), Reprinted with permission from Goodheart HP, Gonzalez ME. *Goodheart's Photoguide to Common Pediatric and Adult Skin Disorders*. 4th ed. Philadelphia, PA: Wolters Kluwer; 2015. Part A (ii-iii) and Part B, Reproduced with permission from Hubiche T, Schuffenecker I, Boralevi F, et al. Dermatological spectrum of hand, foot and mouth disease from classical to generalized exanthema. *Pediatr Infect Dis J*. 2014;33:e92.)

Adults infected with HFMD may not have the typical rash or skin lesions seen on children.

TRANSMISSION

HFMD is spread by ingestion of food or other materials contaminated by infected feces from a person with HFMD or following direct exposure to saliva or vesicular fluid (that then enters into the mouth); indirect exposure can occur via a contaminated environment. Though uncommon, HFMD can also be transmitted from swallowing water from swimming pools if the water is not treated properly with chlorine and becomes contaminated with feces from a person that has HFMD.[59]

Generally, HFMD is the most contagious during the first week of illness. However, people with HFMD can shed potentially infectious virus up to 10 weeks after the onset of symptoms, depending on the virus causing the infection.[60,61]

Outbreaks of HFMD can and do occur regularly. Most published reports of outbreaks are from settings outside of the United States, but the incidence of HFMD in the United States is on the rise. For example, an outbreak of HFMD due to coxsackievirus A6 occurred in 53 basic military trainees in 2015.[62] The patients infected during this outbreak were all young, and almost all were found to have a widespread vesiculopapular rash. A more extensive outbreak occurred on the east coast of the United States in 2016, particularly impacting high-school students in New Jersey and Connecticut.[63] During this outbreak, health departments in these states issued warnings for athletes and parents. Numerous sporting events were canceled or postponed.

Athletes are at risk of acquiring HFMD, given close operating quarters, such as locker rooms. For example, a small outbreak of HFMD recently occurred in a National Football League (NFL) team. Impacted players were in the same practice group (eg, quarterback, center, and wide receiver). Transmission may have occurred via a contaminated football and frequent licking of hands or fingers for grip. Therefore, if one team member acquires HFMD, it can be easily spread to other people in the locker or training room.

PREVENTION MEASURES

Hand hygiene is the most important intervention for preventing the spread of HFMD.[64] People infected with HFMD should wash their hands often, even after symptoms improve. In addition, those affected by HFMD should stay home if they have a fever or do not feel well enough to return to work/school. Finally, frequently touched surfaces and soiled equipment should be cleaned and disinfected frequently.

Influenza

DISEASE BASICS

Influenza is a contagious viral respiratory illness that is readily transmitted from person to person. Influenza infection significantly reduces respiratory capacity and athletic performance even in players with relatively mild infections.[65] A small but important percentage of young and otherwise healthy individuals who acquire influenza may develop severe infections that require hospitalization and, occasionally, intensive care.

TYPICAL PRESENTATION

Influenza is typically characterized by the abrupt onset of symptoms.[66] Specifically, patients develop fevers, chills, muscle aches (myalgias), headache, fatigue, nonproductive cough, sore throat, and rhinorrhea. These symptoms last an average of 3 to 7 days for the majority of afflicted people.

Diagnosing influenza in athletes may be difficult, as the virus mimics other conditions. Specifically, participants may complain of muscle aches or coughing after significant cardiopulmonary activity. Though nonspecific, these symptoms can be signs of influenza. Patients with influenza may also have GI symptoms like vomiting.

TRANSMISSION

Influenza is passed through respiratory droplets when infected people cough, sneeze, or talk. Less often, a person might get flu by touching a surface or object that has flu virus on it and then touching their own mouth, nose, or eyes. People are most contagious 3 or 4 days after symptoms begin. However, players with influenza can continue shedding viral particles for several days after they have symptomatically improved, although the amount of shedding is reduced in this setting.[67]

Athletes are likely at an increased risk for transmission and contraction of the virus because (1) they have increased close contact with others through training and competition, (2) they often travel in close quarters, and (3) they are more likely to share objects such as water bottles, which can act as disease vectors.[68] In addition, intense, long-term exercise may produce more stress-related hormones, which can lead to temporary weakening of the immune system, putting the athlete at risk of infection.[69]

Transmission of influenza has occurred during major sporting events. Influenza was diagnosed in 36 of 188 patients who reported to the Olympic Village medical clinic during the 2002 Winter Olympics. Athletes were found to represent 36% of all flu patients despite accounting for only 24% of those screened for influenza infection.[70]

PREVENTION

Vaccination against influenza is the most effective method to prevent flu.

Vaccination against influenza is the most effective method to prevent flu. Influenza vaccines have proven benefits that are important for athletes. Most importantly, players who receive influenza vaccines are less likely to have fever or influenza-like illness, are less likely to miss work, and are less likely to spread influenza to teammates.[71-73] It is important to recognize, however, that numerous viruses can cause "influenza-like illness"; thus, vaccination will not prevent all episodes of influenza-like illness. This fact should be emphasized when players or skeptics complain "I received influenza vaccine and I got the flu anyway."

From a team perspective, vaccinated players who are exposed to influenza are less likely to spread the virus and are, thus, less likely to cause a locker room–wide outbreak that could potentially devastate a team. In other words, immunization has benefits for individual players and the team.

In addition, individuals who are affected by influenza should remain home and not go to work or school to prevent transmission of influenza to others.

Finally, all team members should perform hand hygiene in order to prevent transmission of influenza virus.

Mononucleosis

DISEASE BASICS

Mononucleosis is a viral illness caused by Epstein-Barr virus (EBV). Nearly 90% of the world's population are infected with EBV before reaching adulthood. Infection rates are highest among children and young adults aged 5 to 25 years. Athletes in their late teens and early 20s are among those at elevated risk, while most older adults are immune due to past infection. The two most significant mononucleosis-related issues for athletes are the risk of splenic rupture and potential for postinfectious fatigue, both of which have significant implications for participation in training or competition.

TYPICAL PRESENTATION

The incubation period for mononucleosis may be as long as 4 to 7 weeks. Infection presents with sore throat, fever, and lymphadenopathy (**Figure 1.8**). Roughly half of people infected will develop splenomegaly. Nonspecific rash is common, especially if a patient receives ampicillin (often due to misdiagnosis as *Strep* throat). Because of the potential risk for splenic rupture, athletes with mononucleosis and splenomegaly are advised to avoid contact sports for 4 weeks after initial illness.[74,75]

A blood count with differential may reveal increased white blood cells, often with lymphocytosis. The presence of atypical lymphocytes (often >10%) or a markedly elevated lymphocyte count (sometimes >50%) are both strongly suggestive of EBV infection.[76] Heterophile antibody testing (including the mononucleosis spot test) yields rapid confirmatory results but has a high false-negative rate in the first week of infection.

There are no specific treatments for mononucleosis. Care is supportive. As noted above, contact sports should be avoided for 4 weeks after onset of illness to minimize risk of splenic rupture. Although infection resolves spontaneously, fatigue may persist for several weeks.

It is important to note that acute HIV can present similarly to mononucleosis. For sexually active patients or those with a mononucleosis-like syndrome but negative confirmatory testing, HIV screening is warranted.

TRANSMISSION

Mononucleosis is transmitted via bodily fluids, including via saliva and sexual contact, leading to its nickname as the "kissing disease."

PREVENTION MEASURES

Infection risk can be reduced by avoiding kissing, sexual contact, or sharing drinks with people who have mononucleosis. There is no specific vaccine for mononucleosis.

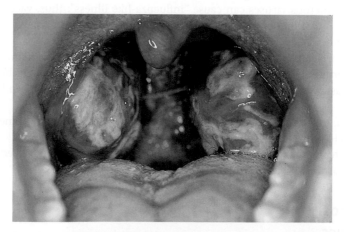

Figure 1.8 Enlarged tonsils due to Epstein-Barr virus (infectious mononucleosis). (Reprinted with permission from Hatfield NT. *Introductory Maternity and Pediatric Nursing*. 3rd ed. Philadelphia, PA: Wolters Kluwer Health; 2013.)

Pertussis

DISEASE BASICS

Pertussis, also known as "whooping cough," is a highly contagious respiratory illness caused by the bacterium *Bordetella pertussis*. Pertussis is erroneously believed to be a rare disease that only impacts infants and children. In fact, pertussis is common. An estimated 2 million Americans acquire pertussis each year. While infants have more severe infections, adolescents and adults account for more than 60% of cases in the vaccination era,[77] likely due to the fact that immunization for pertussis in childhood does not produce durable immunity in adults. Because immunity induced by pertussis vaccine characteristically declines with time, adults who were vaccinated during childhood can and do become infected with *B. pertussis*. For example, 40% of previously immunized adults contract pertussis after exposure to infected children.[78]

Whooping cough is not just a childhood disease. More than 60% of pertussis cases occur in adults.

Though unlikely to cause death, adults with pertussis often have prolonged, significant illnesses. Pertussis infection regularly results in doctor visits, unnecessary use of antibiotics, and most importantly from a team perspective, increased absenteeism from work.[79] Several studies have demonstrated that the majority of adults with pertussis missed between 7 and 10 days of work[80]; 10% to 16% of adults with pertussis missed more than a month of work.

TYPICAL PRESENTATION

Symptoms of pertussis typically present within 5 to 10 days of exposure. In some cases, however, symptoms can be delayed up to 3 weeks.[81]

The clinical course of pertussis has three stages: catarrhal, paroxysmal, and convalescent (**Figure 1.9**). The catarrhal stage is the earliest stage and lasts 1 to 2 weeks. Symptoms in this stage are insidious and often nonspecific: mild cough, fatigue, rhinorrhea, and occasionally fever.[82] The paroxysmal stage occurs during the second week of illness. The symptoms in this phase consist of paroxysms of cough: severe coughing episodes that can occur in rapid succession.[83,84] Following a prolonged cough, a forceful inhalation occurs and causes the characteristic "whooping" sound. This notable sound is more common in infants and smaller children

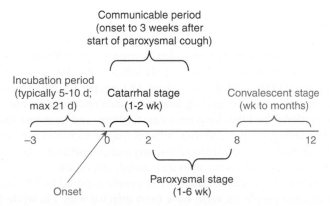

Figure 1.9 Clinical course (in weeks). (Reprinted from Centers for Disease Control and Prevention. https://www.cdc.gov/pertussis/clinical/features.html.)

because of trachea size. Cough paroxysms can be so severe that they lead to vomiting (ie, post-tussive vomiting). The cough paroxysms occur predominantly at night and become more frequent and severe as the illness progresses.[82] However, people are relatively asymptomatic in between coughing. Untreated, the paroxysmal phase lasts 2 to 3 months. The convalescent phase follows the paroxysmal stage. In this final stage, the cough gradually decreases in severity and frequency. This phase lasts 1 to 2 weeks.[84]

Coughing spell so severe it leads to vomiting? Think pertussis.

TRANSMISSION

Pertussis is spread through respiratory droplets emitted during coughing.[85] Of note, mildly symptomatic and asymptomatic infection are common, and asymptomatic individuals can transmit the infection to susceptible people.[86] The incubation period of pertussis is typically 7 to 10 days but can last as long as 3 weeks.[82] Individuals are considered infectious until they have completed 5 days of appropriate antibiotic therapy.[87]

Pertussis is highly contagious. It can spread rapidly, and it frequently causes outbreaks or clusters of infection in populations in close quarters such as sports teams. Large sports meetings and venues provide ample opportunity for transmission of pertussis to and among team members. For example, some high schools have postponed or canceled games due to outbreaks of pertussis among players. While an infection of a single player may be easy to deal with, having a team-wide outbreak can be devastating. An outbreak of pertussis occurred among members of a Polish Sport Shooting National Team in 2015.[88] The outbreak led to significantly decreased exercise performance, interrupted training, and ultimately resulted in failure to win a medal or quota place.

PREVENTION MEASURES

The best way to protect against pertussis is with vaccines. The CDC recommends pertussis vaccination for all infants, children, and adults. Routine initial vaccination is given between the ages of 2 months and 6 years. Adolescents receive a single Tdap "booster" dose between the ages of 11 to 18 years. To ensure durable immunity, all adults should receive at least one additional Tdap "booster" dose in place of the Td (tetanus) immunization given every 10 years.[89]

Tuberculosis

DISEASE BASICS

Tuberculosis, commonly abbreviated TB, is caused by bacteria in the *Mycobacterium tuberculosis* complex. With an estimated 8.9 million new cases in 2017, TB remains one of the most common infections worldwide.[90] TB incidence varies widely by country. Over 80% of cases occur in just 30 high-incidence countries, many of which are in Asia, sub-Saharan Africa, and the Pacific islands. In contrast, TB incidence in the United States is low (2.8 cases per 100,000 persons). The majority of US cases occur in individuals emigrating from high-incidence regions, but TB transmission also occurs in correctional facilities, long-term care facilities, and homeless shelters. While TB risk is generally low among US-born athletes, athletes may be recruited from around the world or may travel extensively during international training and competitions. As recruiting becomes increasingly global, awareness of TB becomes increasingly important.

Unlike many other infections, the majority of people exposed to TB remain asymptomatic. Nearly one in three people on earth have been infected with TB, while fewer than 10% develop active TB disease.[91] Most persons with a healthy immune system who are exposed to TB clear the TB bacillus. In some people, however, macrophages engulf the TB bacillus but are unable to eliminate it. The TB bacillus may persist for many years in these individuals, a condition known as *latent* TB infection. People with latent TB have no symptoms and are not contagious. Latent TB can convert to *active* TB at any time. Roughly 5% of people with latent TB will develop active disease in the first year after infection, and another 5% will develop active TB over the 10 years after initial infection. Smoking, diabetes, HIV, glucocorticoid use, and a compromised immune system all increase the risk of progression to active TB.[92]

TYPICAL PRESENTATION

The diagnosis of TB depends on the stage of disease. Since patients with latent TB lack symptoms, screening to determine if latent TB is present relies on either the purified protein derivative (PPD) skin test or an interferon-gamma release assay (IGRA). The thresholds for a positive skin test vary by host risk factors and immune status. Importantly, people who have received the Bacille Calmette-Guerin (BCG) vaccine, which is more common among people born outside the United States, may have a false-positive response to skin testing. IGRAs are generally favored as they require just a single visit for a blood draw, are less subjective to interpretation, and are not affected by prior BCG vaccination.

In contrast, patients with active TB have signs or symptoms of disease. TB typically affects the lungs (known as pulmonary TB) but can involve almost any organ system. Patients with pulmonary TB classically present with fevers, night sweats, weight loss, cough, and occasionally hemoptysis. While bacterial pneumonia may cause many of the same symptoms, TB tends to be chronic, lasting longer than 2 to 3 weeks, and does not respond to antibiotics typically used for bacterial pneumonias.

All patients with suspected TB should undergo chest x-ray and sputum acid-fast bacilli (AFB) culture. The appearance of TB on chest x-ray varies, but there are a few classic findings strongly suggestive of TB. Characteristic findings include upper-lobe predominant consolidations, cavity formation, a nodular appearance, and enlarged hilar lymph nodes (**Figure 1.10**). Findings consistent with prior resolved TB may include scarring, fibrosis, or calcified granulomas. Sputum AFB culture is essential for confirming the diagnosis; however, the TB bacillus requires specialized media and prolonged incubation periods to culture. It is important to note that skin testing and IGRAs are *not* adequate to diagnose active TB as they may be falsely negative in >30% of cases.[93]

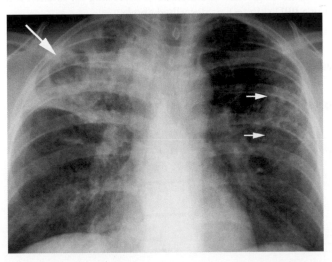

Figure 1.10 Chest x-ray demonstrating upper-lobe infiltrates (small arrows) and cavity formation (large arrow) due to tuberculosis. (Reprinted with permission from Webb RW, Higgins CB. *Thoracic Imaging*. 3rd ed. Philadelphia, PA: Wolters Kluwer Health; 2016.)

Treatment of latent TB and active TB requires input from infectious disease physicians and/or public health officials. Treatment for latent TB is shorter and simpler than treatment for active TB. There are three commonly used regimens in the United States: 9 months of isoniazid per day, 4 months of rifampin per day, or 12 weeks of isoniazid-rifapentine one time a week.[94] The latter two regimens are strongly favored for their shorter duration and lower risk of adverse effects. Treatment of active TB typically requires 6 to 9 months of therapy, depending on sites involved, drug resistance patterns, and response to treatment. In cases of drug-resistant TB, prolonged courses of combination therapy may be required. Most patients begin with four-drug therapy (rifampin, isoniazid, pyrazinamide, and ethambutol) but can step-down to two-drug therapy (isoniazid and rifampin) after the first few months.[95] Because patients with active TB are contagious, treatment of active TB is mandatory in the United States.

TRANSMISSION

TB transmission occurs via the airborne route. Coughing generates small droplets that contain aerosolized TB bacilli. Patients with cavitary disease and positive sputum AFB smears are the most contagious. Transmission risk is highest among people living in the same household or spending long periods of time with one another indoors.[96] Patients with latent TB are not contagious.

PREVENTION MEASURES

Isolation and treatment of individuals with active TB reduces transmission risk. Most individuals are able to complete active TB treatment at home, with appropriate precautions about avoiding public spaces or wearing a surgical mask if they do need to leave home. Transmission risk decreases dramatically after starting treatment, and isolation can be discontinued after sputum AFB smears turn negative.

In addition to treating all active cases of TB, the United States Preventive Services Task Force (USPSTF) currently recommends latent TB screening for all adults at increased risk of TB.[97] This group includes individuals who have immigrated from a high-incidence country (top seven countries by total cases in **Table 1.2**, complete list available at: ***https://www.tbfacts. org/tb-statistics/***), individuals living with HIV, close contacts of an active TB case, healthcare workers, and residents or employees of high-risk congregate settings (eg, correctional institutions, homeless shelters, long-term care facilities). Screening for latent TB involves either an IGRA blood test or a PPD skin test, as described above.

Table 1.2 Top Seven Countries According to Total Tuberculosis Incidence

Countries With Highest Total Burden of TB Cases
India
China
Indonesia
Philippines
Pakistan
Nigeria
South Africa

Modified from TBFacts.org. https://www.tbfacts.org/tb-statistics.

The BCG vaccine is widely used outside of the United States for TB prevention. While partly protective against severe forms of TB in infants, the BCG vaccine is only 50% protective against pulmonary TB in adults.[98] Consequently, even vaccinated individuals remain at risk. The BCG vaccine is not recommended in the United States.

Viral Exanthems and Human Immunodeficiency Virus

Chicken Pox (Varicella)

DISEASE BASICS

Varicella (chicken pox) was once a common childhood disease, though incidence has fallen dramatically since the introduction of an effective vaccine in 1995.[99,100] Without vaccination or prior exposure, the risk for chicken pox persists, and sporadic cases continue to occur in the United States.[101] Although the vaccine is highly effective at preventing chicken pox in childhood, protection is not perfect. One serologic survey of US professional athletes found inadequate immunity to varicella among 7% to 17% of players tested.[102] Consequently, sporadic community cases of chicken pox may still put adults at risk if they have never had chicken pox before. Provider awareness is particularly important, as partial immunity conferred by varicella immunization has been associated with milder or atypical cases of varicella which might otherwise go unrecognized. In contrast, adults who have never been vaccinated and never had prior chicken pox are at risk for more severe illness.

TYPICAL PRESENTATION

The incubation period for varicella can be as long as 2 weeks. Varicella causes an intensively pruritic rash that may involve the skin and mucous membranes.[103] Vesicles develop in groups or crops, and the presence of lesions in varying stages helps to distinguish varicella from smallpox (**Figure 1.11**). While mostly known for its skin lesions, severe complications of varicella infection include encephalitis, thrombocytopenia, hepatitis, arthritis, and glomerulonephritis. While rare overall, adults are more likely to develop varicella pneumonia than children.

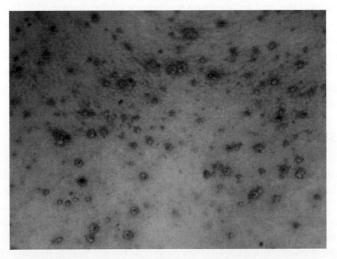

Figure 1.11 Skin rash of chicken pox (varicella). (Reprinted with permission from DeLong L, Burkhart NW. *General and Oral Pathology for the Dental Hygienist*. 3rd ed. Philadelphia, PA: Wolters Kluwer Health; 2018.)

Like other herpes viruses, the varicella virus persists in a latent state and can recur as shingles later in life. Since varicella establishes its latent state in nerve roots, shingles usually presents in limited distributions that match nerve distribution patterns.

While antiviral agents can inhibit replication of the varicella virus, most healthy hosts will control the infection within 2 to 3 days after onset of the rash. Antiviral treatment does not significantly alter the course of chicken pox and is not recommended unless the host is immunocompromised. Care is mostly supportive, with topical applications of calamine or cool bathing with baking soda or oatmeal for symptomatic relief.

TRANSMISSION

Varicella is highly contagious and spreads via both an airborne route and from direct contact with active skin lesions. The virus does not survive for long periods of time outside of the host. Most transmission occurs directly from person to person.

PREVENTION MEASURES

The vaccine for varicella is highly effective at preventing infection. In fact, administration of the vaccine may still offer some protection for unvaccinated individuals if given within 5 days after exposure. In the rare case of the immunocompromised host being exposed to an individual with chicken pox, intravenous immunoglobulin (IVIg) can be given to reduce risk, if available.

Individuals with chicken pox should remain at home until all lesions have fully crusted over.

Individuals with shingles should keep the rash covered until all lesions have fully crusted over.

Measles

DISEASE BASICS

Measles is a highly contagious viral illness that was common in children before the development of the first measles vaccine in 1963. Once on the verge of extinction, misinformation about a link between the measles, mumps, and rubella (MMR) vaccine and autism led to reduced vaccination rates and an alarming resurgence of the disease.[104,105] In reality, the measles vaccine has repeatedly proven safe and effective; multiple large-scale studies have definitively disproven the association between the vaccine and autism.[106-108] As a result of reduced vaccination rates, however, providers need to be increasingly aware of measles as a cause of febrile illnesses accompanied by rash. According to the CDC, the annual number of cases is on the rise (**Figure 1.12**).[109] Measles can spread rapidly among groups of individuals with close contact—including athletes participating in team sports.[110]

TYPICAL PRESENTATION

Measles typically presents in four stages (**Table 1.3**). First, the incubation period, during which the virus has entered the body but is not yet causing symptoms, lasts 7 to 21 days. The second stage, named the "prodrome stage," begins with high fever, cough, rhinorrhea (coryza), and conjunctivitis.[111] The latter three symptoms led to the mnemonic "3 C's" as a way to diagnose measles. At this stage, the symptoms of measles are otherwise nonspecific, making it difficult to distinguish measles from many other viral upper respiratory infections. After 2 to 4 days, small white spots known a Koplik spots may be visible on the buccal mucosa (**Figure 1.13**). For experienced physicians, Koplik spots provide the earliest indication of measles. The third stage begins when the characteristic measles rash appears, 3 to 7 days after first onset of symptoms (**Figure 1.13**). The rash begins as flat red macules, often appearing first in the hairline, before

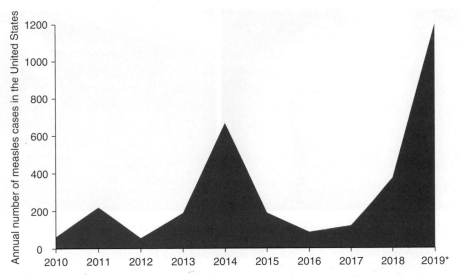

Figure 1.12 Annual number of measles cases in the United States. *Number of cases through August 15, 2019. (Modified from Centers for Disease Control and Prevention. https://www.cdc.gov/measles/cases-outbreaks.html.)

Table 1.3 Stages of Measles Infection

Stage	Duration	Features
Incubation period	7-21 d	Begins with viral entry No symptoms present
Prodrome	2-4 d	Fever, malaise Cough, coryza, conjunctivitis Koplik spots
Exanthem	3-7 d	Characteristic rash High fever Lymphadenopathy
Recovery	1-2 wk	Cough may persist longer

spreading downward over the trunk and limbs. The rash usually blanches to touch and may coalesce as it spreads. The diagnosis can be verified by detection of IgM antimeasles antibodies, though often not detectable until 4 or more days after onset of rash.[111] The fourth stage involves recovery and development of immunity.

Measles is much more severe in adults who have not been vaccinated or did not have the disease in childhood. Rare but severe complications include pneumonia, hepatitis, and encephalitis, which can sometimes be fatal. The measles virus also inhibits the immune system, leaving affected individuals at increased risk for secondary bacterial infections for weeks or even months after measles infection.[112]

No antiviral treatment for measles exists. Since vitamin A deficiency is known to delay recovery, supplementation may help shorten disease duration in children or those at risk of poor nutrition.[113]

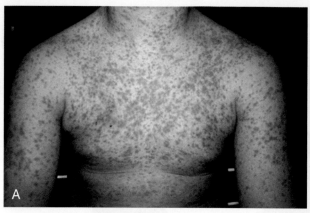
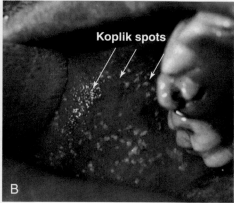

Figure 1.13 Characteristic measles rash (A) and Koplik spots (B). (Part A, Courtesy of Kathleen Cronan, MD. Reprinted with permission from Chung, E. *Visual Diagnosis in Pediatrics*. 3rd ed. Philadelphia, PA: Wolters Kluwer; 2014. *Part B, Reprinted with permission from Harvey RA, et al. Lippincott's Illustrated Reviews: Microbiology. 2nd ed. Philadelphia, PA: Lippincott Williams & Wilkins; 2007.*

TRANSMISSION

Measles spreads via airborne and droplet routes. It is one of the most contagious of all diseases: >90% of unvaccinated individuals having close contact with a measles case will subsequently become infected (**Table 1.4**).[111,114] Complicating matters further, individuals may spread the disease for up to 4 days *before* the rash develops (ie, during the incubation period). Since the diagnosis is often considered only after the rash appears, isolation frequently occurs too late to stop transmission.

PREVENTION MEASURES

Measles vaccination dramatically reduces the likelihood of infection: two doses of the measles vaccine are >97% effective; even a single dose exceeds 90% efficacy. The Advisory Committee on Immunization Practices (ACIP) and American Academy of Pediatrics (AAP) recommend that children in the United States receive two doses of MMR (***https://www.cdc.gov/vaccines/hcp/clinical-resources/mmr-faq-12-17-08.html***). Because the measles vaccine is a live attenuated vaccine, the vaccine is not recommended for individuals with a severely compromised immune system.

Table 1.4 Viral Diseases Ranked by Contagiousness (R_0)

Disease	R_0 (Infection Quotient)
Measles	14.5
Polio	6
Smallpox	4.5
Mumps	4
Zika	2.1
Ebola	1.5

R_0, known as the "reproduction number," is defined as the average number of new infections generated by a single person with the disease.

For any individuals who were not previously immunized, beginning the vaccine series within 72 hours of exposure may reduce the risk of disease. Individuals with measles should remain on isolation out of public spaces until at least 4 days after the appearance of the rash. As humans are the only known host for measles, eradication is possible—however, vaccination rates of >90% are generally necessary for adequate herd immunity.

Mumps

DISEASE BASICS

Mumps is a viral illness that occurs worldwide. The peak incidence is usually from late winter to early spring. Mumps occurs most commonly in older children and college-aged young adults. Since the implementation of routine vaccination, the number of cases of mumps in the United States has decreased by more than 99%.[115] However, since 2006, the number of cases and the number of outbreaks have increased as a direct consequence of declining vaccination rates. The number of cases reported in 2016 and 2017 were the highest in a decade.[116] The highest proportion of these cases occurred in the >30 years age group.

TYPICAL PRESENTATION

People usually develop symptoms 17 days (range 12-25 days) following exposure.[117] Symptoms typically start with a few days of fever, headache, fatigue, and muscle aches. After 1 to 2 days of these symptoms, the characteristic swelling of the parotid salivary glands (cheek, jaw area) develops (**Figure 1.14**). This swelling is called "parotitis." Parotitis can involve one side or both sides of the face. The swelling usually lasts 2 days but can persist up to 10 days.[118]

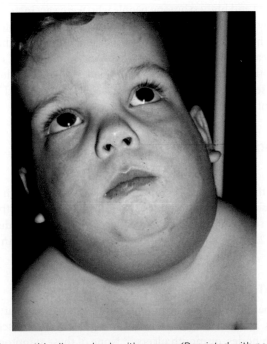

Figure 1.14 Swelling of the parotid salivary glands with mumps. (Reprinted with permission from Kyle T, Carman S. *Essentials of Pediatric Nursing*. 3rd ed. Philadelphia, PA: Wolters Kluwer; 2016.)

TRANSMISSION

Mumps is highly contagious and is transmitted through direct contact with respiratory secretions or saliva of an infected person.[119] Risk of transmission is proportional to duration and proximity of contact with the infected person. Mumps can be transmitted from 2 days prior to the onset of parotitis until 5 days after the onset of parotitis.

Mumps continues to cause periodic outbreaks, particularly among nonimmunized or inadequately immunized young adults and athletes. For example, multiple members of four NHL hockey teams, one NHL referee, and one NHL linesman developed mumps in November 2014.[120] These cases resulted in lost playing time and in at least one case, hospitalization. Mumps outbreaks also occurred in two Canadian hockey teams in 2007, in French rugby league players in 2011, and in European rugby league players in 2013.[89,121-123] These outbreaks are primarily due to low rates of vaccination. For example, only 30% of Canadian adults have been vaccinated against mumps. Other countries, including Russia and Eastern European countries, have similarly low rates of vaccination against mumps. Thus, when one case of mumps occurs in a setting such as the NHL, there is much less "herd immunity" and an outbreak is more likely to occur.

PREVENTION

Vaccination is the best way to prevent mumps. The ACIP currently recommends two doses of MMR. However, proper vaccination (two doses) is only 88% effective at preventing cases; one dose is 78% (range 49%-91%) effective. If someone is diagnosed with mumps, he/she should avoid contact with others from the time of diagnosis until at least 5 days after the onset of parotitis.[117]

Immunity from mumps vaccination wanes over time.

Immunity from mumps vaccination wanes over time. In fact, one outbreak investigation demonstrated that the incidence of mumps was lowest among people who were vaccinated recently (within 2 years) and highest among people who were vaccinated 16 to 23 years prior.[124] Thus, individuals may remain vulnerable even with well-documented vaccination status, especially in athletes that maintain close contact. For example, the Indiana State Department investigated an outbreak of 281 mumps cases involving four Indiana universities in 2016.[125] Eighty-five percent of these cases at the universities had received two doses of MMR, but only 52% of community cases had received a single dose, suggesting the herd immunity of the community was insufficient to prevent transmission.

Human Immunodeficiency Virus

DISEASE BASICS

HIV is a virus spread through certain bodily fluids (blood, semen, vaginal fluids, rectal fluids, breast milk) that attack the body's immune system. If left untreated, the virus depletes CD4 cells, leaving the body susceptible to certain infections. HIV is a global disease that has claimed the lives of more than 22 million people worldwide, including more than 500,000 people in the United States.[126,127]

TYPICAL PRESENTATION

Some people may experience flu-like symptoms within 2 to 4 weeks after becoming infected with HIV. Symptoms include fevers, chills, rash, night sweats, muscle aches, sore throat, fatigue, swollen lymph nodes, or mouth ulcers.[128] None of these symptoms are specific to HIV infection, so diagnosis of acute HIV infection can be difficult. Symptoms resolve on their own after a few days to a few weeks.[129] On the other hand, an estimated 10% to 60% of people acutely infected with HIV will not experience symptoms.[130]

TRANSMISSION

There are many myths about how HIV is transmitted. Specifically, HIV is not transmitted through air, water, saliva, sweat, tears, closed-mouth kissing, or sharing toilets, food, or drinks.[131] Only certain body fluids transmit HIV: blood, semen, preseminal fluid, rectal fluids, vaginal fluids, and breast milk.[131] These fluids must come into contact with a mucous membrane or damaged tissue or be injected directly into the bloodstream for transmission to occur. HIV does not survive for long outside of the human body and cannot replicate outside of the human body.

In sports in which athletes are routinely exposed to blood and open wounds, the risk of HIV transmission is not zero. According to the CDC, the risk of transmission of HIV during sports is small: less than one potential transmission in 1 million games.[132] For example, the risk of transmission in professional football has been conservatively estimated at *less* than one in 1 million games.[133] To date, there are no confirmed cases of spread of HIV through sports activities.[51]

PREVENTION

Education is critical in preventing transmission of HIV. Simply put, athletes must be educated about the risk of HIV transmission through sexual contact and high-risk behaviors including alcohol and drug abuse.[134] Athletes should also be advised not to share personal items that may be contaminated with blood, such as razors, toothbrushes, and nail clippers. Athletes must be trained to follow recommendations of the American Medical Society for Sports Medicine and the American Orthopaedic Society for Sports Medicine[133] to decrease risk of transmission during competition. Athletes must report bleeding injuries in a timely manner and be removed from competition until the bleeding is stopped and blood has been removed from clothing and equipment.

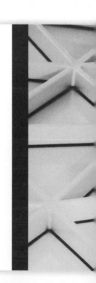

To minimize the risk of bloodborne pathogen transmission, the American Medical Society for Sports Medicine and the American Orthopaedic Society for Sports Medicine recommend the following practices[133]:

1. Existing wounds and skin rashes should be properly prepared.
2. Equipment and supplies should be available for compliance with universal precautions.
3. Those who have uncontrolled bleeding or an uncovered wound should be recognized and removed from competition. Blood-saturated clothing should be removed.
4. The athlete is responsible for wearing protective equipment.
5. Minor cuts and abrasions should be cleaned and dressed.
6. Care providers should follow universal precautions.
7. Personal airway devices should be made available to care providers.
8. Equipment contaminated with blood should be cleaned immediately with disinfecting solution.
9. Wounds should be reevaluated post competition.

REFERENCES

1. Stevens DL, Bisno AL, Chambers HF, et al. Practice guidelines for the diagnosis and management of skin and soft tissue infections: 2014 update by the Infectious Diseases Society of America. *Clin Infect Dis.* 2014;59(2):e10-e52.

2. Raff AB, Kroshinsky D. Cellulitis: a review. *J Am Med Assoc.* 2016;316(3):325-337.

3. Tong SY, Davis JS, Eichenberger E, Holland TL, Fowler VG Jr. Staphylococcus aureus infections: epidemiology, pathophysiology, clinical manifestations, and management. *Clin Microbiol Rev.* 2015;28(3):603-661.

4. Wertheim HF, Melles DC, Vos MC, et al. The role of nasal carriage in *Staphylococcus aureus* infections. *Lancet Infect Dis.* 2005;5(12):751-762.

5. Adams BB. Dermatologic disorders of the athlete. *Sports Med.* 2002;32(5):309-321.

6. Green J. Localized whirlpool folliculitis in a football player. *Cutis.* 2000;65(6):359-362.

7. Adams BB. Transmission of cutaneous infections in athletes. *Br J Sports Med.* 2000;34(6):413-414.

8. Centers for Disease C, Prevention. Methicillin-resistant *Staphylococcus aureus* infections among competitive sports participants–Colorado, Indiana, Pennsylvania, and Los Angeles County, 2000-2003. *MMWR Morb Mortal Wkly Rep.* 2003;52(33):793-795.

9. Stacey AR, Endersby KE, Chan PC, Marples RR. An outbreak of methicillin resistant *Staphylococcus aureus* infection in a rugby football team. *Br J Sports Med.* 1998;32(2):153-154.

10. Lindenmayer JM, Schoenfeld S, O'Grady R, Carney JK. Methicillin-resistant *Staphylococcus aureus* in a high school wrestling team and the surrounding community. *Arch Intern Med.* 1998;158(8):895-899.

11. Adams BB. Skin infections in athletes. *Dermatol Nurs.* 2008;20(1):39.

12. Bradley H, Markowitz LE, Gibson T, McQuillan GM. Seroprevalence of herpes simplex virus types 1 and 2–United States, 1999-2010. *J Infect Dis.* 2014;209(3):325-333.

13. Anderson BJ. The epidemiology and clinical analysis of several outbreaks of herpes gladiatorum. *Med Sci Sports Exerc.* 2003;35(11):1809-1814.

14. Williams C, Wells J, Klein R, Sylvester T, Sunenshine R. Notes from the field: outbreak of skin lesions among high school wrestlers–Arizona, 2014. *MMWR Morb Mortal Wkly Rep.* 2015;64(20):559-560.

15. Belongia EA, Goodman JL, Holland EJ, et al. An outbreak of herpes gladiatorum at a high-school wrestling camp. *N Engl J Med.* 1991;325(13):906-910.

16. White WB, Grant-Kels JM. Transmission of herpes simplex virus type 1 infection in rugby players. *J Am Med Assoc.* 1984;252(4):533-535.

17. Wei EY, Coghlin DT. Beyond folliculitis: recognizing herpes gladiatorum in adolescent athletes. *J Pediatr.* 2017;190:283.

18. Peterson AR, Nash E, Anderson BJ. Infectious disease in contact sports. *Sports Health.* 2019;11(1):47-58.

19. Moriarty B, Hay R, Morris-Jones R. The diagnosis and management of tinea. *Br Med J.* 2012;345:e4380.

20. Ashack KA, Burton KA, Johnson TR, Currie DW, Comstock RD, Dellavalle RP. Skin infections among US high school athletes: a national survey. *J Am Acad Dermatol.* 2016;74(4):679-684.e671.

21. Pickup TL, Adams BB. Prevalence of tinea pedis in professional and college soccer players versus non-athletes. *Clin J Sport Med.* 2007;17(1):52-54.

22. Adams BB. Tinea corporis gladiatorum: a cross-sectional study. *J Am Acad Dermatol.* 2000;43(6):1039-1041.

23. Ely JW, Rosenfeld S, Seabury Stone M. Diagnosis and management of tinea infections. *Am Fam Physician.* 2014;90(10):702-710.

24. Field LA, Adams BB. Tinea pedis in athletes. *Int J Dermatol.* 2008;47(5):485-492.

25. Moris G, Garcia-Monco JC. The challenge of drug-induced aseptic meningitis revisited. *JAMA Intern Med.* 2014;174(9):1511-1512.

26. Logan SA, MacMahon E. Viral meningitis. *Br Med J.* 2008;336(7634):36-40.

27. Yelehe-Okouma M, Czmil-Garon J, Pape E, Petitpain N, Gillet P. Drug-induced aseptic meningitis: a mini-review. *Fundam Clin Pharmacol.* 2018;32(3):252-260.

28. Alexander JP Jr, Chapman LE, Pallansch MA, Stephenson WT, Torok TJ, Anderson LJ. Coxsackievirus B2 infection and aseptic meningitis: a focal outbreak among members of a high school football team. *J Infect Dis.* 1993;167(5):1201-1205.

29. Croker C, Civen R, Keough K, Ngo V, Marutani A, Schwartz B. Aseptic meningitis outbreak associated with echovirus 30 among high school football players–Los Angeles County, California, 2014. *MMWR Morb Mortal Wkly Rep.* 2015;63(51):1228.

30. Moore M, Baron RC, Filstein MR, et al. Aseptic meningitis and high school football players. 1978 and 1980. *J Am Med Assoc.* 1983;249(15):2039-2042.

31. Pons-Salort M, Oberste MS, Pallansch MA, et al. The seasonality of nonpolio enteroviruses in the United States: patterns and drivers. *Proc Natl Acad Sci U S A.* 2018;115(12):3078-3083.

32. Thigpen MC, Whitney CG, Messonnier NE, et al. Bacterial meningitis in the United States, 1998-2007. *N Engl J Med.* 2011;364(21):2016-2025.

33. McGill F, Heyderman RS, Panagiotou S, Tunkel AR, Solomon T. Acute bacterial meningitis in adults. *Lancet.* 2016;388(10063):3036-3047.

34. Ly KN, Klevens RM. Trends in disease and complications of hepatitis A virus infection in the United States, 1999-2011: a new concern for adults. *J Infect Dis.* 2015;212(2):176-182.

35. Foster M, Ramachandran S, Myatt K, et al. Hepatitis A virus outbreaks associated with drug use and homelessness - California, Kentucky, Michigan, and Utah, 2017. *MMWR Morb Mortal Wkly Rep*. 2018;67(43):1208-1210.

36. Sharapov UM, Kentenyants K, Groeger J, Roberts H, Holmberg SD, Collier MG. Hepatitis A infections among food handlers in the United States, 1993-2011. *Public Health Rep*. 2016;131(1):26-29.

37. Teo EK, Lok AS. Epidemiology, transmission, and prevention of hepatitis B virus infection. Post TW, ed. UpToDate. Waltham, MA: *UpToDate Inc*. https://www.uptodate.com. Accessed June 02, 2019.

38. Liaw YF, Tsai SL, Sheen IS, et al. Clinical and virological course of chronic hepatitis B virus infection with hepatitis C and D virus markers. *Am J Gastroenterol*. 1998;93(3):354-359.

39. Fattovich G, Bortolotti F, Donato F. Natural history of chronic hepatitis B: special emphasis on disease progression and prognostic factors. *J Hepatol*. 2008;48(2):335-352.

40. Hoofnagle JH, Di Bisceglie AM. Serologic diagnosis of acute and chronic viral hepatitis. *Semin Liver Dis*. 1991;11(2):73-83.

41. Krugman S, Overby LR, Mushahwar IK, Ling CM, Frosner GG, Deinhardt F. Viral hepatitis, type B. Studies on natural history and prevention reexamined. *N Engl J Med*. 1979;300(3):101-106.

42. Centers for Disease Control and Prevention. Hepatitis B Questions and Answers for Health Professionals. Available at https://www.cdc.gov/hepatitis/hbv/hbv-faq.htm. Accessed July 31, 2019.

43. Lok AS. Hepatitis B virus: Clinical manifestations and natural history. Available at https://www.uptodate.com/contents/hepatitis-b-virus-clinical-manifestations-and-natural-history?search=hepatitis%20b&source=search_result&selectedTitle=4~150&usage_type=default&display_rank=4#H5. Accessed July 2, 2019.

44. Mast EE, Goodman RA, Bond WW, Favero MS, Drotman DP. Transmission of blood-borne pathogens during sports: risk and prevention. *Ann Intern Med*. 1995;122(4):283-285.

45. Beltrami EM, Williams IT, Shapiro CN, Chamberland ME. Risk and management of blood-borne infections in health care workers. *Clin Microbiol Rev*. 2000;13(3):385-407.

46. McGrew C. *Blood-borne pathogens and sports*. In: *Medical Problems Athletes*. Hoboken NJ: Wiley-Blackwell; 1997:64-69.

47. Kashiwagi S, Hayashi J, Ikematsu H, Nishigori S, Ishihara K, Kaji M. An outbreak of hepatitis B in members of a high school sumo wrestling club. *J Am Med Assoc*. 1982;248(2):213-214.

48. Tobe K, Matsuura K, Ogura T, et al. Horizontal transmission of hepatitis B virus among players of an American football team. *Arch Intern Med*. 2000;160(16):2541-2545.

49. FitzSimons D, François G, Hall A, et al. Long-term efficacy of hepatitis B vaccine, booster policy, and impact of hepatitis B virus mutants. *Vaccine*. 2005;23(32):4158-4166.

50. Association NCA. NCAA Sports Medicine Handbook. 2011. Available at http://fs.ncaa.org/Docs/health_safety/2011_12_Sports_Medicine_Handbook.pdf. Accessed July 2011.

51. Kordi R, Wallace W. Blood borne infections in sport: risks of transmission, methods of prevention, and recommendations for hepatitis B vaccination. *Br J Sports Med*. 2004;38(6):678-684.

52. Bond W, Favero M, Petersen N, Gravelle C, Ebert J, Maynard J. Survival of hepatitis B virus after drying and storage for one week. *Lancet*. 1981;1:550-551.

53. Centers for Disease Control and Prevention. Outbreaks of gastroenteritis associated with noroviruses on cruise ships–United States, 2002. *MMWR Morb Mortal Wkly Rep*. 2002;51(49):1112-1115.

54. Bert F, Scaioli G, Gualano MR, et al. Norovirus outbreaks on commercial cruise ships: a systematic review and new targets for the public health agenda. *Food Environ Virol*. 2014;6(2):67-74.

55. Repp KK, Keene WE. A point-source norovirus outbreak caused by exposure to fomites. *J Infect Dis*. 2012;205(11):1639-1641.

56. Glass RI, Parashar UD, Estes MK. Norovirus gastroenteritis. *N Engl J Med*. 2009;361(18):1776-1785.

57. Matthews JE, Dickey BW, Miller RD, et al. The epidemiology of published norovirus outbreaks: a review of risk factors associated with attack rate and genogroup. *Epidemiol Infect*. 2012;140(7):1161-1172.

58. Centers for Disease Control and Prevention. Notes from the field: severe hand, foot, and mouth disease associated with coxsackievirus A6-Alabama, Connecticut, California, and Nevada, November 2011-February 2012. *MMWR Morb Mortal Wkly Rep*. 2012;61(12):213.

59. Wong S, Yip C, Lau S, Yuen K. Human enterovirus 71 and hand, foot and mouth disease. *Epidemiol Infect*. 2010;138(8):1071-1089.

60. Teng S, Wei Y, Zhao SY, Lin XY, Shao QM, Wang J. Intestinal detoxification time of hand-foot-and-mouth disease in children with EV71 infection and the related factors. *World J Pediatr*. 2015;11(4):380-385.

61. Teng S, Zhao SY, Wei Y, et al. Observation on virus shedding periods of enterovirus-71 and coxsackievirus A 16 monitored by nucleic acids determination in stool samples of children with hand, foot and mouth disease. *Zhonghua Er Ke Za Zhi*. 2013;51(10):787-792.

62. Banta J, Lenz B, Pawlak M, et al. Notes from the field: outbreak of hand, foot, and mouth disease caused by coxsackievirus A6 among basic military trainees—Texas, 2015. *MMWR Morb Mortal Wkly Rep*. 2016;65:678-680.

63. Stanmyre, M. (2016, September 15). 'Unprecedented' hand-foot-and-mouth disease outbreak reaches fourth school district. Available at https://www.nj.com/highschoolsports/article/unprecedented-hand-foot-and-mouth-disease-outbreak-reaches-fourth-school-district/. Accessed July 7, 2019.

64. Ruan F, Yang T, Ma H, et al. Risk factors for hand, foot, and mouth disease and herpangina and the preventive effect of hand-washing. *Pediatrics*. 2011;127(4):e898-904.

65. Friman G, Wesslén L. Infections and exercise in high-performance athletes. *Immunol Cell Biol*. 2000;78(5):510-522.

66. Centers for Disease Control and Prevention. Clinical Signs and Symptoms of Influenza. 2019. Available at https://www.cdc.gov/flu/professionals/acip/clinical.htm. Accessed July 8, 2019.

67. Ip DK, Lau LL, Leung NH, et al. Viral shedding and transmission potential of asymptomatic and paucisymptomatic influenza virus infections in the community. *Clin Infect Dis*. 2016;64(6):736-742.

68. Lautermilch J, Doyle-Baker P. The athlete and the flu vaccine: melodrama, common sense or ignorance?. *J Sci Med Sport*. 2014;18:e54.

69. Schwellnus M, Soligard T, Alonso J-M, et al. How much is too much?(Part 2) International Olympic Committee consensus statement on load in sport and risk of illness. *Br J Sports Med*. 2016;50(17):1043-1052.

70. Gundlapalli AV, Rubin MA, Samore MH, et al. Influenza, Winter Olympiad, 2002. *Emerg Infect Dis*. 2006;12(1):144-146.

71. Bridges CB, Thompson WW, Meltzer MI, et al. Effectiveness and cost-benefit of influenza vaccination of healthy working adults: a randomized controlled trial. *J Am Med Assoc*. 2000;284(13):1655-1663.

72. Nichol KL, Mendelman PM, Mallon KP, et al. Effectiveness of live, attenuated intranasal influenza virus vaccine in healthy, working adults: a randomized controlled trial. *J Am Med Assoc*. 1999;282(2):137-144.

73. Wilde JA, McMillan JA, Serwint J, Butta J, O'riordan MA, Steinhoff MC. Effectiveness of influenza vaccine in health care professionals: a randomized trial. *J Am Med Assoc*. 1999;281(10):908-913.

74. Auwaerter PG. Infectious mononucleosis: return to play. *Clin Sports Med*. 2004;23(3):485-497, xi.

75. Kinderknecht JJ. Infectious mononucleosis and the spleen. *Curr Sports Med Rep*. 2002;1(2):116-120.

76. Ebell MH, Call M, Shinholser J, Gardner J. Does this patient have infectious mononucleosis?: the rational clinical examination systematic review. *J Am Med Assoc*. 2016;315(14):1502-1509.

77. Burgess MA, McIntyre PB, Heath TC. Pertussis re-emerging: who is responsible?. *Aust N Z J Public Health*. 1998;22(1):9-10.

78. Storsaeter J, Hallander HO, Gustafsson L, Olin P. Low levels of antipertussis antibodies plus lack of history of pertussis correlate with susceptibility after household exposure to Bordetella pertussis. *Vaccine*. 2003;21(25-26):3542-3549.

79. Forsyth KD, Wirsing von Konig CH, Tan T, Caro J, Plotkin S. Prevention of pertussis: recommendations derived from the second Global Pertussis Initiative roundtable meeting. *Vaccine*. 2007;25(14):2634-2642.

80. Kretsinger K, Broder KR, Cortese MM, et al. Preventing tetanus, diphtheria, and pertussis among adults: use of tetanus toxoid, reduced diphtheria toxoid and acellular pertussis vaccine recommendations of the Advisory Committee on Immunization Practices (ACIP) and recommendation of ACIP, supported by the Healthcare Infection Control Practices Advisory Committee (HICPAC), for use of Tdap among health-care personnel. *MMWR Recomm Rep*. 2006;55(RR-17):1-37.

81. Heininger U, Cherry JD, Stehr K, et al. Comparative Efficacy of the Lederle/Takeda acellular pertussis component DTP (DTaP) vaccine and Lederle whole-cell component DTP vaccine in German children after household exposure. Pertussis Vaccine Study Group. *Pediatrics*. 1998;102(3 pt 1):546-553.

82. Mattoo S, Cherry JD. Molecular pathogenesis, epidemiology, and clinical manifestations of respiratory infections due to Bordetella pertussis and other Bordetella subspecies. *Clin Microbiol Rev*. 2005;18(2):326-382.

83. Rutledge RK, Keen EC. Images in clinical medicine. Whooping cough in an adult. *N Engl J Med*. 2012;366(25):e39.

84. Centers for Disease Control and Prevention. Pertussis (Whooping Cough). Available at https://www.cdc.gov/pertussis/clinical/features.html. Accessed July 7, 2019.

85. Warfel JM, Beren J, Merkel TJ. Airborne transmission of Bordetella pertussis. *J Infect Dis*. 2012;206(6):902-906.

86. Deen JL, Mink CA, Cherry JD, et al. Household contact study of Bordetella pertussis infections. *Clin Infect Dis*. 1995;21(5):1211-1219.

87. Tiwari T, Murphy TV, Moran J. National Immunization Program CDC. Recommended antimicrobial agents for the treatment and postexposure prophylaxis of pertussis: 2005 CDC Guidelines. *MMWR Recomm Rep*. 2005;54(RR-14):1-16.

88. Skrzypiec-Spring M, Krzywanski J, Karlikowska-Skwarnik M, et al. Pertussis outbreak in Polish shooters with adverse event analysis. *Biol Sport*. 2017;34(3):243-248.

89. Centers for Disease Control and Prevention. Pertussis: Summary of Vaccine Recommendations. 2017. Available at https://www.cdc.gov/vaccines/vpd/pertussis/recs-summary.html. Accessed July 8, 2019.

90. James SL, Abate D, Abate KH, et al. Global, regional, and national incidence, prevalence, and years lived with disability for 354 diseases and injuries for 195 countries and territories, 1990-2017: a systematic analysis for the Global Burden of Disease Study 2017. *Lancet*. 2018;392(10159):1789-1858.

91. Getahun H, Matteelli A, Chaisson RE, Raviglione M. Latent *Mycobacterium tuberculosis* infection. *N Engl J Med*. 2015;372(22):2127-2135.

92. Dheda K, Barry CE III, Maartens G. Tuberculosis. *Lancet*. 2016;387(10024):1211-1226.

93. Zumla A, Raviglione M, Hafner R, von Reyn CF. Tuberculosis. *N Engl J Med*. 2013;368(8): 745-755.

94. Menzies D, Adjobimey M, Ruslami R, et al. Four months of rifampin or nine months of isoniazid for latent tuberculosis in adults. *N Engl J Med*. 2018;379(5):440-453.

95. Horsburgh CR Jr, Barry CE III, Lange C. Treatment of tuberculosis. *N Engl J Med*. 2015;373(22):2149-2160.

96. Churchyard G, Kim P, Shah NS, et al. What we know about tuberculosis transmission: an overview. *J Infect Dis*. 2017;216(suppl_6): S629-S635.

97. Bibbins-Domingo K, Grossman DC, Curry SJ, et al. Screening for latent tuberculosis infection in adults: US preventive services task force recommendation statement. *J Am Med Assoc*. 2016;316(9):962-969.

98. Colditz GA, Brewer TF, Berkey CS, et al. Efficacy of BCG vaccine in the prevention of tuberculosis. Meta-analysis of the published literature. *J Am Med Assoc*. 1994;271(9):698-702.

99. Marin M, Watson TL, Chaves SS, et al. Varicella among adults: data from an active surveillance project, 1995-2005. *J Infect Dis*. 2008;197 suppl 2:S94-S100.

100. Guris D, Jumaan AO, Mascola L, et al. Changing varicella epidemiology in active surveillance sites–United States, 1995-2005. *J Infect Dis*. 2008;197 suppl 2:S71-S75.

101. Glanz JM, McClure DL, Magid DJ, Daley MF, France EK, Hambidge SJ. Parental refusal of varicella vaccination and the associated risk of varicella infection in children. *Arch Pediatr Adolesc Med*. 2010;164(1):66-70.

102. Conway JJ, Toresdahl BG, Ling DI, Boniquit NT, Callahan LR, Kinderknecht JJ. Prevalence of inadequate immunity to measles, mumps, rubella, and varicella in MLB and NBA athletes. *Sports Health*. 2018;10(5):406-411.

103. Heininger U, Seward JF. Varicella. *Lancet*. 2006;368(9544):1365-1376.

104. McCarthy M. Measles outbreak linked to Disney theme parks reaches five states and Mexico. *Br Med J*. 2015;350:h436.

105. Zipprich J, Winter K, Hacker J, Xia D, Watt J, Harriman K. Measles outbreak–California, December 2014-February 2015. *MMWR Morb Mortal Wkly Rep*. 2015;64(6):153-154.

106. Jain A, Marshall J, Buikema A, Bancroft T, Kelly JP, Newschaffer CJ. Autism occurrence by MMR vaccine status among US children with older siblings with and without autism. *J Am Med Assoc*. 2015;313(15):1534-1540.

107. Taylor B, Miller E, Farrington CP, et al. Autism and measles, mumps, and rubella vaccine: no epidemiological evidence for a causal association. *Lancet*. 1999;353(9169):2026-2029.

108. Taylor LE, Swerdfeger AL, Eslick GD. Vaccines are not associated with autism: an evidence-based meta-analysis of case-control and cohort studies. *Vaccine*. 2014;32(29):3623-3629.

109. Centers for Disease Control and Prevention. Measles Cases and Outbreaks. 2019. Available at https://www.cdc.gov/measles/cases-outbreaks. html. Accessed July 6, 2019.

110. Ehresmann KR, Hedberg CW, Grimm MB, Norton CA, MacDonald KL, Osterholm MT. An outbreak of measles at an international sporting event with airborne transmission in a domed stadium. *J Infect Dis*. 1995;171(3):679-683.

111. Moss WJ. Measles. *Lancet*. 2017;390(10111):2490-2502.

112. Griffin DE. Measles virus-induced suppression of immune responses. *Immunol Rev*. 2010;236:176-189.

113. Glasziou PP, Mackerras DE. Vitamin A supplementation in infectious diseases: a meta-analysis. *Br Med J*. 1993;306(6874):366-370.

114. van den Driessche P. Reproduction numbers of infectious disease models. *Infect Dis Model*. 2017;2(3):288-303.

115. Centers for Disease Control and Prevention. Available at https://www.cdc.gov/mumps/outbreaks.html. Accessed July 8, 2019.

116. Marin M, Marlow M, Moore KL, Patel M. Recommendation of the Advisory Committee on Immunization Practices for use of a third dose of mumps virus-containing vaccine in persons at increased risk for mumps during an outbreak. *MMWR Morb Mortal Wkly Rep*. 2018;67(1):33-38.

117. Centers for Disease Control and Prevention. Updated recommendations for isolation of persons with mumps. *MMWR Morb Mortal Wkly Rep*. 2008;57(40):1103-1105.

118. Hviid A, Rubin S, Muhlemann K. Mumps. *Lancet*. 2008;371(9616):932-944.

119. Gupta RK, Best J, MacMahon E. Mumps and the UK epidemic 2005. *Br Med J*. 2005;330(7500):1132-1135.

120. Reisz B, Capitals AW. *Somebody's Got a Case of the MumpDays: A Review of the Mumps Outbreak in the NHL*: Washington Capitals; 2014.

121. Newstaff C. Mumps outbreak continues in Alberta. 2007. Available at https://www.ctvnews.ca/mumps-outbreak-continues-in-alberta-1.265769. Accessed June 30, 2019.

122. Pretot J. Mumps epidemic forces French to postpone games. 2011. Available at https://www.moneycontrol.com/news/business/wire-news/-1940187.html. Accessed July 1, 2019.

123. Rubin SA, Link MA, Sauder CJ, et al. Recent mumps outbreaks in vaccinated populations: no evidence of immune escape. *J Virol*. 2012;86(1):615-620.

124. Cardemil CV, Dahl RM, James L, et al. Effectiveness of a third dose of MMR vaccine for mumps outbreak control. *N Engl J Med*. 2017;377(10):947-956.

125. Golwalkar M, Pope B, Stauffer J, Snively A, Clemmons N. Mumps outbreaks at four universities—Indiana, 2016. *MMWR Morb Mortal Wkly Rep*. 2018;67(29):793.

126. Centers for Disease Control and Prevention. Twenty-five years of HIV/AIDS–United States, 1981-2006. *MMWR Morb Mortal Wkly Rep*. 2006;55(21):585.

127. Centers for Disease Control and Prevention. Epidemiology of HIV/AIDS–United States, 1981-2005. *MMWR Morb Mortal Wkly Rep*. 2006;55(21):589.

128. Crowell TA, Colby DJ, Pinyakorn S, et al. Acute retroviral syndrome is associated with high viral burden, CD4 depletion, and immune activation in systemic and tissue compartments. *Clin Infect Dis*. 2018;66(10):1540-1549.

129. Centers for Disease Control and Prevention. About HIV/AIDS. HIV Basics Web site. Available at https://www.cdc.gov/hiv/basics/whatishiv.html. Accessed July 1, 2019.

130. Services DoHaH. Panel on Antiretroviral Guidelines for Adults and Adolescents. Guidelines for the use of antiretroviral agents in HIV-1-infected adults and adolescents. Department of Health and Human Services. Available at https://aidsinfo.nih.gov/contentfiles/lvguidelines/adultandadolescentgl.pdf. Accessed July 9, 2019.

131. Centers for Disease Control and Prevention. HIV Transmission. HIV Basics Web site. Available at https://www.cdc.gov/hiv/basics/transmission.html. Accessed June 30, 2019.

132. Centers for Disease Control and Prevention. HIV/AIDS and Sports. 1996. Available at www.ed.state.nh.us/HealthHIVAIDS/HIVPolicyTrainingResources.pdf. Accessed July 3, 2019.

133. Human immunodeficiency virus (HIV) and other blood-borne pathogens in sports. Joint position statement. The American Medical Society for Sports Medicine (AMSSM) and the American Academy of Sports Medicine (AASM). *Am J Sports Med*. 1995;23(4):510-514.

134. Clem KL, Borchers JR. HIV and the athlete. *Clin Sports Med*. 2007;26(3):413-424.

135. Hasbun R. The acute aseptic meningitis syndrome. *Curr Infect Dis Rep*. 2000;2(4):345-351.

136. Kupila L, Vuorinen T, Vainionpää R, Hukkanen V, Marttila R, Kotilainen P. Etiology of aseptic meningitis and encephalitis in an adult population. *Neurology*. 2006;66(1):75-80.

2

The Athlete's Perspective—Reduce Your Risk of Infection

Tori Kinamon | Deverick J. Anderson

Introduction

The content within this chapter is unique. It has been specifically designed for you, the athlete, and your support group, parents, and coaches. The material in this chapter is intended to provide practical, useful, and easily digestible information to reduce your risk of infection and stay in the game.

Throughout this manual, we provide information on strategies to reduce risk. **We provide numerous recommendations for team medical staff in Chapters 3-6.** *These recommendations are provided as Best Practices for prevention followed by recommendations to meet the Best Practices. In this chapter, we first describe a risk factor for you, the athlete; we then provide recommendations and action points about how you can reduce that risk, and finally we provide insight into why you should care about these behaviors and recommendations. It's important to note, however, that no interventions exist to reduce your risk of infection to zero. As a result, you always must remain vigilant for high-risk scenarios or, better yet, diligently practice preventative techniques.*

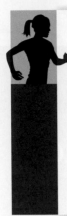

Tips From Tori

Do you experience any of these as an athlete?

- **Contact:** skin to skin
- **Compromised skin** (cuts or scrapes)
- Difficulty with **cleanliness** (think: washing your hands or showering immediately after practice because of time constraints)
- **Crowded** areas or shared personal items (think: locker rooms!)
- **Contaminated** equipment or surfaces shared between players

These "5 C's" of transmission increase your risk for infection. I should know—my collegiate gymnastics career was threatened by an MRSA infection. Three months and eight surgeries later, I made it back to my team.

As an athlete, you take precautions to protect yourself on the court, field, or mat. You engage in physical therapy for musculoskeletal injuries, receive pre- and postpractice treatments from athletic trainers, and build muscle mass in the weight room. However, did you know that being an athlete places you at increased risk for common infectious diseases? Athletes have increased risk of several infections, including norovirus, influenza, skin and soft-tissue infections due to methicillin-resistant *Staphylococcus aureus* (MRSA), and herpes gladiatorum. **These infections not only have the potential to sideline you from athletic participation but can also place the entire team at risk if not managed appropriately.** It is important for you to, first, be aware of your risk for infection as an athlete and, second, adhere to basic infection prevention strategies to help protect yourself and your teammates from these infections.

Infection risk for athletes falls into four broad categories: (1) personal and social behaviors, (2) medical care, (3) interactions with other athletes, and (4) use of facilities and equipment (**Figure 2.1**). The 5 C's outlined above contribute to all of these categories. We outline specific risks within each of these categories in **Table 2.1**. Of course, team medical personnel

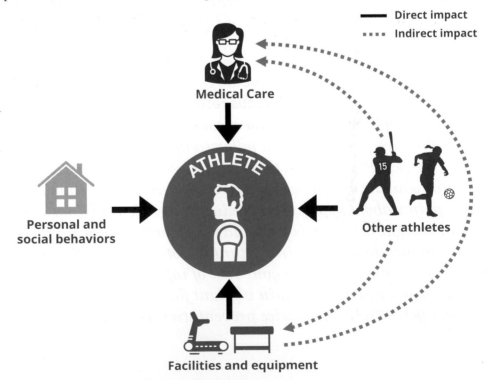

Figure 2.1 Framework for infection transmission in athletes.

Table 2.1 Summary of Risk Factors for Infections in Athletes—Behaviors, Risks, and Recommendations to Stay Infection Free

Personal and Social Behaviors

Behavior	Risk	Recommendation
Player knowledge and education	Lack of knowledge, unaware of risk for infection Poor team culture	Actively participate in preseason athlete health meetings. Recognize symptoms of infection and present these symptoms to your athletic trainer ASAP. Notify your athletic trainer when you have vomiting or diarrhea. Recognize the signs of "athlete's foot" and present symptoms to athletic trainer. Recognize the signs of herpes gladiatorum and present symptoms to athletic trainer. Notify your athletic trainer if you develop flu-like symptoms. Become an infection prevention champion.
Hand hygiene practices	Regular skin-to-skin contact Lack of hand cleanliness	Increase use of hand hygiene while in athletic environments. Locate and use alcohol-based hand hygiene dispensers throughout the facility. Promote hand hygiene among your teammates. Clean hands with soap and water if they are visibly soiled.
Body hygiene	Regular skin-to-skin contact Skin contact with contaminated surfaces Lack of body cleanliness	Shower immediately after practice. Do not use bar soap in the shower. Use soap dispensers that utilize prepackaged liquid soap. Bathe with chlorhexidine gluconate 3x/week.
Body shaving	Compromised skin	Avoid cosmetic body shaving. If hair removal is necessary, remove with individual- or single-use clippers. If hair must be removed through shaving, shave clean skin with a fresh razor. Never share a razor.

Medical Care

Type of Medical Care	Risk	Recommendation
Basic medical care	Insufficient knowledge of fundamental infection prevention practices	Talk with your athletic trainer about infection prevention protocols utilized in your athletic training facility. Take an active role in disinfecting the materials that you use in the athletic training room during and after treatments. Practice good hand hygiene in the athletic training facilities.

(Continued)

Table 2.1 Summary of Risk Factors for Infections in Athletes—Behaviors, Risks, and Recommendations to Stay Infection Free   (Continued)

Cut care	Compromised skin from routine athletic activities High rate of colonization with *Staphylococcus aureus* and methicillin-resistant *Staphylococcus aureus* (MRSA)	Monitor skin on a daily basis for skin wounds, including cuts, scrapes, and any suspicious lesions. Show all wounds to your athletic trainer for cleaning and treatment as soon as you notice them. Be knowledgeable of the policy for cut care in your athletic training facility and discuss with your athletic trainer.
Hydrotherapy	Use of hydrotherapy pools	Do not enter the hydrotherapy pool with an open wound unless the wound is covered by an impermeable dressing. Shower prior to using hydrotherapy pools. Do not use the hydrotherapy pools if you have a known MRSA infection until the infection is completely resolved. Use a clean, laundered, individual use towel after exiting the whirlpool.
Antimicrobial stewardship	Inappropriate use of antibiotics	Understand the risk of taking unnecessary antibiotics. Do not expect to receive antibiotics for viral illnesses.
Travel medicine and emerging infections	Crowding on planes, buses Tight living quarters Novel exposures	Discuss travel medicine requirements with team medical personnel prior to traveling abroad for an athletic event. Attend travel medicine clinic in order to reduce your risk of contracting an infectious disease while abroad.
Nonmedical wellness practices	Insufficient knowledge of infection risk associated with nonmedical wellness practices	Understand the risk of "alternative therapies" such as acupuncture, home IV therapy, cupping, and massage. Use facilities that have licensed practitioners and are inspected by the health department if you choose to engage in an alternative therapy and receive treatment outside of your athletic facility. Ensure that single-use instruments are used when engaging in a therapy (such as acupuncture, home IV therapy) that punctures the skin.
Medical care–involving procedures	Compromised skin Poor injection practices	Ask your provider if they are using aseptic techniques and "safe injection practices." Observe the provider washing their hands and using a single-use needle and vial.
Surgical procedures	Compromised skin from the incision High rate of colonization with *Staphylococcus aureus* and MRSA	Discuss what symptoms might indicate an early infection at the surgical site with your athletic trainer and physician. Monitor surgical incision on a daily basis for symptoms of potential infection. If deemed necessary, follow decolonization protocols as instructed by your physician.

Table 2.1 Summary of Risk Factors for Infections in Athletes—Behaviors, Risks, and Recommendations to Stay Infection Free   (Continued)

Other Athletes

Behavior	Risk	Recommendation
Direct contact	Transmission of germs through direct contact (skin to skin) with other athletes	Understand how and when direct transmission may occur during athletic participation and take necessary precautions. Practice consistent and frequent hand hygiene.
Shared equipment	Indirect transmission of germs through equipment or surfaces contaminated by other athletes	Do not share personal equipment that comes into contact with the skin, such as towels or razors. Make a habit of disinfecting shared equipment prior to use in the treatment room, training room, and weight room.
Crowding in shared spaces	Vaccine-preventable illnesses	Receive all required vaccinations. Make sure to receive influenza vaccination annually.

Facilities and Equipment

Location	Risk	Recommendation
Weight room	Contaminated surfaces and equipment Crowding	Use an alcohol-based hand sanitizer upon entering the weight room. Pick up a clean towel upon entering the weight room. Place "barriers" (such as a clean towel) over equipment. Wipe down equipment after each use.
Athletic training room	Contaminated surfaces and equipment Crowding	Ask your athletic trainer about cleaning and disinfection protocols in place in your athletic training environment. Ensure that treatment equipment is appropriately disinfected before and after your individual use. Disinfect cardiovascular, rehabilitation, and other training equipment after each use. Be sure that the electrostimulation pads you are using have not been used by another player. Reusable athletic equipment should be appropriately disinfected after it is used, visibly soiled, or otherwise dirty.
Visiting team locker room	See above. The same risks that you face at your home facilities are present at away facilities	Abide by your athletic trainer's guidelines for infection prevention and follow the recommendations outlined above.

have important roles to play and tasks to complete to keep you safe, but **you** play a critically important role in maintaining your own health and safety. As you read these sections, consider how and when you might face these risks in your routine as an athlete.

Team medical personnel have important roles to play and tasks to complete to keep you safe, but you play a critically important role in maintaining your own health and safety.

Personal and Social Behaviors

Your personal and social behaviors can increase your risk for infection. However, you have the direct ability to modify behavior, improve habits, and decrease risk. One key strategy highlighted throughout is hygiene.

A key strategy to prevent infection: hygiene

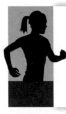

Tips From Tori

You study game film to prepare for your opponent. Infectious diseases, however, can be an opponent that defeats your team before you even exit the locker room.

To mount an adequate defense against these germs, you should be aware of your risk for infection and knowledgeable about how you can reduce this risk.

Player Knowledge and Education

⊙ **Risk** Lack of knowledge.

If you are unaware of your risk for athletically acquired infections, you may be missing opportunities to protect yourself and your teammates from these preventable infections.

⊘ **Recommendation 1** Participate in preseason athlete health meetings and ask athletic trainers and medical staff for additional information about infection prevention and control protocols in your athletic facility.

Rationale: Athletes are at increased risk for infection for several reasons. Primarily, athletes are often in close quarters and have frequent, close contact with other athletes. Athletic activities often lead to skin abrasions, cuts, and scrapes. Finally, athletes often have inadequate access to clean equipment/facilities and/or simply don't practice good hand and body hygiene. During just 1 day of training, you will be repeatedly exposed to these risks not only on the court, field, or mats but also in the athletic training room, weight room, and locker room.

You know the cliché—"knowledge is power." Cliché or not, education is a critical and effective component of infection prevention. In preseason meetings, you should be educated about recognizing and preventing several types of infection, such as skin and soft-tissue infections. One such example, MRSA, is of particular importance. These infections occur commonly among athletes and may produce outbreaks or clusters of infection that consequently impact numerous players.[1]

Tips From Tori

When in doubt, point it out!

Athletic trainers agree; it is much better to be safe than sorry when it comes to potential infections.

✓ Recommendation 2 Recognize the signs and symptoms of skin infection and present these symptoms to your athletic trainer.

Rationale: You know your body better than anyone, and you know when something might be wrong. So, it's important that you know of and remain vigilant for early signs of infection. Symptoms of an early infection include but are not limited to a skin lesion with:

- Redness
- Swelling
- Warmth
- Excessive pain
- Pus or other drainage

These symptoms may also be accompanied by fever, chills, and generalized malaise. Notify your athletic trainer immediately if you develop any of these symptoms.

More specifically, present any concerning issues or symptoms to your athletic trainer immediately if they occur. We've spoken to hundreds of athletic trainers, and we know they agree: when in doubt, point it out. Proper diagnosis and prompt treatment could prevent these infections from becoming more severe. The earlier you receive treatment, the less likely the infection will cause serious problems.

Additionally, you should communicate with your athletic trainer about the infection prevention policies that are in place in your athletic facility. These may include but are not limited to protocols regarding hydrotherapy room usage, cut care, laundry services, and hand hygiene. Understanding and abiding by these policies can help you avoid preventable infections.

✓ Recommendation 3 Notify your athletic trainer when you have vomiting and/or diarrhea.

Rationale: If you have vomiting AND diarrhea, you could potentially have norovirus. Norovirus is the most common cause of outbreaks of acute gastroenteritis in the United States. It is highly contagious and is easily spread from person to person and via aerosols, food, or contact with contaminated environmental surfaces.

Outbreaks among athletes have been documented. For instance, an outbreak of norovirus infections occurred during a football game between Duke and Florida State University. The original source of infection was thought to be turkey sandwiches in box lunches served to the Duke team 50 hours before the game. 50% of the team personnel became ill before and during the game. 11 Florida State players then developed norovirus infection after the game.[2] A similar team-to-opposing team transmission occurred in the National Basketball Association (NBA).

Wash your hands thoroughly with soap and water if norovirus is suspected. Norovirus is not inactivated by alcohol-based sanitizers.

Due to the highly contagious nature of norovirus, it is very important that you are transparent with your athletic trainer about your symptoms. Doing so could save all members of your team from missed game time. Your athletic trainers and athletic facility will use special disinfection strategies when a case of norovirus has been identified. You should do the same. At home, wash your hands frequently and disinfect your bathroom with a bleach or hydrogen peroxide–containing disinfectant.

✓ Recommendation 4 Recognize the signs of "athlete's foot" and present these symptoms to your athletic trainer.

Rationale: Tinea pedis or "athlete's foot" is a fungal infection of the skin, typically between the toes. Athlete's foot can be easily diagnosed by its appearance, which your athletic trainer will be able to evaluate. Your athletic trainer will likely advise you to apply a topical antifungal cream for 4 weeks. Athlete's foot should be treated for two reasons. First, the presence of athlete's foot, and the resulting damage to the skin, can put you at risk for skin infection in the foot and lower leg. Second, athlete's foot can be spread to other athletes. When an athlete has tinea pedis, the spore-like cells of the fungus are shed on the training floor. Other athletes in the facility can then acquire tinea pedis through contact with that training floor. If untreated, the infection could persist indefinitely.

✓ Recommendation 5 Recognize the signs of herpes gladiatorum and present these symptoms to your athletic trainer. Know that you are at particularly increased risk for these infections in contact sports, such as wrestling, rugby, and football.

Rationale: Herpes gladiatorum is a viral skin infection caused by the herpes simplex virus (HSV). Most people are familiar with herpes-related cold sores, as almost two-thirds of adults have HSV. HSV is classified into two broad types, HSV-1 and HSV-2. Nearly all reported outbreaks of herpes gladiatorum involve HSV-1, the same virus responsible for nearly 80% of cold sores.

Since the virus gains entry to the body via small breaks in the skin, athletes involved in contact sports are at increased risk. While the majority of outbreaks have been described among wrestlers, transmission between rugby players has also been described (informally called "scrum pox"). The same mechanisms of transmission described above—frequent abrasions and skin-to-skin contact between athletes—put athletes at risk. Sometimes mistaken for other common skin infections, delayed diagnosis contributes to ongoing transmission.

✓ Recommendation 6 Notify your athletic trainer if you develop flu-like symptoms.

Rationale: Flu-like symptoms typically include the sudden onset of fever, chills, myalgias, headache, cough, loss of appetite, and a generalized feeling of weakness. These symptoms can be caused by different viral infections, but influenza should be suspected during the "flu season," especially when flu levels are high in your area. Your athletic trainer may want to have you tested for influenza and other respiratory viruses. If you test positive for influenza, you can be treated with oseltamivir to shorten the duration of the symptoms. As importantly, your athletic trainer can initiate a layered response to help prevent you from spreading the flu to other teammates.

▶ Risk Poor team culture.

✓ Recommendation 1 Become an infection prevention champion to improve the "culture" of infection prevention and accountability.

Rationale: As an athlete, you are well aware of how team culture affects performance, and likely, the final outcome of a game, match, or competition. Just as you, your teammates, and coaches try to build a culture of athletic excellence, you can and need to create a "culture" of quality in infection prevention. Accountability is a key component of both your culture of athletic excellence and the culture of quality in infection prevention.

Who do you identify as a leader in your team? Are you the leader? Leaders play a critical role in developing team culture. In quality improvement initiatives, leaders are often labeled as "champions." Infection prevention champions serve as role models for effective infection prevention practices and hold other members of the team accountable. In order to be an infection prevention champion, you must be familiar with specific infection prevention policies used at the facilities and integrate them into your daily routine. What can you do to lead the way?

Infection prevention champions serve as role models for effective infection prevention practices and hold other members of the team accountable.

Here is a list of suggested **actions** that will demonstrate to your teammates that you are committed to creating a safe environment and upholding a culture of quality:

- Shower immediately after practice
- Don't use whirlpools with open wounds
- Perform hand hygiene in the weight room
- Get up-to-date with recommended vaccinations

By adhering to these recommendations, you can motivate and stimulate others to embrace and follow good infection prevention practices (**Figure 2.2**). Lead by example! You also can effectively reeducate and remind teammates who violate infection prevention principles by positively motivating them to change their behaviors. For example, teammates are less likely to enter a whirlpool with open wounds if they see you, a leader on your team, adhering to team-based protocols and good practices.

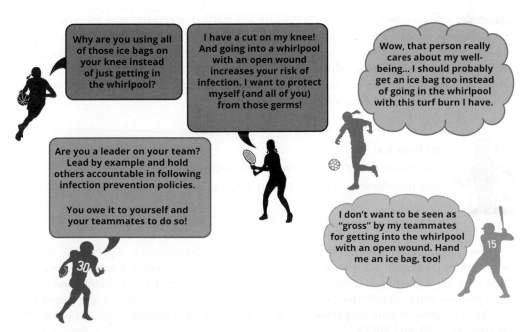

Figure 2.2 Infection prevention champions model behavior for other athletes.

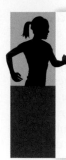

Tips From Tori

Let's list examples of skin-to-skin contact we might have as athletes:

- Tackling an opponent
- Jockeying for a position
- Receiving treatment from an athletic trainer
- Shaking hands or high-fiving your teammates and coaches

Those add up over the course of a day in the life of an athlete!

▶ **Risk** **Poor hygiene.**

As in any athletic endeavor, focusing on the fundamentals is critical to success. Hygiene is a fundamental component of health and one that you can directly control. This subsection includes specific strategies to help you improve and maintain your hygiene through hand washing, showering, and using appropriate strategies for hair removal, as necessary. You have a responsibility to yourself and your teammates to adhere to these strategies!

Hand Hygiene

▶ **Risk Factors** **Regular hand contact (skin to skin); hand cleanliness (or lack thereof).**

✓ **Recommendation 1** Increase use of hand hygiene while in all athletic environments.

✓ **Recommendation 2** Locate and use alcohol-based hand hygiene dispensers throughout the facility.

✓ **Recommendation 3** Be an infection prevention champion by promoting hand hygiene.

Rationale: Skin-to-skin transmission is the primary method of transmission for most bacterial pathogens, such as MRSA, and viruses (**Figure 2.3**). These pathogens may temporarily be present on the hands of other athletes or athletic trainers. As a result, these pathogens are most commonly transmitted through direct contact. Since this type of interaction is universal, how do you eliminate this type of exposure? Frequent, consistent hand washing is your best strategy to stop the infection cycle (**Figure 2.4**).

Tips From Tori

Hygiene can prevent the progression from exposure to skin colonization.

Break the infection cycle by following good hand hygiene!

Overall, hand hygiene is the #1 method for preventing transmission of germs and should be integrated frequently into your daily routine. Simply utilizing alcohol-based hand hygiene dispensers upon entering and exiting facilities can decrease your risk of infection **and** effectively position you as an infection prevention champion. Alcohol-based hand hygiene products are highly effective in reducing person-to-person transmission in pathogens such as influenza, the common cold, and MRSA.

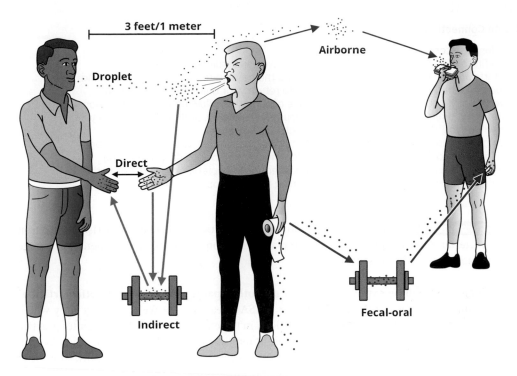

Figure 2.3 Methods for microbe transmission between athletes.

✅ **Recommendation 4** Clean hands with soap and water instead of alcohol-based products after using the toilet, when visibly soiled, or when heavily contaminated with dirt, debris, body fluids, or blood.

Rationale: Alcohol-based hygiene products are not effective when hands are soiled with dirt or other materials such as oils, blood, or other body fluids.

Showering After Athletic Participation

▶ **Risk Factors** **Body cleanliness (or lack thereof). Body contact (skin to skin). Skin contact with contaminated items or surfaces.**

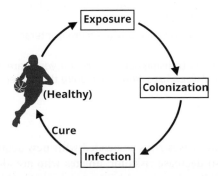

Figure 2.4 Cycle of transmission and infection in athletes.

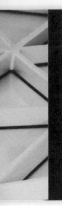

Athlete Connection

Consider this scene.

You finish a 3-hour practice at 6:00 PM and have an examination review session that starts at 6:30 PM. You rush off the field, into the training room to do a foam rolling session or ice bath, then into the locker room to return your uniform. No time for a shower! Finally, you're off to the academic side of campus. Following the study session, you go to the dining hall, put in a few more hours at the library, and finally return to your dorm where you shower hours after your athletic participation.

During that time, you've had bacteria sitting on your skin that you acquired through interacting with other athletes during practice. Any cuts or scrapes may already be contaminated. In addition, you may have deposited those bacteria onto surfaces in the athletic training room, locker room, library, dining hall, and your dorm room.

⊘ Recommendation 1 Immediately shower after practice to decrease your risk of infection and bacterial transmission from player to player and from player to environment. Encourage your teammates to do the same.

Rationale: You will be exposed to MRSA and other pathogens during athletic participation. Humans are the natural reservoirs for MRSA, meaning that we are the agent by which the bacteria are spread and the source for MRSA in the environment. Showering after practice decreases the risk of MRSA infection because it removes the bacteria from the skin. As with hand hygiene, this intervention stops the infection cycle for you. More specifically, showering after practice can remove MRSA and other pathogens acquired during practice.

You will be exposed to MRSA and other pathogens during athletic participation.

Removal of these bacteria decreases risk of infection in two ways. First, with fewer bacteria present, the risk of infection in compromised skin is decreased in the short term. Second, removing bacteria will prevent long-term colonization on the skin. Colonization means that a person carries the bacteria on their skin without showing signs of infection. However, colonization increases the risk of infection in the long term. That is, the germ is present and ready to cause trouble when an opportunity occurs later on (eg, a subsequent scratch or cut).

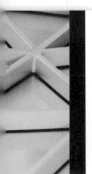

Key Terms

Primary transmission: transmission occurs when there is direct skin-to-skin contact.
• Athlete connection: primary transmission can occur during the skin-to-skin contact that happens when you tackle an opponent.

Secondary transmission: transmission occurs when there is interaction with a contaminated surface.
• Athlete connection: secondary transmission can occur if you share athletic equipment without disinfecting it in between uses. You can acquire the bacteria from contaminated surfaces!

As above, showering decreases risks associated with **new** acquisition of a pathogen like MRSA. Showering will also decrease risks for athletes who are already colonized. A recent study showed that 13% of US collegiate athletes are colonized with MRSA without showing signs of infection.[3] In other words, on a 50-member team, nearly 7 players are silently colonized with MRSA. The study also demonstrated that players with MRSA colonization were 7.3 times more likely to experience a subsequent MRSA infection. In comparison, only 2% of people in the general American public carry the bacteria on their skin. So, to relate to the hypothetical team we described above, that means that out of 50 people, only 1 person would be silently colonized with MRSA. Showering after practice improves skin health and decreases the risk that MRSA (or some other germ) will enter a skin abrasion, even if the MRSA is already on the skin.

Finally, showering after practice will decrease the risk of secondary transmission to your teammates both by direct contact (primary transmission) and through contamination of the environment (secondary transmission). By reducing the amount of MRSA on the skin, you will reduce the amount of MRSA in the environment. This intervention will reduce contamination of a training facility and athletic environment, ultimately protecting other athletes from contamination as well.

REMEMBER—contact with MRSA is inevitable in team settings. MRSA exposure increases the risk of subsequent infection as well, particularly in the setting of skin abrasions and cuts acquired through athletic participation. Simple interventions can help you decrease this risk.

✓ Recommendation 2 Do not use bar soap present in the shower. Use soap dispensers that utilize prepackaged liquid soap in the shower.

Rationale: Bar soap has previously been implicated as a potential source of MRSA transmission. Specifically, sharing bar soap was associated with MRSA infections during an outbreak among football players and in an outbreak in a prison.[4]

✓ Recommendation 3 Bathe with chlorhexidine gluconate three times each week.

Tips From Tori
Think back to our "Infection Cycle." Bathing with chlorhexidine gluconate can also block the progression from exposure to contamination.

Rationale: As noted above, MRSA colonization among athletes is six times higher than the rate of colonization in the community. Chlorhexidine gluconate is a topical disinfectant that is included in some soaps. It effectively reduces potentially disease-causing bacteria on the skin and has prolonged antibacterial effects after application.[5] In fact, chlorhexidine-containing soap is used throughout health care as a strategy to decrease risk of infection. For example, surgical patients often use chlorhexidine-containing soap prior to their surgical procedures. Chlorhexidine has also been used to decrease risk of infection outside of the hospital. For instance, when army recruits (another population with increased risk of MRSA infection) bathed with chlorhexidine three times each week, MRSA acquisition and infection was reduced.[6] We believe athletes can also take advantage of this strategy. *We recommend that your athletic trainers add chlorhexidine-containing soap dispensers in the showers of the training facility in Chapter 4.* If you purchase chlorhexidine-containing soap for use at home, be sure to buy a product with 2% to 4% chlorhexidine.

Don't forget, any type of chemical (dye, perfume, or disinfectant) can potentially cause allergic reactions. As with many other soaps, some (though very few) people are allergic to chlorhexidine. Always watch for allergic reactions when starting to use a new product.

Body Shaving

▶ **Risk Factor** Compromised skin.

✓ **Recommendation 1** Avoid cosmetic body shaving (shaving below the neck).

✓ **Recommendation 2** If hair removal is necessary, remove with individual- or single-use clippers.

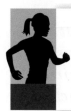

Tips From Tori

Many of us choose to shave for personal reasons. Make sure to always use a fresh razor on clean skin and NEVER share a razor.

However, know that shaving does put you at risk for infection. So, monitor your skin accordingly!

✓ **Recommendation 3** If hair is removed with clippers, dispose the clipper head after each use. Do not share clipper head with another player. Certainly, do not shave before surgical procedures.

✓ **Recommendation 4** If hair must be removed by shaving, shave clean skin with a fresh razor, soap, and lubricant away from the athletic training facility.

Rationale: Intact skin is the most important defense against skin infections, such as MRSA. Shaving creates microabrasions in the skin, which decrease the body's ability to fight off infection. Pathogenic organisms, such as MRSA and group A streptococci, are capable of accessing these tiny skin defects and can, in turn, lead to long-term skin colonization and/or increased risk of subsequent infection.

We recognize that cosmetic body is largely a personal matter. However, cosmetic body shaving has been linked to MRSA outbreaks in athletes. Therefore, it is important for you to consider the potential consequences of a skin infection on your season or even athletic career and weigh these against the benefits of cosmetic body shaving.

We also acknowledge that certain athletes (swimmers, cyclists) may practice body shaving for aerodynamic improvement. Similarly, athletes may shave legs and armpits for social reasons. If shaving for these reasons is required, NEVER share a razor. Ideally, you should shave for these purposes at home with soap and a skin lubricant away from the training facility.

Medical Care

You frequently receive medical care at the hands of your athletic trainer or team physician. It is important to be an advocate for your own health and an infection prevention champion anytime you receive medical care. We believe that athletic training facilities are medical facilities. So, for our purposes, we also include physical therapy, massage therapy, and pre- and posttreatment sessions as medical care. Basically, if someone on the medical team (physician, athletic trainer, therapist) needs to examine you, perform a procedure, provide therapy, or, basically, put their hands on you, then you are receiving medical care!

How could medical care put you at risk for infection? Unfortunately, all medical procedures that involve cutting or puncturing the skin have some, albeit small, risk of infection. In addition, any patient can be exposed to germs if medical personnel fail to perform recommended infection prevention practices.

Basic Medical Care

⊙ **Risk Factor** Insufficient knowledge of fundamental infection prevention practices.

⊘ **Recommendation 1** Talk with your athletic trainer about infection prevention protocols utilized in the athletic training facility.

⊘ **Recommendation 2** Take an active role in disinfecting the materials that you use in the athletic training room during and after treatments.

⊘ **Recommendation 3** Practice good hand hygiene in the athletic training facilities.

> **Tips From Tori**
> It's okay to ask your athletic trainer to wash their hands before starting treatment.

Rationale: Receiving health care in the athletic training environment is a potentially "high-risk scenario" for pathogen transmission due to the direct contact you have with the trainer/physician and with shared surfaces, such as treatment tables.

Given that hand-to-skin contact is the primary method of bacterial transmission, it is critical that you inquire about hand hygiene practices among team medical personnel. Keenly observe or speak with your athletic trainer or physician about hand hygiene practices. It's ok to ask them to wash their hands before starting treatment.

Additionally, you should ensure that the space or equipment you plan to use has been appropriately disinfected. Though this should mainly be handled by athletic trainers, your athletic trainer is also forced to manage many other tasks in the fast-paced, high-traffic training room. You can take an active role in protecting yourself from infection by disinfecting shared surfaces. *Chapter 6 provides extensive information for your athletic trainers on the most effective strategies for disinfection of equipment and surfaces.* In a nutshell, disinfection is most effective when

1. The right disinfectant chemical is used.
2. The disinfectant is allowed to remain wet on the surface for the appropriate "contact time," typically 1 to 2 minutes.
    a. **In other words, DON'T spray and wipe! Spray and leave wet!**

You can take an active role in protecting yourself from infection by disinfecting shared surfaces.

These recommendations are applicable anytime you receive care in the athletic training facility, including your daily pre- and postpractice treatment sessions and additional medical care.

CUT CARE

▶ **Risk Factor** Compromised skin from routine athletic activities.

✓ **Recommendation 1** Monitor skin on a daily basis for skin wounds, including cuts, scrapes, and any suspicious lesions.

✓ **Recommendation 2** Show all wounds to your athletic trainer for cleaning and treatment as soon as you notice them.

✓ **Recommendation 3** Be knowledgeable of the policy for "cut care" in your athletic training facility and discuss with your athletic trainer.

Rationale: Healthy, intact skin is your body's #1 defense against infection. Any break in the skin—even turf burn or shaving nicks—can be large enough for bacteria to enter the body and cause infection. **Though most abrasions or cuts are uncomplicated, these injuries are common antecedents of subsequent infection.** Keep in mind, bacteria will most commonly access these skin wounds during practice, but bacteria can also be introduced through improperly disinfected equipment or improper hand hygiene by medical personnel.

Tips From Tori
You know your body better than anyone else. If something (a wound or skin lesion) doesn't look "right," report it to your athletic trainer ASAP!

It is therefore necessary to monitor your skin for lesions on a daily basis. Prompt recognition, diagnosis, and treatment will help minor cuts or wounds from becoming infected and prevent minor infections from becoming more severe. Again, you can take an active role in your skin health and hygiene by noting how the wound changes over time and reporting these changes to your athletic trainer.

Your athletic training room should have protocols in place outlining specific details of wound cleaning, the use of antibacterial ointments, and wound dressings. Follow these procedures as recommended. Although soap and water are adequate cleaning agents, your athletic trainer may want to clean the wound with additional agents designed to kill bacteria that colonize skin and could lead to infection. They may also apply antibacterial ointment prior to placing a clean, dry dressing over the wound.

Make sure to ask your athletic trainer about how to care for the wound and about what signs or symptoms could indicate the start of a potential infection. Continue communicating with your athletic trainer about the status of the wound on a daily basis. Do not enter the hydrotherapy pools with an open, uncovered wound.

HYDROTHERAPY

▶ **Risk Factor** Use of hydrotherapy pools.

✓ **Recommendation 1** Do not enter the hydrotherapy pool with an open wound unless the wound is covered by an impermeable dressing.

⊘ **Recommendation 2** Shower prior to using the hydrotherapy pools.

⊘ **Recommendation 3** Do not use the hydrotherapy pools if you have a known MRSA infection until the infection is completely resolved.

Questions to Ask Yourself Before Entering a Whirlpool

- Has this pool been cleaned appropriately?
- Do I have any open wounds?
  - If yes, are they covered appropriately?
- Do I have an active MRSA infection?
  - If yes, DO NOT USE THE WHIRLPOOL.
- Have I showered?
- Is there a clean towel available for me upon exit?

Rationale: MRSA has been shown to be present in and around whirlpools.[7] Therefore, it is important that you are aware of your risk not only upon entering the hydrotherapy room but also upon using the pool (**Figure 2.5**). Open sores or breaks in the skin can become infected by bathing in contaminated pool water. Other body fluids can also contaminate pools.

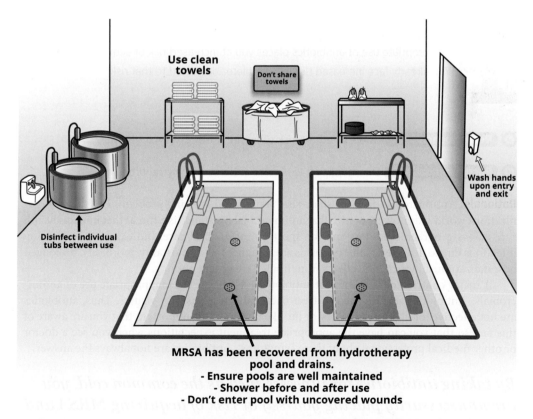

Figure 2.5 Infection risks in the hydrotherapy room. Some areas of the hydrotherapy are higher risk (red) than others.

Whirlpools can harbor MRSA and have been implicated in previous MRSA outbreaks. As a result, it is essential for players to shower PRIOR to using the pools in order to reduce or remove bacteria from their skin. One MRSA outbreak of 10 college football players (2 of whom required hospitalization) was linked to a whirlpool. Players who used whirlpools during or after players with MRSA infections entered the water had a 12-fold higher risk of MRSA infection.[8]

However, hydrotherapy is viewed as an essential aspect of athlete rehabilitation. Therefore, if you do have an open wound and want to utilize the pool, make sure that the wound is covered with an impermeable dressing. If you or one of your teammates enters the hydrotherapy pool with an open wound, notify a trainer so that the pool can be drained, dried, and disinfected appropriately.

⊘ Recommendation 4 Use a clean, laundered, individual-use towel after exiting the whirlpool.

Rationale: Sharing towels places athletes at higher risk for developing MRSA and other infections. In one outbreak investigation, athletes who shared towels were over eight times more likely to develop MRSA than those who did not.[9] This recommendation follows a core tenet of infection prevention: individual-use equipment eliminates transmission.

ANTIMICROBIAL STEWARDSHIP

⊙ Risk Inappropriate use of antibiotics.

Tips From Tori
Inappropriate use of antibiotics places you at increased risk of acquiring MRSA. You already face increased risk as an athlete...don't add to that risk!

⊘ Recommendation 1 Understand the risk of taking unnecessary antibiotics.

⊘ Recommendation 2 Do not expect to receive antibiotics for viral illnesses.

Rationale: Antimicrobial drug resistance is a serious and growing problem. Healthcare organizations worldwide now recognize that antimicrobial resistance is a threat that impacts health care across geographic borders and the spectrum of medical care. Individuals who develop infections due to drug-resistant organisms are at higher risk of mortality, morbidity, prolonged hospitalization, and toxic side effects from limited treatment options.

A major contributor to the rise of antibiotic resistance is the inappropriate use of antimicrobials. Antibiotics are designed to treat bacterial infections, not viruses. Thus, antibiotics are not effective for upper respiratory or flu-like illnesses. It is important that you are aware of this fact so that you can have the appropriate treatment expectations when you see a doctor or other medical professional about these symptoms—antibiotics are not always the answer!

By taking antibiotics for illnesses such as the common cold, you are unnecessarily placing yourself at risk of acquiring MRSA and experiencing other adverse events.

TRAVEL MEDICINE AND EMERGING INFECTIONS

⊙ **Risk Factors** Crowding (on planes, buses, tight living quarters) and novel exposures.

⊘ **Recommendation 1** Discuss travel medicine requirements with team medical personnel prior to traveling abroad for an athletic event.

⊘ **Recommendation 2** Attend travel medicine clinic in order to reduce your risk of contracting an infectious disease while abroad.

Rationale: You may face different types of infection when you travel outside of the United States (eg, traveler's diarrhea). Your risk for these infections depends on the travel destination, duration of the visit, activities planned, and each individual traveler's other existing health conditions.

Nonmedical Wellness Practices

Athletes may also use "nonmedical" wellness practices to help them achieve their peak performance levels. However, these practices confer an infection risk as well.

⊙ **Risk Factor** Insufficient knowledge of risk of infection associated with nonmedical wellness practices.

⊘ **Recommendation 1** Understand the risk of "alternative therapies" such as acupuncture, home IV therapy, cupping, and massage.

⊘ **Recommendation 2** Use facilities that have licensed practitioners and are inspected by the health department if you choose to engage in an alternative therapy and receive treatment outside of your athletic facility.

⊘ **Recommendation 3** Ensure that single-use instruments are used when engaging in a therapy (such as acupuncture, home IV therapy, etc.) that punctures the skin.

Rationale: Some of these "alternative medicine" therapies involve directly puncturing the skin, such as acupuncture, home IV therapy, and wet cupping (also known as "Hijama"). Any skin puncture can potentially expose you to the same bloodborne pathogens that injection drug users are at high risk of contracting, such as HIV, hepatitis B, hepatitis C, and MRSA skin and soft-tissue infections.[10-12]

Additionally, remember that an intact skin barrier is your #1 defense against pathogens. Dry cupping can cause microabrasions and localized burns that break that defense and therefore place you at increased risk of local skin and soft-tissue infection.[13,14] Massage and reiki are relatively low risk as long as your practitioner washes their hands between clients. Again, know that it is ok (and smart!) to ask your practitioner if they have washed their hands before your session.

Medical Care Involving Procedures

INJECTIONS

⊙ **Risk Factors** Compromised skin; poor injection practices.

⊘ **Recommendation 1** Ask your provider if they are using aseptic techniques and "safe injection practices."

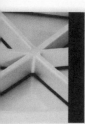

✅ **Recommendation 2** Observe the provider washing their hands and using a single-use needle.

Questions to Ask Your Medical Professional When Receiving an Injection

1. Are you using aseptic techniques?
2. Is this a single-use needle/syringe?
3. Is this a single-use medication vial?
4. Have you washed your hands?

Rationale: Injections are commonly used in athletics for pain relief and treatment. In fact, injections are the most common medical procedure performed in the United States. However, unsafe injection practices put patients and providers at risk for infectious (and noninfectious) events. For example, injections can lead to skin infections, joint infections, and in cases when unsafe injection practices are used, infections such as hepatitis B, hepatitis C, and HIV. Failure of providers to adhere to safe injection practices has led to numerous outbreaks of infections and patient suffering. Your provider should always use **one needle, one syringe, only one time.**[15]

SURGICAL PROCEDURES

▶ **Risk Factor** Compromised skin from the incision.

✅ **Recommendation 1** Discuss what symptoms might indicate an early infection at the surgical site with your athletic trainer and physician.

✅ **Recommendation 2** Monitor surgical incision on a daily basis for symptoms of potential infection.

Rationale: Surgical sites have the potential to become infected. Even when all best practices are used, 1% to 3% of surgical procedures are complicated by a surgical wound infection or "surgical site infection" (SSI).[16] Most orthopedic procedures have even lower risk. However, the severity of a SSI can range from a nuisance to a career-threatening injury. These infections occur due to germs entering the surgical site either during or after surgery (**Figure 2.6**). It is therefore important that you monitor the surgical incision and surrounding area for signs of infection, including

- Redness
- Swelling
- Warmth
- Excessive pain
- Pus or other drainage

These symptoms may also be accompanied by fever, chills, and generalized malaise. Notify your athletic trainer immediately if you develop any of these symptoms.

You can reduce the likelihood of postoperative infections from occurring by following adequate wound care guidelines, cleaning and monitoring the incision site frequently, and avoiding body shaving prior to the procedure.

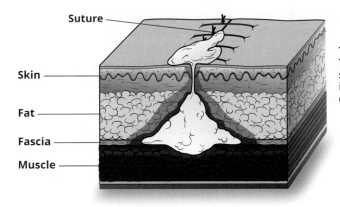

Suture

Skin

Fat

Fascia

Muscle

The wound is not opened. The infection begins within the subcutaneous space, making the skin incision and fascia vulnerable to dehiscence (splitting open).

Figure 2.6 Signs and symptoms of a wound infection.

Tips From Tori

A surgery already takes you out of the game...you definitely don't want an infection to hinder and extend your recovery process.

✓ **Recommendation 3** If deemed necessary, follow decolonization protocols as instructed by your physician.

Rationale: Injuries sustained during athletic activities may require surgical repair. While germs that cause SSIs can be introduced during or after the surgical procedure, the majority of SSIs are caused by germs already present on the patient at the time of the procedure. Athletes are at higher risk for MRSA colonization than the general population, making it critical to have appropriate interventions in place to promote skin hygiene and decrease colonization with pathogens when the athlete is undergoing an elective surgical procedure. Your physician or athletic trainer might provide you with treatment to "decolonize" you prior to a surgical procedure.

Other Athletes

All athletes are well aware that it takes a team to tackle an opponent. Preventing infection in your athletic facilities is no exception!

As previously mentioned, direct contact (person-to-person transmission) is the primary method of transmission of bacterial pathogens (such as MRSA) and viruses (such as the common cold). Indirect transmission (via a contaminated environment or surface) occurs as well.

Key Terms

- Direct transmission: transmission of pathogen from person to person (eg, through skin-to-skin contact).
- Indirect transmission: transmission via a contaminated environment or surface (eg, a contaminated weight bench).

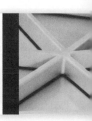

Consider how often you are exposed to direct or indirect transmission situations during athletic participation (**Figure 2.7**). Your frequent and repeated skin-to-skin contact with other athletes and contact with shared surfaces place you at high risk for infection.

The busier the training facility and locker room, the more likely these transmissions can occur. In other words, infections are more easily spread when people crowd in the same location. In fact, a crowded location is a perfect setup for an outbreak of infections.

▶ **Risk** **Transmission of germs through direct contact (skin to skin) with other athletes.**

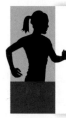

Tips From Tori

Think of instances of skin-to-skin contact during athletic participation...anything from a game-saving tackle to a motivational team huddle!

These interactions present risks for direct transmission to occur.

Should you stop these activities? No! Just know the rules and respond accordingly.

✓ **Recommendation 1** Understand how and when direct transmission may occur during athletic participation and take necessary precautions.

✓ **Recommendation 2** Practice consistent and frequent hand hygiene.

Rationale: Direct person-to-person exposure has been the primary cause of infection transmission for millennia. Many infections are most easily spread through direct contact and direct exposure, including norovirus, measles, chicken pox, sexually transmitted infections, and influenza.

For athletes, MRSA provides an excellent case example of how infections can be spread through direct contact. Humans are the natural reservoir for MRSA. Humans with MRSA infection or colonization deposit the bacteria into their environments and can transfer the bacteria to other humans.

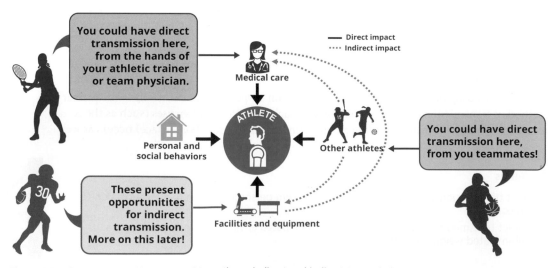

Figure 2.7 Infections spread between athletes through direct and indirect transmissions.

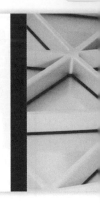

Athlete Connection

Not surprisingly, different sports present different amounts of skin-to-skin contact.

High contact/collision sports include football, rugby, and wrestling. These sports have the most skin-to-skin contact.

Medium- to high-risk contact sports include soccer, basketball, and hockey.

Limited contact sports include squash, volleyball, and gymnastics.

Noncontact sports, such as running, dancing, or swimming, have the lowest amount of skin-to-skin contact.

However, athletes share equipment and surfaces, especially in the athletic training environment. **This means that all athletes—not just contact sport athletes—are at risk for infection.**

You may not have MRSA now, but you will be exposed to MRSA during your athletic activities. Almost 7 out of every 50 US collegiate athletes are colonized with MRSA, meaning that they carry the bacteria on their skin without showing signs of infection. In comparison, only 1 out of 50 people of the general population carries the bacteria on their skin.

We place a heavy emphasis on hygienic practices after exposure to other athletes (eg, during practice), as hygiene is the key strategy to prevent an MRSA exposure from turning into MRSA colonization. Why is that important? Athletes colonized with MRSA are 7.3 times more likely to experience a subsequent infection. While contact sport athletes, such as football players and wrestlers, are more likely to be colonized with the bacteria, noncontact sport athletes are also at risk for infection because of shared spaces and equipment. These germs, therefore, are not confined to specific teams or sports. **You are primarily at increased risk for infection because you are an athlete, not because of the specific sport that you play.**[17]

Due to the nature of pathogen transmission, your hygiene practices not only affect you but also directly impact your teammates. Similarly, your teammates' hygiene practices can affect you. Keep this in mind before foregoing an after-practice shower or handing off a used piece of equipment to one of your teammates! If you notice poor hygiene practices among teammates, be an infection prevention champion and remind them to help the team and help reduce risk of infection for everyone.

▶ **Risk** **Equipment or surfaces contaminated by other athletes (surfaces that come into contact with the skin of multiple athletes such as shared athletic equipment or athletic training rehabilitation equipment).**

✓ **Recommendation 1** Do not share personal equipment that comes into contact with the skin, such as towels or razors.

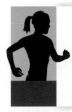

Tips From Tori

Just because a surface doesn't *look* dirty, doesn't mean that there aren't any bacteria or other pathogens present.

Make sure to wipe down equipment prior to use. You are protecting yourself by doing so!

Rationale: Sharing towels places athletes at higher risk of developing MRSA and other infections. In one outbreak, athletes who shared towels were over eight times more likely to develop MRSA infections than those who did not.[9] Thus, make sure to use a clean, laundered towel after exiting the hydrotherapy pools and after you shower. Never share razors.

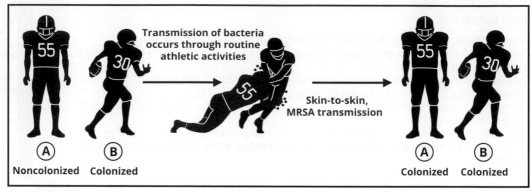

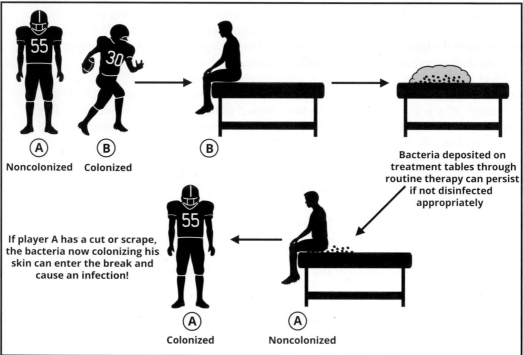

Figure 2.8 Methicillin-resistant *Staphylococcus aureus* (MRSA) moves from athlete to athlete through direct and indirect transmissions.

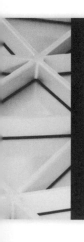

Show What You Know!

Here, we illustrate how MRSA spreads by **direct** and **indirect transmission**.

1. In the first figure, we show a **colonized** individual, who carries MRSA on their skin. Colonized individuals can spread bacteria to noncolonized individuals through skin-to-skin contact, resulting in **direct transmission.**

2. In the second figure, we show how this **colonized** individual can spread the bacteria to the environment when they touch surfaces or equipment via **indirect transmission.** Noncolonized individuals, then, can acquire the bacteria when their skin comes into contact with these contaminated surfaces.

Though colonized individuals can certainly spread the bacteria to others and to the environment, individuals with active infections are most likely to spread the bacteria to others (**Figure 2.8**).

✅ **Recommendation 2** Make a habit of disinfecting shared equipment prior to use in the treatment room, training room, and weight room.

Rationale: Can you tell which bacteria are present on the treatment table before you receive therapy? *No.* Who was on it before you? *Sometimes you won't know.* So, assume the worst, and ensure the treatment table surface has been disinfected before you use it. That way, the surface will not be a source of infection transmission to you, regardless of what prior athletes might have left behind.

Vaccine-Preventable Illnesses

▶ **Risk Factor** Crowding.

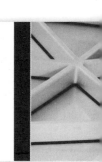

Athlete Connection

Infectious diseases spread easily in athletics because there are commonly a large number of people in a confined space.[18]

Let's consider a well-known vaccine-preventable illness: influenza. Flu commonly spreads through droplet transmission. When people infected with flu cough or sneeze, flu virus is spread via respiratory droplets that can float up to 6 feet away from the infected person. Think about your team bus or locker room during flu season—you are rarely, if ever, more than 6 feet away from your teammates or a potential source of infection.

✅ **Recommendation 1** Receive all required vaccinations.

Rationale: Several transmissible and potentially serious infections, such as pertussis, meningococcal meningitis, measles, mumps, or chicken pox, can be prevented through safe vaccines. In fact, vaccination against these germs is the best strategy for preventing infection in you **and** preventing an outbreak in the team. Effective vaccination strategies against these pathogens may take one or two shots. While they are all part of routine childhood vaccination recommendations, adherence to vaccination recommendations is waning. Be prepared to review your vaccination history with your medical team.

✅ **Recommendation 2** Make sure to receive influenza vaccination annually.

Rationale: Influenza is a common and partially preventable respiratory infection that is readily transmitted from person to person. Influenza significantly reduces your respiratory capacity and athletic performance even in the case of mild infections. A small but important percentage of young and otherwise healthy individuals who acquire influenza may develop severe infections requiring hospitalization.

Vaccination is the most effective flu prevention strategy. Players who receive influenza vaccines are less likely to have fever or influenza-like illnesses, are less likely to miss school or sport, and are less likely to spread influenza to teammates.

Don't hurt your team or your playing time—get an annual influenza vaccine.

Facilities and Equipment

As discussed throughout this chapter, germs such as bacteria and viruses can spread indirectly among athletes due to contamination of the environment or equipment. There are opportunities for indirect transmission from any surface that comes into contact with skin.

Tips From Tori

Think of all the surfaces or pieces of equipment you touch in the athletic setting! There are plenty of opportunities for indirect transmission...

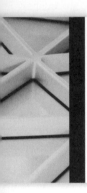

Athlete Connection

Let's talk about the peak business hours in an athletic training room: just before and just after practice! You know the scene—there are a number of athletes (maybe even from different teams and sports) waiting to have their ankles taped, their muscle injuries massaged, and to use the bike and foam rollers for a quick warm-up.

Disinfecting surfaces is challenging during a high-traffic time. There are likely opportunities, then, for indirect pathogen transmission to occur. As athletes use equipment and have contact with surfaces for extended periods of time during treatment sessions, they are unknowingly contaminating the equipment.

What can you do to reduce this contamination?

Your medical team, athletic trainers, and facilities managers are provided specific information on best practices for cleaning and disinfection in Chapter 6. While you may not have the primary responsibility for cleaning surfaces and equipment in the facility, you still play a critical role in decreasing the risk of indirect transmission through contaminated equipment.

Bacteria and viruses can survive on nonporous surfaces (eg, vinyl, formica, metal, counters, etc.) for extended periods of time. For example, bacteria can live on vinyl surfaces in the weight room (padding of benches). Bacteria can survive on these surfaces even longer if the vinyl is damaged or cracked. In extreme cases, spores from some bacteria can survive for years!

Key Terms

Microbiome: microorganisms, including bacteria and viruses, that live in and around you.

Why do surfaces become contaminated? Every time a human (or any animal) enters an environment or touches a surface, it leaves germs behind (**Figure 2.9**). The term "**microbiome**" is often used to describe the incredible amount and diversity of microorganisms (including bacteria and viruses) that live in and on you. Essentially, each of us leaves part of our "microbiome" behind wherever we go. As a result, you are regularly interacting with other peoples' microbiomes and they are interacting with yours.

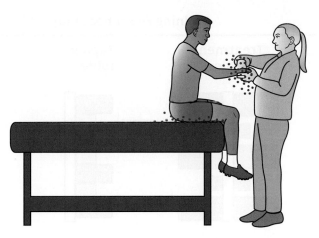

Figure 2.9 Interaction of the athlete (blue) and athletic trainer's (red) microbiomes.

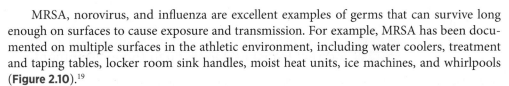

Athlete Connection

Consider the following scenario that commonly occurs during one weight training session:

Let's say that player 1 is colonized with MRSA—he carries that bacteria on his skin but does not show any signs of infection. Player 1 uses a weight set to complete 3 × 10 bench presses. His partner, player 2, spots him and then alternates with player 1, using the same bench and weights. After this group finishes their sets, player 3 and player 4 approach the weight set and complete their exercises. Due to time constraints, the bench is not wiped off in-between uses and the players do not place towels or other coverings over the seat. Three athletes, then, have been exposed to MRSA (and most likely other germs) while completing just one exercise!

MRSA, norovirus, and influenza are excellent examples of germs that can survive long enough on surfaces to cause exposure and transmission. For example, MRSA has been documented on multiple surfaces in the athletic environment, including water coolers, treatment and taping tables, locker room sink handles, moist heat units, ice machines, and whirlpools (**Figure 2.10**).[19]

Two different strategies for cleaning and disinfection are used for equipment (**Table 2.2**). If nonporous (vinyl, plastic, ceramic, metal), then it needs to be sprayed with an EPA-registered surface disinfectant. If porous (textiles like cotton, polyester, or performance clothing or towels, hydrocollator pads), then stick it in the laundry. However, some equipment has both nonporous and porous components, such as suspension straps, or may be made of neither, such as elastic straps or battle ropes. Appropriate disinfection of these equipment is difficult. What should you do? Wash your hands after use!

In the remainder of this section, we provide specific recommendations to minimize indirect transmission in different parts of the athletic training facility.

Weight Room

▶ **Risks** Contaminated surfaces and equipment (**Figure 2.11**); crowding.

✓ **Recommendation 1** Use an alcohol-based hand sanitizer upon entering the weight room.

✓ **Recommendation 2** Pick up a clean towel upon entering the weight room.

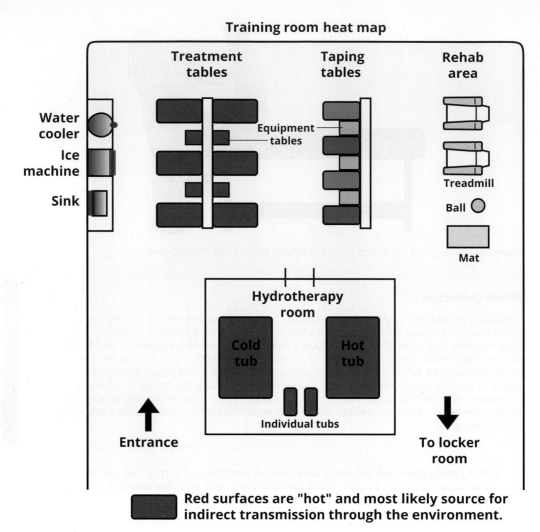

Figure 2.10 Heat map of high-risk areas for indirect transmission in the training room.

Table 2.2 Type of Material Determines How the Item Should Be Cleaned and Disinfected

Nonporous	Porous
For example, vinyl, plastic, ceramic, metal	For example, cotton, polyester, clothing, or towels
Spray it with an EPA-registered disinfectant!	Stick it in the laundry!

✅ **Recommendation 3** Place "barriers" (such as a clean towel) over equipment.

✅ **Recommendation 4** Wipe down equipment after each use.

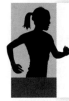

> **Tips From Tori**
> Sometimes, it's just not realistic to disinfect equipment between each use when you're in a team weight training session. But, by wiping off the surface with a towel, you can at least decrease some of the sweat you leave on the bench! And don't forget: wash your hands when the session is complete!

✅ **Recommendation 5** Use an alcohol-based hand sanitizer upon exiting the weight room.

Rationale: Players should use clean towels when using weight room equipment to decrease direct skin contact with surfaces. It's not really practical for athletes or strength and conditioning coaches to disinfect surfaces after each player during high-volume workout sessions. Instead, strength and conditioning coaches should disinfect surfaces in between sessions. We suggest that players should wipe equipment down with towels after each use to decrease the amount of sweat. This action does not disinfect the surface but can help decrease the amount of bioburden present for the next player.

Equipment Etiquette

• Wipe down equipment with a towel after use.
• Notify a strength coach if the surface is visibly dirty.
• Notify a strength coach if a vinyl surface is damaged

If equipment becomes visibly soiled, however, athletes should notify a strength coach so that they can appropriately clean and disinfect the equipment.

Bacteria and viruses can survive for extended time periods on vinyl surfaces. This longevity may be prolonged further if vinyl surfaces are damaged. If a vinyl surface is damaged, notify your strength coach so that the item can be repaired.

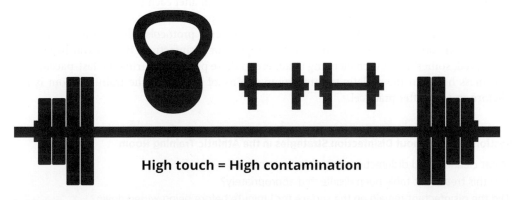

High touch = High contamination

Figure 2.11 High-touch surfaces are highly contaminated.

Tips From Tori
Going by the statistics, you will be exposed to MRSA during a strength training session. You can respond to this risk by practicing good hand hygiene before, during, and after weight training.

The number of surfaces that players may potentially contact in the weight room is extraordinary. Some athletes, particularly athletes who play contact sports such as football and rugby, are more likely to have MRSA colonization on hands; as a result, weights, equipment, and surfaces in the weight room may serve as a source of transmission. Therefore, we ask that you recognize the risk for transmission during a weight training session. Make sure to practice good hand hygiene frequently during and after weight training sessions and abide by the recommendations above.

Athletic Training Room

▶ **Risk** Contaminated items or surfaces; crowding.

✓ **Recommendation 1** Ask your athletic trainer about the cleaning and disinfection protocols in place in your athletic training environment.

✓ **Recommendation 2** Ensure that treatment equipment is appropriately disinfected before and after your individual use.

Rationale: Treatment tables and treatment equipment are "noncritical" items, meaning that these are surfaces or equipment that come into contact with intact skin but not mucous membranes. While sterility of these items is not required, they should be disinfected between uses.

Did the athletic trainer spray the treatment table and immediately wipe it?
Wait a minute! Literally ask the athletic trainer to try again. Most disinfectants need to remain wet on the surface for **at least a minute** in order to correctly disinfect the surface.

Intact skin is an effective barrier against most bacteria and viruses, but the prolonged exposure and surface contact with skin mean that risk of transmission is still present. Therefore, these surfaces should be cleaned with an appropriate disinfectant after each player's treatment session.

In most training facilities, athletic trainers are responsible for cleaning the surfaces and equipment in the treatment area through facility-specific protocols. These protocols include instructions on how to use appropriate techniques for disinfection. But, as you have likely observed, sometimes it is challenging to adhere to these protocols during the fast-paced, peak business hours in the athletic training room—think of how busy the training room is just before and just after practice!

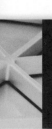

Questions to Ask About Disinfection Strategies in the Athletic Training Room
- What cleaning and disinfecting protocols are in place?
- Has this treatment table been disinfected appropriately?
- Did the disinfectant remain on the surface for 1 minute before being wiped down?
- Was the taping table or chair disinfected after the last taping session?

You can be an infection prevention champion by taking an active role in cleaning and disinfecting the equipment that you use. Ask your athletic trainer if the treatment table you are about to use has been disinfected appropriately. Or, observe them doing so. Alternatively, ask your athletic trainer if there is anything that you can do to help disinfect and prepare additional treatment tables, rehabilitation equipment, or taping tables during these times.

In contrast to treatment tables and equipment, taping tables in the training room pose less risk of a transmission. Though *ideally* these surfaces would be disinfected after each use, we realize that it usually is not practical to disinfect taping tables and chairs between each player during high-volume taping sessions. Fortunately, routine taping sessions pose minimal risk to players due to short exposure time; however, taping tables should be disinfected, at minimum, after each taping session. Additional disinfection should be performed after any player contacts surfaces with skin that is not intact, such as an open or uncovered wound.

✓ **Recommendation 3** Disinfect cardiovascular, rehabilitation, and other training equipment after each use.

Rationale: Similar to equipment used in the training room, rehabilitation equipment should be disinfected after each use. Look for wipes or surface sprays in the surrounding area and clean the equipment appropriately before you return it or discontinue using it. If you do it routinely, chances are high that others will do the same! Lead by example as an infection prevention champion.

✓ **Recommendation 4** Be sure that the electrostimulation pads you are using have not been used by another player.

Rationale: Electrostimulation pads cannot be routinely disinfected and consequently should be used by only one player.

✓ **Recommendation 5** Reusable athletic equipment should be appropriately disinfected after it is used, visibly soiled, or otherwise dirty.

Rationale: Fortunately, reusable athletic equipment (such as helmets or shoulder pads) presents a minimal risk of transmission of infectious agents, particularly if this equipment is used repeatedly by a single player. Routine drying, cleaning, and disinfection (wiping with a disinfectant) of such equipment are most likely safe and satisfactory.

Laundry Service Recommendations

Many athletic training facilities provide laundry services for athletic clothing, towels, and other porous materials. If available, we strongly recommend utilizing these services; wash your uniforms and practice equipment on a daily basis. The equipment team has been provided with specific protocols and instructions to ensure laundered items are appropriately cleaned, dried, and disinfected *(see Chapter 6)*.

However, some athletes may not have access to these laundry services. If not, you can mirror the recommendations for equipment teams at home or in your dorm room when you launder your personal towels, sheets, or other clothes and apparel.

Briefly, routine disinfection of laundry is not necessary. In general, risk of transmission of germs through contaminated laundry is very low. However, disinfection of laundry used in health care is recommended. Since we consider athletic training facilities to be healthcare facilities, we recommend that laundry in athletic training facilities follow recommendations used in other healthcare settings. Laundry can only be disinfected with hot water (>160°F) or through use of a chemical disinfectant. In our experience, no washing machines consistently use water >160°F, even industrial washers used in athletic training facilities. As a result, we recommend that equipment managers use a chemical disinfectant in all laundry cycles in the athletic training facility. By extension, it is reasonable for you, the athlete, to follow similar recommendations when you wash your own laundry.

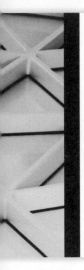

Quick Instructions and Considerations for Laundry Habits

- If clothes are visibly soiled with blood or heavy amounts of dirt, wash separately from other, less soiled clothes. Once washed alone, add into routine loads for a second wash.
- Add a chemical disinfectant to the load. You can purchase one of the three types of laundry disinfectants for use:
  ○ Bleach—highly effective, but can't be used on all types of clothes. Most people are familiar with bleach. It can be damaging to fragile textiles.
  ○ Quaternary ammonium—highly effective, can be used on all clothes. Highly effective disinfectant, though doesn't work against many diarrhea-causing illnesses.
  ○ Hydrogen peroxide—highly effective, can be used on all clothes. Typically purchased as "color safe bleach," but be sure to read the label and make sure it contains hydrogen peroxide as the active ingredient.
- Disinfectant concentration matters. Be sure to follow manufacturer's instructions for use.
- Dry clothes completely in the dryer.

Visiting Team Locker Room

Infection prevention is still an important part of your health as an athlete on the road. You can maintain your high quality of prevention and care even as an away team.

Remember that the same risks that you face at your home facility are present at away facilities. Additionally, you should have increased vigilance for infection prevention opportunities while traveling. Essentially, you don't know how well visiting facilities have been cleaned and disinfected. So, be sure to abide by your athletic trainer's guidelines for infection prevention and to follow the recommendations we've outlined in this chapter for the personal and social behaviors you should aim to model.

Summary—It's All About You

There are four categories of infection risk for athletes: (1) personal and social behaviors, (2) medical care, (3) interactions with other athletes, and (4) use of facilities and equipment. Using the information provided above, **you** should now have a game plan for how **you** can minimize these risks and intercept opportunities for pathogen transmission or infection.

Consider a few examples in **Figure 2.12**.

We hope that **you** now understand why **you** are at increased risk for infection as an athlete. Information in this chapter has been designed to help **you** know how, when, and where germs are likely to spread in athletic settings. Armed with this knowledge, **you** can take an active role in **your** health and the health of **your** teammates. In other words, **you** now have more power and knowledge to protect **your** career as a student athlete.

We challenge **you** to "go the extra mile" and become an infection prevention champion. By doing so, **you** can help establish a culture of infection prevention and accountability within **your** athletic department and keep **yourself** and **your** teammates safe from these preventable infections.

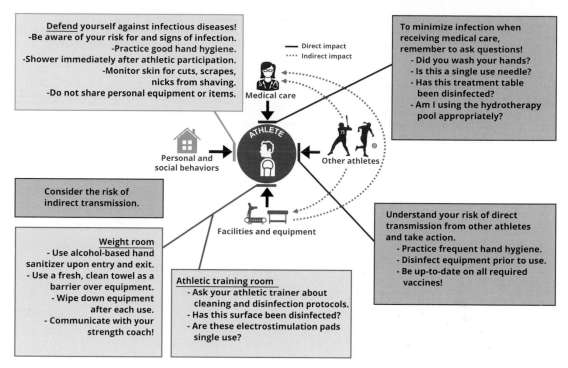

Figure 2.12 Example strategies for stopping the transmission of infections in athletes.

REFERENCES

1. Kazakova SV, Hageman JC, Matava M, et al. A clone of methicillin-resistant *Staphylococcus aureus* among professional football players. *N Engl J Med*. 2005;352:468-475.

2. Becker KM, Moe CL, Southwick KL, MacCormack JN. Transmission of Norwalk virus during a football game. *New Engl J Med*. 2000;343(17):1223-1227.

3. Karanika S, Kinamon T, Grigoras C, Mylonakis E. Colonization with methicillin-resistant Staphylococcus aureus and risk for infection among asymptomatic athletes: a systematic review and metaanalysis. *Clin Infect Dis*. 2016;63(2):195-204.

4. Nguyen DM, Mascola L, Brancoft E. Recurring methicillin-resistant *Staphylococcus aureus* infections in a football team. *Emerg Infect Dis*. 2005;11(4):526-532.

5. McDonnell G, Russell AD. Antiseptics and disinfectants: activity, action, and resistance. *Clin Microbiol Rev*. 1999;12(1):147-179.

6. Whitman TJ, Schlett CD, Grandits GA, et al. Chlorhexidine gluconate reduces transmission of methicillin-resistant *Staphylococcus aureus* USA300 among Marine recruits. *Infect Control Hosp Epidemiol*. 2012;33(8):809-816.

7. Kahanov L, Kim YK, Eberman L, et al. *Staphylococcus aureus* and community-associated methicillin-resistant *Staphylococcus aureus* (CA-MRSA) in and around therapeutic whirlpools in college athletic training rooms. *J Athl Train*. 2015;50(4):432-437.

8. Begier EM, Frenette K, Barrett NL, et al. A high-morbidity outbreak of methicillin-resistant *Staphylococcus aureus* among players on a college football team, facilitated by cosmetic body shaving and turf burns. *Clin Infect Dis*. 2004;39(10):1446-1453.

9. Centers for Disease Control and Prevention. Methicillin-resistant *Staphylococcus aureus* among players on a high school football team—New York City, 2007. *MMWR Morb Mortal Wkly Rep*. 2009;58:52-55.

10. Rehman A, Ul-Ain Baloch N, Awais M. Practice of cupping (Hijama) and the risk of bloodborne infections. *Am J Infect Control*. 2014;42(10):1139.

11. Lemos MA Jr, Silva JB, Braga AC, et al. Acupuncture needles can carry hepatitis C virus. *Infect Control Hosp Epidemiol*. 2014;35(10):1319-1321.

12. Xu S, Wang L, Cooper E, et al. Adverse events of acupuncture: a systematic review of case reports. *Evid Based Complement Alternat Med*. 2013;2013:581203.

13. Lee SY, Sin J, Yoo HK, et al. Cutaneous Mycobacterium massiliense infection associated with cupping therapy. *Clin Exp Dermatol*. 2014;39(8):904-907.

14. Hon KL, Luk DCK, Leong KF, Leung AKC. Cupping therapy may be harmful for Eczema: a PubMed search. *Case Rep Pediatr*. 2013;2013:605829.

15. Safe Injection Practice Coalition. One and Only Campaign website. 2017. Available at https://www.one-andonlycampaign.org. Accessed September 1, 2019.

16. Anderson DJ, Arduino JM, Reed SD, et al. Variation in the type and frequency of postoperative invasive *Staphylococcus aureus* infections according to type of surgical procedure. *Infect Control Hosp Epidemiol.* 2010;31(7):701-709.

17. Rice SG. Medical conditions affecting sports participation. *Am Acad Pediatr.* 2008;121(4):841-848.

18. How Flu Spreads. Centers for Disease Control and Prevention Website. Available at https://www.cdc.gov/flu/about/disease/spread.htm. Accessed September 1, 2019.

19. Stanforth B, Krause A, Starkey C, Ryan TJ. Prevalence of community-associated methicillin-resistant *Staphylococcus aureus* in high school wrestling environments. *J Environ Health.* 2010;72(6):12-16.

Infection Risks Due to Athletes' Personal and Social Behaviors

Daniel J. Sexton | Christopher J. Hostler

Introduction

This chapter focuses on explaining how personal and social behaviors affect an athlete's risk of infection. Several best practices and recommendations have been included to help team medical personnel mitigate these risks and behaviors. Simple interventions and player education can substantially and effectively reduce these risks for athletes.

Basic Premises

Consistent use of best practices related to personal hygiene is the primary method of infection prevention among athletes. Such practices are simple and effective. For example, direct contact between athletes (hand-to-skin, skin-to-skin, and mucous membranes-to-skin) is how most bacterial and many viral pathogens are transmitted in athletic facilities. Bacterial pathogens such as methicillin-resistant *Staphylococcus aureus* (MRSA) are frequently present on the hands of players and athletic trainers and, if personal hygiene is not scrupulously practiced, these microbes can be transmitted to other players and staff. This sequence of transmission can in turn lead to clinical infection, especially if other players have abraded or damaged skin. Athletes train and interact with one another in facilities that allow unusually close contact. If personal hygiene is ignored, these interactions and close contact in turn facilitate and increase the risk of transmission of pathogens such as MRSA, respiratory viruses, and numerous other potential pathogens.

Basic personal hygiene practices such as hand hygiene, prompt showering after practice, and avoidance of sharing personal equipment such as towels and razors can prevent transmission of infectious agents in team settings. Other measures such as keeping cut or abraded skin clean, dry, and covered are also important. All the personal hygiene practices discussed below should be ingrained and regularly practiced by all team members and staff even when all individuals seem to be and feel perfectly healthy.

Basic personal hygiene practices such as hand hygiene, prompt showering after practice, and avoidance of sharing personal equipment such as towels and razors can prevent transmission of infectious agents in team settings.

As discussed elsewhere, asymptomatic colonization of staff and players is common, and transmission of pathogens such as MRSA can occur from a healthy team member to a team mate. Such transmission from asymptomatic staff or patients occurs regularly in healthcare facilities throughout the world when lapses in personal hygiene occur.

Finally, personal and social behaviors of individual athletes may have direct or indirect adverse effect on the health of their teammates. For example, athletes with skin, gastrointestinal, or respiratory infections who fail to report and seek immediate treatment from athletic trainers or team physicians before participating in practices or competition can expose their teammates, opponents, and other staff members to transmissible pathogenic viruses or bacteria.

Hand Hygiene

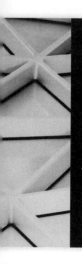

Tips and Advice

- Athletes should be educated about basic hygienic practices that reduce their and fellow team members' risk of becoming ill.
- Hand hygiene and access to hand cleaning agents should be facilitated and promoted in all athletic training facilities.
- Signage and other types of reminders can be helpful in promoting basic knowledge about and adherence to basic personal hygienic practices such as hand hygiene, prompt showering after practices, and other strategies that reduce the risk of transmission of common pathogens.
- Identify strategic locations for hand hygiene stations, including all entry and exit points in the training room, treatment room, locker room, exercise rooms, weight rooms, meeting rooms, and the cafeteria (see **Figure 3.1**).
- Encourage athletes to perform hand hygiene any time they pass a dispenser.

▶ **Best Practice** Educate athletes to routinely perform hand hygiene with alcohol-based hand hygiene cleaning agents before eating, when players and staff enter the training facility and treatment areas and when hands are visibly soiled or contaminated.

✓ **Recommendation 1** Use alcohol-containing dispensers to promote hand hygiene.

Rationale: Direct (skin-to-skin) transmission is the primary method by which most bacterial pathogens (such as MRSA) are transmitted in athletic facilities. Similar direct transmission is also important in the spread of viruses causing influenza and the common cold. Pathogens such as MRSA are often temporarily present on the hands of team players and team medical personnel; these agents can be transmitted to others if hand hygiene is not performed correctly. Alcohol-based hand hygiene products are highly effective in reducing person-to-person transmission of almost all pathogens including MRSA.[1,2] Alcohol-based

EXAMPLE TRAINING FACILITY
-Place hand hygiene dispensers in strategic locations ("Pinch Points")

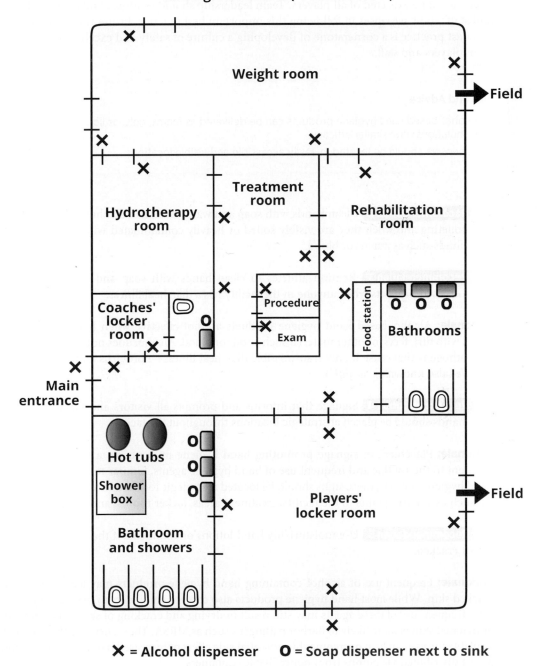

✗ = Alcohol dispenser   O = Soap dispenser next to sink

Figure 3.1 Hand hygiene stations can be placed in strategic locations throughout the facility.

hand hygiene products are as effective as traditional handwashing with soap and water in most situations. Use of alcohol-containing hand cleaning agents takes less time and causes less skin irritation than soap and water. Adherence to hand hygiene protocols and best practices should be expected of all players. Team leadership should reinforce and correct players and staff who have lapses in following this important best practice. Promoting adherence to this best practice is a cornerstone of developing a culture of safety and excellence among all team players and staff.

Tips and Advice

- Alcohol-based hand hygiene products can be delivered as foams, gels, or liquids. All of these formulations have similar efficacy.
- Dispensers should be located in easily accessible and visible locations.

⊘ Recommendation 2 Clean hands with soap and water instead of alcohol-based products after toileting and when they are visibly soiled or heavily contaminated with dirt, debris, or body fluids such as mucus or blood.

⊘ Recommendation 3 Remind athletes to clean hands with soap and water instead of alcohol-based products when anyone in the facility has a diarrheal illness.

Rationale: Alcohol-based hand hygiene products are not effective when hands are heavily soiled with dirt, feces, or other material such as oils or blood. Alcohol does not kill two important pathogens that cause highly transmissible diarrheal illness—norovirus and *Clostridioides difficile* (also known as "*C. diff*").

⊘ Recommendation 4 Signage that informs and prompts all visitors and players to clean their hands should be placed at strategic locations throughout the facility.

Rationale: Placement of signage promoting hand hygiene underscores a team-wide commitment to the routine and frequent use of hand hygiene agents. Similar to the placement of hand hygiene stations, these signs should be located at strategic location throughout the facility, such as at entry points to the facility, treatment areas, locker rooms, and weight rooms.

⊘ Recommendation 5 Use moisturizing hand lotions or emollients if the skin on hands is dry or cracked.

Rationale: Frequent use of alcohol-containing hand hygiene products may lead to dry and cracked skin. While most hand hygiene products also contain emollients to prevent drying of skin, frequent use of these agents may still result in drying and cracking of skin. Dry, cracked, or irritated skin is more likely to harbor pathogens such as MRSA. Thus, ensuring that lotion is available for use can help overcome this potential side effect of increased hand hygiene. Lotion is best distributed via pumps from nonrefillable containers.

Tips and Advice

When possible, lotion should be dispensed via pumps from nonrefillable containers. Refillable containers can become contaminated with bacteria.

⊘ **Recommendation 6** Use hospital-grade soap from prefilled/prepackaged dispensers in the training, treatment, and examination/procedure rooms.

Rationale: Handwashing with soap and water rather than alcohol-based products is necessary in selected situations as discussed above. There is no compelling evidence that antibacterial soaps prevent infection in the community better than plain soap and water.[3] Antibacterial soaps are recommended for use in medical facilities. However, we currently **do not** recommend the use of soaps containing triclosan. Instead, we recommend using hospital-grade liquid soaps containing chloroxylenol, benzalkonium, or chlorhexidine in prefilled dispensers. Triclosan, the active ingredient of most commercially available household antibacterial liquid soaps, may disrupt reproductive or thyroid function in aquatic life and laboratory animals.[4,5] In fact, the Food and Drug Administration (FDA) recently concluded that the majority of chemicals used in the over-the-counter antiseptic soap, including triclosan, were "not generally recognized as safe and effective."[6]

Finally, refillable soap dispensers have a small but known risk of becoming contaminated with potential pathogens such as *Pseudomonas* and *Serratia*. Thus, prefilled/prepackaged dispensers that can be replaced when the soap content becomes empty or low are recommended.

Skin Hygiene

⊙ **Best Practice** Shower after practice to decrease the risk of bacterial transmission from player to player and player to environment.

⊘ **Recommendation 1** All players should shower immediately after practice sessions or games.

Rationale: MRSA exposure in the setting of skin abrasions and cuts acquired through routine team activities such as practice or workouts substantially increases the risk of subsequent infection. The highest risk of transmission of important pathogens such as MRSA from one player to another likely occurs during and immediately after practice. Approximately 1% to 3% of the general American population is colonized with MRSA,[7,8] but as many as 10% to 20% of competitive athletes are colonized either transiently or for longer time periods.[9,10] Thus, periodic contact with MRSA is inevitable in team settings. Such exposures occur "silently," and players and staff have no way to know when such exposures occur.

In other words, there is no amount of infection prevention interventions that will eliminate all exposures during athletic endeavors. As a result, players must assume they have been and will be exposed to MRSA and other potential pathogens during practices and games. Showering immediately after practice or games is a critical step to prevent long-term skin colonization with MRSA particularly if there are minor skin cuts or abrasions (**Figure 3.2**). Showering also reduces the density and number of MRSA bacteria on the skin of colonized players which further reduces the risk of a true skin infection if minor cuts or skin abrasions are present. Finally, showering also reduces the density and amount of MRSA bacteria in the environment of the team training facility and locker room.

There is no amount of infection prevention interventions that will eliminate all exposures during athletic endeavors.

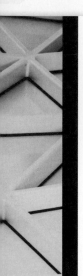

Educate players—"you will be exposed to MRSA during routine athletic activities."
  Showering immediately after practice will decrease the risk of MRSA infections in three specific ways:

1. **Prevents long-term colonization.** Showering removes bacteria before long-term colonization occurs and before low-grade colonization (following an exposure) results in infection in skin transiently damaged by minor cuts or abrasions. Prompt showering after games or practice is also an effective way to prevent long-term colonization in players who had direct skin-to-skin contact with other players who have long-term colonization with MRSA.

2. **Reduces the density and number of MRSA bacteria in colonized players.** Players who are colonized with MRSA are at increased risk of subsequent MRSA infection.[11] Showering immediately after practice reduces the amount of MRSA on the skin in patients previously colonized with MRSA, thereby also decreasing the risk that any cuts or skin abrasions sustained during practice become infected.

3. **Reduces the amount of MRSA in the environment.** Players who are heavily or transiently colonized with MRSA on the skin are more likely to contaminate the environment. Postpractice showers reduce the amount of MRSA on the skin and, thus, secondarily reduce contamination of the training facility and its equipment.

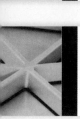

Tips and Advice

- Use of bar soap in showers is not recommended. Bar soap has been implicated as a potential source of MRSA transmission in athletes and in prisons.[12]
- Soap dispensers that utilize prefilled/prepackaged liquid soap are preferable.

⊙ **Best Practice** Educate athletes to NEVER share razors.

⊙ **Best Practice** Discourage cosmetic body shaving, particularly among athletes in contact sports.

⊘ **Recommendation 1** Discourage cosmetic body shaving (ie, shaving below the neck).

⊘ **Recommendation 2** If hair removal is necessary, remove hair with individual- or single-use clippers.

⊘ **Recommendation 3** If hair is removed with clippers, dispose of the clipper head after each use or ensure that each player has a dedicated clipper head.

⊘ **Recommendation 4** If body hair is electively removed by shaving, shave clean skin with a fresh razor using soap and lubricants at locations separate from the athletic training facility.

Rationale: Shaving causes small, frequently invisible abrasions and cuts in the skin.[13] Pathogenic microorganisms such as MRSA and group A streptococci can access these tiny skin defects. This sequence, in turn, often leads to long-term skin colonization and/or an increased risk of subsequent skin and soft-tissue infections.[14] This phenomenon is directly responsible for the well-known fact that preoperative skin shaving of the operative site significantly increases the risk of wound infections after surgery. As a result, shaving of hair prior to a surgical procedure is strongly discouraged.[15]

  Cosmetic shaving has been implicated in outbreaks of MRSA infections in athletes. For example, 10 players on a college football team developed MRSA cellulitis or skin abscesses

Cycle of transmission in athletes

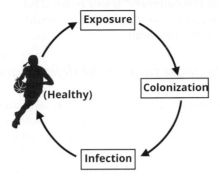

Team-spread among athletes

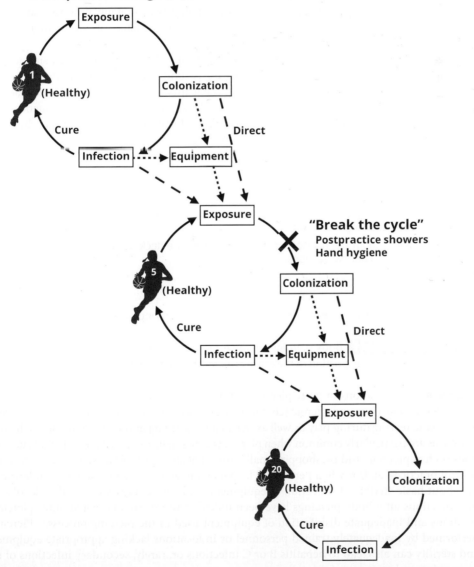

Figure 3.2 Break the transmission cycle—shower after practice to prevent exposure leading to colonization.

during a 2-month period; body shaving was strongly and significantly associated with increased MRSA infection risk in this outbreak.[16] If hair removal below the neck is required for medical reasons or for personal preferences of a player, hair should be removed using clippers that have a disposable rather than reusable head.

Intact skin is the most important defense against skin infections

We acknowledge that certain athletes (such as swimmers, cyclists) may practice body shaving for aerodynamic improvement. Similarly, athletes may shave legs and armpits for social reasons. If shaving for these reasons is required, athletes must be educated to NEVER share a razor. Ideally, shaving for these purposes should be performed at home with a skin lubricant after the skin has been cleaned with soap. Ultimately, the decision to use cosmetic body shaving is largely a personal matter beyond the control of team physicians and athletic trainers. Thus, bans on such practices are, in most instances, neither practical nor absolutely necessary in healthy players. Temporary bans on cosmetic body shaving, however, can be reasonably used by teams as secondary control measure when clusters of two or more MRSA infections occur over a short time period.

Signage may be useful in educating players about the risks associated with cosmetic body shaving and may reduce the number of players who use body shaving or the frequency of such shaving. Similarly, these risks should be part of the team's annual or new-player educational programs on infection prevention. Players should be reminded that the consequences of a skin infection on their career or on their performance during an individual season should be weighed against the benefits of cosmetic body shaving.

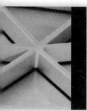

Tips and Advice

- Place signage in the team training facility to educate and remind players about the risk of cosmetic body shaving.
- Educate players about the risks of body shaving below the neck during the team's annual or new-player educational sessions.

▶ **Best Practice** Discourage body piercing and tattoos among athletes.

✓ **Recommendation 1** Body piercings of the tongue, lips, nose, eyebrows, nipples and "high piercing" of the cartilage portion of the ear in athletes should be avoided due to risk of infection.

Rationale: Complications of body piercing can be severe. These complications include local and systemic infections and allergic (contact) reactions; keloid formation; and secondary risks of traumatic tearing during play as well as permanent scarring and disfigurement. Such complications are particularly common when piercing occurs in unregulated and often unsafe locations such as piercing studios, shopping mall kiosks that lack appropriate sterility and infection control practices, and/or when performed by personnel who lack education and understanding about basic sterility, disinfection of equipment, and sterile technique. Outbreaks of serious infections after body piercings have been linked to use of contaminated "after-piercing" solutions and inadequate disinfection of equipment used in the piercing process.[17] Piercings performed by inadequately trained personnel or in locations lacking appropriate equipment and sterility can also lead to hepatitis B or C infections or, rarely, secondary infections of the heart valves or brain abscesses.

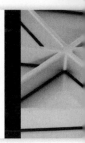

Tips and Advice

- Athletes who have piercings should remove all jewelry from pierced body parts while competing or training.
- Athletes who decide to have piercings should visit the studio or facility prior to the procedure to examine and understand the availability of sterile equipment and to be certain that the personnel performing the piercing have a full understanding of sterile technique, proper disinfection, and proper storage of equipment.

⊘ **Recommendation 2** Educate athletes about the risks and potential health hazards of tattooing.

Rationale: Permanent tattoos can occasionally result in serious complications including keloid formation, localized infections with bacteria such as MRSA, and various mycobacteria that can be difficult to treat, hepatitis B and C infections, and both major and minor hypersensitivity reactions related to the various metallic salts used in tattoo pigments.

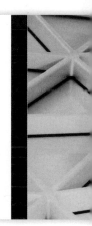

Tips and Advice

- We acknowledge "discouraging" body piercing and tattoos is an uphill battle for medical personnel, as both are increasingly a part of sports culture and society in general. Nevertheless, we recommend providing important information about infection risks related to these practices to athletes before they elect to participate in them.
- Athletes should be educated about the potential risks of tattoos and provided basic information about how to avoid or minimize these risks.
- Athletes who are contemplating getting a new tattoo should be counseled to avoid tattoo parlors or tattoo artists that fail to properly use sterile and aseptic techniques or work in studios that lack appropriate infection control products, supplies, and processes (eg, gloves, hand hygiene sterile materials, and storage facilities).
- Athletes should receive hepatitis B vaccine before getting a tattoo.

Drug Use Habits

In this section, we discuss athletes' drug use habits—legal and illegal—and how those habits potentially put athletes at risk of infectious diseases. The term "drug use" invokes thoughts about illicit drugs such as cocaine and heroin in many people. While illicit drug use certainly increases risk of infection, it's important to note that inappropriate use of legal drugs such as antibiotics (even when well-intentioned) can also predispose athletes to infectious diseases.

Prescription Medications

▶ **Best Practice** Practice good "antimicrobial stewardship."

⊘ **Recommendation 1** Follow principles of antimicrobial stewardship whenever antibiotic treatment is considered in order to reduce the risk of antimicrobial resistance and adverse drug events.

Rationale: Antimicrobial drug resistance is a serious and growing problem. Healthcare organizations worldwide now recognize that antimicrobial resistance is a threat that impacts health care across geographic borders and the spectrum of medical care.[18,19] Patients who develop infections due to drug-resistant organisms are at higher risk of mortality, morbidity, prolonged hospitalization, and toxic side effects from limited treatment options.[20] To make matters worse, the antimicrobial "pipeline" for new drugs is running dry, especially for gram-negative multidrug-resistant organisms.[21] A major contributor to the increase of drug resistance is inappropriate use of available antimicrobials.[22]

A major contributor to the increase of drug resistance is inappropriate use of available antimicrobials.

In addition to driving drug resistance, inappropriate use of antimicrobials predisposes individuals to the risk of developing a *C. difficile* infection. Inappropriate antibiotic use also leads to higher hospital costs (both indirect drug costs and prolonged hospital length of stay) and increased risk of one or more adverse drug reactions.[20] Transmission of antimicrobial-resistant organisms within a medical facility can also affect the successful treatment of other patients. In response to this growing issue, most healthcare institutions have developed "antimicrobial stewardship" programs to guide the judicious and appropriate use of antibiotics.[23] While these programs are not feasible in athletic training facilities, following basic antimicrobial stewardship practices will reduce the frequency of unnecessary use of antibiotics and help prevent acquisition and transmission of infectious diseases in athletic facilities. As an example of the principles of antimicrobial stewardship, in general, treatment of upper respiratory or influenza-like illness or uncomplicated acute sinusitis in a team member should *NOT* include antibacterial therapy with an oral antibiotic.

Treatment of upper respiratory or influenza-like illness or uncomplicated acute sinusitis in a team member should NOT include antibacterial therapy with an oral antibiotic.

⊘ **Recommendation 2** Educate players about the risk of taking unnecessary antibiotics.

⊘ **Recommendation 3** Do not use antibiotics to treat infections that are known or likely to be caused by viral pathogens such as acute pharyngitis, acute rhinosinusitis, acute bronchitis, or the common cold.

Rationale: Antibiotic treatment of an uncomplicated upper respiratory tract infection causes more harm than benefit. Use of antibiotic therapy in this or similar situations may lead to colonization or infections with resistant organisms (such as MRSA), allergic reactions, and *C. difficile* infection. A systematic review of randomized trials in people with upper respiratory symptoms for less than 7 days found no difference in the duration of symptoms in individuals who received antibiotics compared to individuals who received placebos; however, individuals who received antibiotics had a threefold greater risk of developing one or more adverse effects.[24]

Don't treat colds with antibiotics.

Many patients and physicians place considerable emphasis upon the color of nasal discharge when making decisions about antibiotic use.[25] However, colored nasal discharge is a normal self-limited phase of the common cold and acute sinusitis. While the authors of the systematic review cited above found that the relative risk for persistent acute purulent rhinitis was decreased in subjects who received antibiotic treatment compared to placebo, the increased risk of adverse effects from antibiotic use outweighed these minimal and clinically insignificant benefits.[24]

We realize that many players or staff may "expect" to receive antibiotics when any symptoms of illness occur. In addition to explaining the results of the studies cited above, we believe it is often useful to explain that players and staff are unnecessarily placing themselves at risk of acquiring MRSA and other adverse events if they take antibiotics for illnesses such as the common cold or other viral upper respiratory tract infections. For example, the FDA updated their "black box warning" for fluoroquinolones in 2016, stating that these medications should be used for true bacterial sinusitis, urinary tract infections, and acute bacterial exacerbation of chronic bronchitis only when there are no other options available.[26] Similarly, the FDA warned practitioners that azithromycin may lead to increased risk of fatal heart rhythms.[27] Finally, many different classes of antibiotics, including cephalosporins or fluoroquinolones, are strongly correlated with increased risk of *C. difficile* infection and MRSA colonization and infection.

Unnecessary antibiotics put players at risk for MRSA infections.

Illicit Drugs

⊙ **Best Practice** Recognize the infection risks of illicit or performance-enhancing drug use among players and staff.

⊘ **Recommendation 1** Educate players and staff about the infection risks of illicit drug use, including the risk of transmissible infections.

⊘ **Recommendation 2** Offer testing for infectious diseases that can be transmitted through illicit drug use, such as human immunodeficiency virus (HIV), hepatitis B, and hepatitis C.

Rationale: A proportion of athletes at all levels of competition and all types of sports use illicit substances and performance-enhancing drugs. For example, self-reported survey data from the National Athletic Trainers' Association (NATA) suggest that up to 6.6% of high school athletes, 5% of male college athletes, and 1.6% of female college athletes have used anabolic steroids in the last year.[28] Nine percent of professional football players and 67% of competitive power lifters reported using anabolic steroids at some point in their career.[28] Fifty-two percent of professional football players also reported using opiates at some point in their career, and of those, 71% admitted to misusing opiates (or taking other than as directed by a physician).[29] These numbers are likely underestimated since the data were acquired through self-reporting and not biochemical verification.[30]

Athletes who use subcutaneous injection drugs such as anabolic steroids can be exposed to bloodborne pathogens such as HIV, hepatitis B, and hepatitis C if unsafe injection practices are used.[31-35] Furthermore, use of anabolic steroids is associated with a significantly higher risk of use of other illicit substances as well as risky sexual behavior (eg, unprotected intercourse), which further increase the likelihood of contracting a bloodborne pathogen.[36,37] Athletes who use intravenous injection drugs (opiates, amphetamines) also have significant risks of contracting HIV, hepatitis B, and hepatitis C through sharing of needles or syringes. However even if single-use sterile needles and syringes are used, injection drug use itself carries a high risk of developing both bloodstream infections and/or endocarditis (a potentially fatal heart-valve infection). The rate of IV heroin use in the United States has more than doubled in the last decade,[38] and during that time-frame, the incidence of drug use–associated infective endocarditis has increased 12-fold.[39]

All athletes should be counseled about the risks of illicit drug use. However, given the illegal nature of injection drug use, counseling alone is insufficient to identify at-risk individuals. We recommend offering all athletes testing for hepatitis B, hepatitis C, and HIV when routine lab work is done (or upon request).

Athletes who use injection drugs are also at significantly greater risk of MRSA skin and soft-tissue infections at the site of injection.[40] Athletes who have abscesses (from intravenous or subdermal injections of drugs or other evidence of injection drug use such as track marks) (**Figure 3.3**) should be encouraged to have HIV, hepatitis B, and hepatitis C testing in conjunction with therapy for their skin and soft-tissue infection.

Athletes who use injection drugs are at high risk for infection.

Social Behaviors

⊙ **Best Practice** Ensure athletes are aware of the risk of contracting infectious diseases outside the athletic facility.

⊘ **Recommendation 1** Counsel athletes on the risks of sharing toiletries.

Rationale: Athletes' behavior or activities while outside athletic facilities can potentially put them at risk for infection. In general, any behavior that involves potentially sharing bodily fluids with another person puts the athlete at risk of contracting an infectious disease. All athletes should be counseled about these potential risks even though the risks of some of these behaviors are obvious. For instance, most people know that having sexual intercourse without barrier protection can lead to sexually transmitted infections such as syphilis, chlamydia, HIV, hepatitis B, or hepatitis C. Other behaviors may not be obvious, such as sharing a razor or toothbrush. These behaviors may put an athlete at risk of hepatitis B or C if the person with whom they're sharing toiletries has unrecognized or asymptomatic infection with either of those viruses.[41-43] Sharing a toothbrush may also put athletes at risk of contracting respiratory viruses, though ostensibly anyone who is sharing a toothbrush with another person is likely in close enough contact to that person to be at risk for their respiratory viruses anyway. In general, we recommend advising athletes not to share toiletries with anyone.

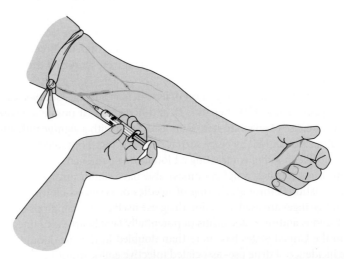

Figure 3.3 Track marks on skin imply potential injection drug use. (Reprinted with permission from Timby BK, Smith NE. *Introductory Medical-Surgical Nursing.* 12th ed. Philadelphia, PA: Wolters Kluwer; 2017.)

⊘ **Recommendation 2** Counsel athletes on the risks of unprotected sexual intercourse and means to protect themselves and their partners.

⊘ **Recommendation 3** Make barrier protection such as condoms available to athletes to increase the likelihood that they will practice safe sex.

⊘ **Recommendation 4** Offer testing for sexually transmitted diseases (or referral to health-care facilities that can perform testing) routinely and upon request.

Rationale: Sexually transmitted infections remain relatively common in all sexually active individuals in the United States. The most recent data from the Centers for Disease Control and Prevention (CDC) show that syphilis, gonorrhea, and chlamydia continue to increase in prevalence among all demographic groups.[44] Infection with HIV continues to be a personal risk and a societal problem because of widespread complacence related to the availability of highly effective therapy. Recent estimates suggest that approximately 1.1 million people aged 13 years and older are living in the United States with HIV.[45] Athletes who engage in unprotected intercourse put themselves at risk for sexually transmitted infections. While athletic staff will not be able to directly intervene on risky sexual behavior, we nevertheless recommend counseling players on the risks of unprotected sexual intercourse. "Make it easy to do the right thing" is a fundamental principle of infection prevention, so having condoms readily available is a great way to encourage safe sex. If you have medical staff working directly with your athletes, they may also be able to counsel athletes about additional means of preventing some sexually transmitted infections. For instance, preexposure prophylaxis (or PrEP) is recommended for persons who engage in behaviors that put them at high risk for contracting HIV, such as men who have sex with men (MSM), HIV-uninfected individuals in an HIV-discordant couple, and injection drug users.[46] Additionally, we recommend offering annual or upon-request testing for sexually transmitted infections, as early treatment can reduce morbidity related to these diseases.

Alternative and Nonmedical "Wellness" Practices

▶ **Best Practice** Make athletes aware of the risks of infection associated with alternative and nonmedical wellness practices.

⊘ **Recommendation 1** Educate athletes about the risks of "alternative therapies" such as acupuncture, home IV therapy, cupping, massage, and use of improperly disinfected or monitored whirlpools.

⊘ **Recommendation 2** Advise athletes to use facilities that have licensed practitioners (if your state has a licensing board) and that are inspected by the health department (if your state requires health department inspection) when possible.

⊘ **Recommendation 3** Athletes should demand single-use instruments when engaging in any nonmedical wellness therapy (acupuncture, home IV therapy, etc.) that punctures or impairs skin.

Rationale: Athletes commonly seek care with nonmedical practitioners to treat one or more of the myriad physical ailments that come hand in hand with their athletic endeavors. Some of these "alternative medicine" therapies involve directly puncturing the skin, such as acupuncture or "dry needling," home IV therapy, and wet cupping (also known as "hijami"). Any skin puncture can potentially expose athletes to the same bloodborne pathogens that injection drug users are at high risk of contracting, such as HIV, hepatitis C, and MRSA skin and soft-tissue infections.[47-49] Dry cupping can cause microabrasions and localized burns that increase the risk of local skin and soft-tissue infection.[50,51] Massage and reiki are relatively low risk as long as the practitioner washes their hands between clients.

Home IV infusions or "IV drip bars" may increase risk of infection for athletes.

Nonmedically indicated intravenous (IV) infusions have become increasingly popular due to publicity from celebrities and social media marketing campaigns by "IV drip bars." These unregulated services confer some risk of infection to recipients, though it's difficult to quantify this risk. The two primary potential etiologies of infection related to nonmedically indicated IV infusions are inadequate skin preparation when inserting the catheter and contamination of the infused fluids. Medical personnel who place IVs receive regular training on appropriate methods of skin disinfection and catheter placement. Even with this routine training, prospective studies have demonstrated that catheter insertion by personnel other than dedicated IV therapists resulted in a 1.6-fold increased risk of infection related to the IV catheter.[52] In other words, placement of IVs by personnel who are not highly trained increases the risk of infection related to the infusion. Finally, many services are adding "special blends of vitamins and electrolytes" to IV fluids that, if not compounded in a sterile fashion, could pose a significant infectious risk to athletes receiving IV therapies from these unregulated sources.[53]

This book includes several recommendations for decreasing risk of infection related to use of whirlpools in athletic training facilities **(see Chapters 4 and 6)**. However, many athletes use hydrotherapy and whirlpools outside of the training facility. Even in treated recreational water, outbreaks of infectious diseases occur. Public health officials from 46 states and Puerto Rico reported 493 outbreaks between 2000 and 2014 associated with treated recreational water; these outbreaks resulted in at least 27,219 affected individuals and 8 deaths.[54] The most common pathogens associated with these outbreaks were *Cryptosporidium* (58%), which causes a diarrheal illness, *Legionella pneumophila* (16%), which causes severe pneumonia and Pontiac fever, and *Pseudomonas aeruginosa* (13%), which causes folliculitis or focal areas of cellulitis ("hot tub rash").[54]

Travel Medicine and Emerging Infections

(▶) **Best Practice** Ensure that players traveling outside the United States receive appropriate travel medicine counseling.

(✓) **Recommendation 1** Identify a physician or clinic to perform travel counseling for players.

(✓) **Recommendation 2** Ensure players are aware that travel medicine visits are available and may reduce their risk of contracting infectious diseases.

Rationale: Infectious diseases remain the #1 cause of mortality in many parts of the world.[55] The type of infection to which a traveler may be exposed depends on the travel destination, the duration of visit, the types of activities planned, and the traveler's individual comorbidities. Accordingly, travel counseling must be tailored to each player's travel itinerary. Family practitioners, internists, and infectious diseases specialists commonly perform this type of counseling and screening in the community. We discuss specific travel counseling recommendations common to areas frequented by American travelers below, but this information should not replace formal travel medicine counseling.

▶ **Best Practice** Counsel players traveling to tropical areas with endemic mosquito-borne illnesses such as Zika virus, dengue, and malaria about methods to reduce the likelihood of infection.

✓ **Recommendation 1** Counsel players to use EPA-registered insect repellents such as DEET when traveling to tropical areas with mosquito-borne illnesses and reapply as directed by the product label instructions.

✓ **Recommendation 2** Counsel players to treat clothing and gear with permethrin when heavy mosquito exposure is anticipated.

✓ **Recommendation 3** Counsel players to use condoms when engaging in sexual intercourse during and after travel to Zika-endemic areas.

Rationale: Mosquitoes that transmit Zika virus are endemic to Central America, the Caribbean, South America, Southeast Asia, and Sub-Saharan Africa.[56] Transmission occurs through the bite of an infected *Aedes* species mosquito but can be spread between humans through sexual intercourse. While most cases of Zika virus infection are asymptomatic or produce mild respiratory symptoms, Zika virus infection has been associated with birth defects (microcephaly) and fetal loss in women infected during pregnancy.[57] The most effective way to avoid getting sick from mosquito-borne illnesses is to prevent mosquito bites. Using mosquito repellents such as DEET spray and permethrin-treated clothing can prevent mosquito bites and are recommended by the CDC when traveling to areas with mosquito-borne illnesses.[58] Condoms should be used when engaging in sexual intercourse during travel to endemic areas and for 3 months after return to the United States, as Zika can remain viable in semen for an extended period of time.[59]

▶ **Best Practice** Counsel players about methods to prevent and manage travelers' diarrhea.

✓ **Recommendation 1** Counsel players about the importance of prudently selecting food and drink while traveling.

✓ **Recommendation 2** Provide players traveling to resource-poor settings with antibiotics to be taken in the event they experience severe travelers' diarrhea.

Rationale: Between 10% and 40% of travelers contract travelers' diarrhea, depending on their destination.[60] Common high-risk (>20% incidence) destinations for American travelers include Mexico, South and Central America, and Southeast Asia.[60] Travelers' diarrhea is most commonly caused by enterotoxigenic *Escherichia coli* (ETEC), enteroaggregative *E. coli* (EAEC), *Salmonella* spp., or *Campylobacter jejuni*.[61,62] Symptoms include anorexia and cramps followed by the sudden onset of watery or bloody diarrhea. Nausea, vomiting, and low-grade fevers are also common.

The most important intervention to prevent travelers' diarrhea is to make educated choices in selecting food and drinks. Beverages should be bottled or disinfected (boiled water), and players should be reminded not to ask for ice in their drinks, as it is commonly made with tap water. Hot tea and coffee are usually safe since they are made with boiled water. Alcoholic beverages may still be contaminated despite the fact that alcohol itself is a disinfectant. Fruit salads, lettuce, chicken salads, steam table buffet foods, and condiments left on the table are high risk to be contaminated with pathogens that can cause travelers' diarrhea. Players should be advised to avoid these foods.[63]

Players who are traveling to resource-poor settings can be given antibiotics in case they develop severe travelers' diarrhea. Players should be instructed not to take antibiotics unless they develop severe diarrhea, defined as diarrhea that is incapacitating/completely prevents planned activities, or dysentery (passage of grossly bloody stools). The preferred regimen is azithromycin 1000 mg by mouth one time or 500 mg by mouth per day for 3 days. Ciprofloxacin is an acceptable alternative (750 mg by mouth one time or 500 mg by mouth two times per day for 3 days). However, resistance to fluoroquinolones is rising worldwide, and this class of drugs has an increased risk of *C. difficile* infection and tendon injury. Therefore, ciprofloxacin should not be used unless the player has a contraindication to azithromycin therapy. Players should be cautioned not to take antibiotics for mild or moderate travelers' diarrhea, as the risks associated with antibiotic therapy may outweigh the benefits.[64]

REFERENCES

1. WHO Guidelines on Hand Hygiene in Health Care: First Global Patient Safety challenge; Clean Care Is Safer Care; 2009. Available at https://apps.who.int/iris/bitstream/handle/10665/44102/9789241597906_eng.pdf;jsessionid=0893B316AC321139F-C84042D3BFCE9A6?sequence=1. Accessed September 6, 2019.
2. Allegranzi B, Pittet D. Role of hand hygiene in healthcare-associated infection prevention. *J Hosp Infect.* 2009;73(4):305-315.
3. Aiello AE, Larson EL, Levy SB. Consumer antibacterial soaps: effective or just risky? *Clin Infect Dis.* 2007;45(suppl 2):S137-S147.
4. Crofton KM, Paul KB, Devito MJ, Hedge JM. Short-term in vivo exposure to the water contaminant triclosan: evidence for disruption of thyroxine. *Environ Toxicol Pharmacol.* 2007;24(2):194-197.
5. Hwang J, Suh SS, Chang M, et al. Effects of triclosan on reproductive prarmeters and embryonic development of sea urchin, *Strongylocentrotus nudus*. *Ecotoxicol Environ Saf.* 2014;100:148-152.
6. FDA Issues Final Rule on Safety and Effectiveness of Antibacterial Soaps [press release]; September 2, 2016.
7. Kuehnert MJ, Kruszon-Moran D, Hill HA, et al. Prevalence of *Staphylococcus aureus* nasal colonization in the United States, 2001-2002. *J Infect Dis.* 2006;193(2):172-179.
8. Salgado CD, Farr BM, Calfee DP. Community-acquired methicillin-resistant *Staphylococcus aureus*: a meta-analysis of prevalence and risk factors. *Clin Infect Dis.* 2003;36(2):131-139.
9. Creech CB, Saye E, McKenna BD, et al. One-year surveillance of methicillin-resistant *Staphylococcus aureus* nasal colonization and skin and soft tissue infections in collegiate athletes. *Arch Pediatr Adolesc Med.* 2010;164(7):615-620.
10. Oller AR, Province L, Curless B. *Staphylococcus aureus* recovery from environmental and human locations in 2 collegiate athletic teams. *J Athl Train.* 2010;45(3):222-229.
11. Huang SS, Platt R. Risk of methicillin-resistant *Staphylococcus aureus* infection after previous infection or colonization. *Clin Infect Dis.* 2003;36(3):281-285.
12. Nguyen DM, Mascola L, Brancoft E. Recurring methicillin-resistant *Staphylococcus aureus* infections in a football team. *Emerg Infect Dis.* 2005;11(4):526-532.
13. Hamilton HW, Hamilton KR, Lone FJ. Preoperative hair removal. *Can J Surg.* 1977;20(3):269-271, 274-265.
14. Briggs M. Principles of closed surgical wound care. *J Wound Care.* 1997;6(6):288-292.
15. Anderson DJ, Podgorny K, Berrios-Torres SI, et al. Strategies to prevent surgical site infections in acute care hospitals: 2014 update. *Infect Control Hosp Epidemiol.* 2014;35(6):605-627.
16. Begier EM, Frenette K, Barrett NL, et al. A high-morbidity outbreak of methicillin-resistant *Staphylococcus aureus* among players on a college football team, facilitated by cosmetic body shaving and turf burns. *Clin Infect Dis.* 2004;39(10):1446-1453.
17. Evans H, Bolt H, Heinsbroek E, et al. National outbreak of *Pseudomonas aeruginosa* associated with an aftercare solution following piercings, July to September 2016, England. *Euro Surveill.* 2018;23(37):1700795.
18. Edwards LD. The epidemiology of 2056 remote site infections and 1966 surgical wound infections occurring in 1865 patients: a four year study of 40,923 operations at Rush-Presbyterian-St. Luke's Hospital, Chicago. *Ann Surg.* 1976;184(6):758-766.

19. Ehrenkranz NJ. Antimicrobial prophylaxis in surgery: mechanisms, misconceptions, and mischief. *Infect Control Hosp Epidemiol.* 1993;14(2):99-106.

20. Dellit TH, Owens RC, McGowan JE Jr, et al. Infectious diseases Society of America and the Society for Healthcare Epidemiology of America guidelines for developing an institutional program to enhance antimicrobial stewardship. *Clin Infect Dis.* 2007;44(2):159-177.

21. Boucher HW, Talbot GH, Bradley JS, et al. Bad bugs, no drugs: no ESKAPE! an update from the Infectious Diseases Society of America. *Clin Infect Dis.* 2009;48(1):1-12.

22. Society for Healthcare Epidemiology of America, Infectious Diseases Society of America, Pediatric Infectious Diseases Society. Policy statement on antimicrobial stewardship by the Society for Healthcare Epidemiology of America (SHEA), the Infectious Diseases Society of America (IDSA), and the Pediatric Infectious Diseases Society (PIDS). *Infect Control Hosp Epidemiol.* 2012;33(4):322-327.

23. Barlam TF, Cosgrove SE, Abbo LM, et al. Implementing an antibiotic stewardship program: guidelines by the Infectious Diseases Society of America and the Society for Healthcare Epidemiology of America. *Clin Infect Dis.* 2016;62(10):e51-e77.

24. Arroll B, Kenealy T. Antibiotics for the common cold and acute purulent rhinitis. *Cochrane Database Syst Rev.* 2005;(3):CD000247.

25. Mainous AG III, Hueston WJ, Eberlein C. Colour of respiratory discharge and antibiotic use. *Lancet.* 1997;350(9084):1077.

26. FDA updates warnings for fluoroquinolone antibiotics [press release]. U.S. Food and Drug Administration; July 26, 2016.

27. FDA Drug Safety Communication: Azithromycin (Zithromax and Zmax) and the risk of potentially fatal heart rhythms [press release]. U.S. Food and Drug Administration; March 12, 2013.

28. Kersey RD, Elliot DL, Goldberg L, et al. National Athletic Trainers' Association position statement: anabolic-androgenic steroids. *J Athl Train.* 2012;47(5):567-588.

29. Cottler LB, Ben Abdallah A, Cummings SM, Barr J, Banks R, Forchheimer R. Injury, pain, and prescription opioid use among former National Football League (NFL) players. *Drug Alcohol Depend.* 2011;116(1-3):188-194.

30. Petroczi A, Uvacsek M, Nepusz T, et al. Incongruence in doping related attitudes, beliefs and opinions in the context of discordant behavioural data: in which measure do we trust? *PLoS One.* 2011;6(4):e18804.

31. Aitken C, Delalande C, Stanton K. Pumping iron, risking infection? Exposure to hepatitis C, hepatitis B and HIV among anabolic-androgenic steroid injectors in Victoria, Australia. *Drug Alcohol Depend.* 2002;65(3):303-308.

32. Bolding G, Sherr L, Elford J. Use of anabolic steroids and associated health risks among gay men attending London gyms. *Addiction.* 2002;97(2):195-203.

33. Larance B, Degenhardt L, Copeland J, Dillon P. Injecting risk behaviour and related harm among men who use performance- and image-enhancing drugs. *Drug Alcohol Rev.* 2008;27(6):679-686.

34. Midgley SJ, Heather N, Best D, Henderson D, McCarthy S, Davies JB. Risk behaviours for HIV and hepatitis infection among anabolic-androgenic steroid users. *AIDS Care.* 2000;12(2):163-170.

35. Rich JD, Dickinson BP, Feller A, Pugatch D, Mylonakis E. The infectious complications of anabolic-androgenic steroid injection. *Int J Sports Med.* 1999;20(8):563-566.

36. Buckman JF, Farris SG, Yusko DA. A national study of substance use behaviors among NCAA male athletes who use banned performance enhancing substances. *Drug Alcohol Depend.* 2013;131(1-2):50-55.

37. McCabe SE, Brower KJ, West BT, Nelson TF, Wechsler H. Trends in non-medical use of anabolic steroids by U.S. college students: results from four national surveys. *Drug Alcohol Depend.* 2007;90(2-3):243-251.

38. *Heroin.* National Institutes of Health; 2018. Available at https://www.drugabuse.gov/publications/research-reports/heroin/overview. Accessed September 7, 2019.

39. Schranz AJ, Fleischauer A, Chu VH, Wu LT, Rosen DL. Trends in drug use-associated infective endocarditis and heart valve surgery, 2007 to 2017: a study of statewide discharge data. *Ann Intern Med.* 2018;170(1):31-40.

40. Lloyd-Smith E, Hull MW, Tyndall MW, et al. Community-associated methicillin-resistant *Staphylococcus aureus* is prevalent in wounds of community-based injection drug users. *Epidemiol Infect.* 2010;138(5):713-720.

41. Eroglu C, Zivalioglu M, Esen S, Sunbul M, Leblebicioglu H. Detection of hepatitis B virus in used razor blades by PCR. *Hepat Mon.* 2010;10(1):22-25.

42. Lock G, Dirscherl M, Obermeier F, et al. Hepatitis C - contamination of toothbrushes: myth or reality? *J Viral Hepat.* 2006;13(9):571-573.

43. Valois RC, Maradei-Pereira LM, Crescente JA, Oliveira-Filho AB, Lemos JA. HCV infection through perforating and cutting material among candidates for blood donation in Belem, Brazilian Amazon. *Rev Inst Med Trop Sao Paulo.* 2014;56(6):511-515.

44. Sexually Transmitted Disease Surveillance 2017: Centers for Disease Control and Prevention; September 2018, 2017. Available at https://www.cdc.gov/std/stats17/default.htm. Accessed January 23, 2020.

45. Estimated HIV incidence and prevalence in the United States, 2010-2016. Centers for Disease Control and Prevention. HIV Surveillance Supplemental Report Web site. Available at https://www.cdc.gov/hiv/statistics/overview/index.html. Accessed July 12, 2019.

46. *Preexposure Prophylaxis for the Prevention of HIV Infection in the United States - 2017 Update: A Clinical Practice Guideline.* Centers for Disease Control and Prevention; 2018. Available at https://www.cdc.gov/hiv/pdf/risk/prep/cdc-hiv-prep-guidelines-2017.pdf. Accessed September 9, 2019.

47. Rehman A, Ul-Ain Baloch N, Awais M. Practice of cupping (Hijama) and the risk of bloodborne infections. *Am J Infect Control.* 2014;42(10):1139.

48. Lemos MA Jr, Silva JB, Braga AC, Carneiro BM, Rahal P, Silva RC. Acupuncture needles can carry hepatitis C virus. *Infect Control Hosp Epidemiol.* 2014;35(10):1319-1321.

49. Xu S, Wang L, Cooper E, et al. Adverse events of acupuncture: a systematic review of case reports. *Evid Based Complement Alternat Med.* 2013;2013:581203.

50. Lee SY, Sin JI, Yoo HK, Kim TS, Sung KY. Cutaneous mycobacterium massiliense infection associated with cupping therapy. *Clin Exp Dermatol.* 2014;39(8):904-907.

51. Hon KL, Luk DC, Leong KF, Leung AK. Cupping therapy may be harmful for eczema: a PubMed search. *Case Rep Pediatr.* 2013;2013:605829.

52. Lee WL, Chen HL, Tsai TY, et al. Risk factors for peripheral intravenous catheter infection in hospitalized patients: a prospective study of 3165 patients. *Am J Infect Control.* 2009;37(8):683-686.

53. Shmerling RH. Drip Bar: Should You Get an IV on Demand. Harvard Health Publishing; 2018. Available at https://www.health.harvard.edu/blog/drip-bar-should-you-get-an-iv-on-demand-2018092814899. Accessed September 9, 2019.

54. Hlavsa MC, Cikesh BL, Roberts VA, et al. Outbreaks associated with treated recreational water - United States, 2000-2014. *MMWR Morb Mortal Wkly Rep.* 2018;67(19):547-551.

55. *Global Health Estimates 2016: Deaths by Cause, Age, Sex, by Country, and by Region, 2000-2016.* World Health Organization; 2018. Available at https://www.who.int/news-room/fact-sheets/detail/the-top-10-causes-of-death. Accessed September 9, 2019.

56. Travelers' Health: World Map of Areas With Risk of Zika. Centers for Disease Control and Prevention. Available at https://wwwnc.cdc.gov/travel/page/zika-travel-information. Accessed September 9, 2019.

57. Staples JE, Martin SW, Fischer M. Zika. Centers for Disease Control and Prevention. Travel-related infectious diseases Web site. Available at https://wwwnc.cdc.gov/travel/yellowbook/2020/travel-related-infectious-diseases/zika. Accessed September 9, 2019.

58. Prevent Mosquito Bites. Centers for Disease Control and Prevention. Available at https://www.cdc.gov/features/stopmosquitoes/index.html. Accessed September 9, 2019.

59. Zika Virus: Sexual Transmission and Prevention. Centers for Disease Control and Prevention. Available at https://www.cdc.gov/zika/prevention/sexual-transmission-prevention.html. Accessed September 9, 2019.

60. Steffen R, Hill DR, DuPont HL. Traveler's diarrhea: a clinical review. *J Am Med Assoc.* 2015;313(1):71-80.

61. Steffen R, Collard F, Tornieporth N, et al. Epidemiology, etiology, and impact of traveler's diarrhea in Jamaica. *J Am Med Assoc.* 1999;281(9):811-817.

62. Adachi JA, Jiang ZD, Mathewson JJ, et al. Enteroaggregative *Escherichia coli* as a major etiologic agent in traveler's diarrhea in 3 regions of the world. *Clin Infect Dis.* 2001;32(12):1706-1709.

63. LaRocque R, Harris JB. *Travelers' Diarrhea: Microbiology, Epidemiology, and Prevention.* UpToDate; 2019. Available at http://www.uptodate.com. Accessed September 9, 2019.

64. Riddle MS, Connor BA, Beeching NJ, et al. Guidelines for the prevention and treatment of travelers' diarrhea: a graded expert panel report. *J Trav Med.* 2017;24(suppl 1):S57-S74.

4

Medical Care of Athletes and Infection Risk

Deverick J. Anderson | Samuel Hume

Introduction

Team medical personnel play a critical role in infection prevention among athletes. Primarily, medical personnel are responsible for practicing rigorous infection control strategies while providing medical care, preventative strategies, and appropriate education to athletes. Secondarily, team medical personnel must help promote best practices for infection prevention as part of a culture of safety.

This chapter provides best practices, recommendations, and information for infection prevention while performing direct medical care. Many of the recommendations included in this chapter are based on the premise that the athletic training facility and treatment rooms are medical facilities. In addition to strategies for direct medical care, we also provide several recommendations on indirect strategies for prevention, including standardization and building a culture of safety in the facility.

The athletic training facility is a medical facility. The same infection prevention practices used in hospitals and clinics must be used in the training facility.

General Information

Medical personnel interact with athletes on multiple levels. In addition to providing direct care, medical personnel are responsible for "setting the tone" in the facility. Adherence to key infection prevention principles improves care in real time and provides an example to others in the facility. Basic principles like standardization and building a culture of safety are proven strategies to improve care and adherence to best practices. More practical principles include single-use items (when possible) and simply put, making it easy to do the right thing. Examples of all of these principles are provided throughout this chapter.

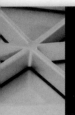

Basic Infection Prevention Principles Can Be Summarized in a Few Simple Statements

- Use a systematic approach to implementation
- Develop a culture of safety
- Use single-use disposable medical equipment
- Make it easy to do the right thing

Standardization

▶ **Best Practice** Standardize infection prevention approaches throughout the facility.

✓ **Recommendation 1** Develop and use specific, written policies to guide infection prevention efforts.

Rationale: Standard practice guidelines improve patient care in the hospital setting[1,2] and are a cornerstone in the fight to prevent healthcare-associated infections.[3] Successful infection prevention methods often combine a number of evidence-based interventions into an easy-to-follow "bundle" or checklist.[4,5] Despite the success of these standardized interventions, each healthcare facility must critically analyze and tailor standard practice guidelines to their local environment.

Sample policies provided in the appendices can be directly used or further modified to fulfill this recommendation. Ideally, athletic trainers, team physicians, coaches, and administration participate in the creation of their local infection prevention policies.

In addition to standardizing practices through policies, materials should be standardized throughout the facility when possible. For example, we recommend using the same types of surface disinfectants in all areas of the training facility (eg, training room, equipment room, weight room, and even offices). This approach ensures users are familiar with the products and ensures that materials are more easily ordered and stocked. Other materials that can be standardized include hand hygiene products (gel, foam, or liquid) and soap.

✓ **Recommendation 2** Ensure that policies are readily available for review and reference.

Rationale: Standard practice guidelines are most helpful when they are easily accessible.[6] Many professional medical societies post best practice guidelines online to improve accessibility and adherence. All teams should disseminate infection prevention guidelines to their staff. Readily accessible documents not only help to improve standardization but also can be easily referenced if/when specific questions arise. Electronically available guidelines improve adherence to policies in hospitals.

However, easy and convenient access to electronic guidelines is not a practical solution in most training facilities. Thus, we recommend creating and placing a policy folder in treatment rooms where it can be readily accessed when needed.

Training in Infection Prevention

▶ **Best Practice** Ensure team medical personnel know basic and advanced infection prevention strategies and recommendations.

✓ **Recommendation 1** Athletic trainers must review educational materials regarding infection prevention annually.

⊘ **Recommendation 2** Document review of infection prevention policies by athletic trainers annually.

Athletic trainers are the most important members of the infection prevention team for athletes.

Rationale: Team athletic trainers have the most interaction with and provide the most care to players. Athletic trainers are important and key members of the infection prevention team. As a result, athletic trainers must stay up-to-date with standards of infection prevention and team infection prevention policies.

Annual review of educational materials concerning common infections among players, such as skin and soft-tissue infections due to methicillin-resistant *Staphylococcus aureus* (MRSA), will improve the care that athletic trainers provide for players. A study of more than 150 athletic trainers revealed conflicting viewpoints about MRSA, hand hygiene, and the use of disinfectants.[7] These discrepancies highlight the need for ongoing education and standardization among athletic trainers. Furthermore, infection prevention is a dynamic field. The epidemiology of infectious agents changes over time, and advances in infection prevention principles and technology lead to continually evolving standards of care.

⊘ **Recommendation 3** Provide team physicians with infection prevention policies.

⊘ **Recommendation 4** Ensure team physicians know of changes to infection prevention policies when changes are made.

Rationale: Annual infection prevention training is required of all physician staff at most medical institutions. Thus, we assume that most, if not all, team physicians receive formal training and education in basic infection prevention strategies each year. However, specific components of infection prevention policies at one institution may vary significantly from components at a different institution (eg, the types of antiseptic agent used preoperatively). Thus, we recommend that team physicians thoroughly understand and periodically review infection prevention policies written specifically for your team (and outlined in this manual). First, this approach will ensure that the physicians are aware of potential differences in policy components. Second, this approach will simultaneously promote discussion when differences in infection prevention approaches are identified. These discussions may help identify the best approaches to use at the training facility.

Culture of Safety

▷ **Best Practice** Implement a culture of safety in the athletic training facility.

⊘ **Recommendation 1** Engage leadership to ensure player safety is a top priority.

Rationale: When a culture of safety is in place, all members of the athletic training staff and team are actively engaged in monitoring and improving safe practices. Pressure to improve practices comes from peers and, more importantly, leaders. According to the Institute for Healthcare Improvement, an organization can develop a culture of safety only when leaders are openly and visibly committed to change, improvement, and open sharing of information. The sum of our proposed best practices and recommendations will augment this culture of safety, but this culture must ultimately be generated and fostered within each facility and training staff.

Pressure to improve practices comes from peers and, more importantly, leaders.

✓ **Recommendation 2** Use proven strategies to "make it easy to do the right thing."

Rationale: Knowledge of best practices is easier to achieve than rigorous implementation of best practices. Thus, additional effort is required to ensure adherence to best practices and recommendations. One basic approach to assist implementation is to ensure **easy access** to materials necessary to implement best practices. For example, all athletic trainers know hand hygiene is important, but washing hands is a more difficult task if the only available alcohol dispenser or sink is located across the training room. Similarly, using a **systematic approach** improves implementation. For example, we recommend that facilities identify a single agent for disinfection and use it throughout the facility instead of using a unique disinfectant agent in every setting. Following a systematic approach improves understanding of the why *and* how practices must be completed. Finally, while athletes inevitably will be exposed to potentially infectious organisms, exposure can be limited by the use of **single-use items**. Use of single-use items eliminates the risk of cross-transmission *and* simplifies processes (making it easier to do the right thing).

▶ **Best Practice** Provide visual reminders about the importance of infection prevention strategies and policies.

✓ **Recommendation** Add signs or posters throughout the facility to improve infection prevention practices.

Rationale: Signs increase awareness of important infection prevention policies. Such signs are routinely placed in most medical facilities. Educational signage improves the culture of safety by providing constant reminders of core principles to players and athletic trainers. Their presence demonstrates the team's acknowledgment of the importance of these policies.

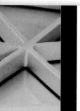

Signs Improve the Culture of Safety

Avoid "sign fatigue" with simple strategies.

1. Move signs on a rotating basis
2. Change the physical appearance of the signs (though not necessarily changing the content)
3. Changing the content or wording of signs while retaining the same message

Signs are recommended to improve hand hygiene, discourage cosmetic body shaving, improve infection prevention in the hydrotherapy room, and promote safe injection policies. *For examples of these type of signs, visit the e-book version of this book.*

Basic Medical Care

Best practices and recommendations provided throughout this book are founded on one major tenet: **athletic training facilities are medical facilities**. Many of the same infection prevention practices and recommendations related to medical care provided in hospitals and outpatient clinics are applicable guides for infection prevention in athletic training facilities. Overall, these infection prevention approaches can be categorized as (1) strategies that decrease the inherent risk of infection *from medical care* or (2) strategies that decrease the inherent risk of infection *from athletic activities*.

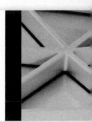

Athletic training facilities are medical facilities.

Basic Strategies to Decrease Risk of Infection in Athletes

1. Hygiene—emphasize skin care with regular hand and body hygiene
2. Use protocols to guide treatment of common infections
3. Safe injection practices
4. Vaccination

Vaccination is a critical component of infection prevention. **See Chapter 6** *for detailed information about which vaccines are most important for athletes.*

Decrease Risk of Infection From Medical Care

Simply put, **medical care involves risk of infection**. Any time skin is disrupted during a procedure—even simply drawing blood or administering an IV—risk of infection occurs. In fact, the biggest culprit for transmission of infection while providing medical care is contaminated, unwashed hands of medical personnel. Simple but effective strategies can reduce these risks.

Medical care involves risk of infection.

HAND HYGIENE

▶ **Best Practice** Actively promote and increase the use of hand hygiene as the primary method of infection prevention in the facility.

✓ **Recommendation 1** Increase the number and locations of alcohol-based hand hygiene dispensers throughout the facility.

✓ **Recommendation 2** Ensure hand hygiene stations (ie, sink and soap dispensers and/or alcohol-based hand cleaning agents) are located at convenient locations in all medical treatment areas and at entry and exit doors in other areas of the facility.

Rationale: Direct (hand-to-skin) transmission is the primary method by which most bacterial pathogens (such as MRSA) are transmitted in healthcare facilities. Similar direct transmission also plays an important role in the spread of viruses such as those causing influenza or the common cold.[8,9] Common pathogens that are temporarily present on the hands of athletic trainers or players can be transmitted to others through direct skin contact if hand washing is omitted, inadequate, or performed with an inappropriate agent.[10] Put another way, your hands are contaminated with potential pathogens **every time** you provide player treatment.

Hand hygiene is the #1 method for preventing transmission.

Alcohol-based hand hygiene products are highly effective in reducing direct, person-to-person transmission of almost all of these pathogens, including MRSA.[11,12] In fact, alcohol-based products are as effective as traditional hand washing with soap and water in most situations *(see Recommendation 4 for important exceptions)*. Use of these products takes less time and results in less skin irritation than soap or other antiseptic agents that require water.[13]

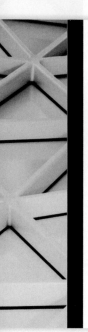

Increasing the number and use of hand hygiene product dispensers has two positive effects. First and most importantly, placing hand hygiene products close to the point of care makes it both convenient and easy for athletic trainers and players to perform hand hygiene. Second, increasing the number of hand hygiene dispensers underscores, highlights, and makes overt the team's commitment to hand hygiene as the cornerstone of all infection prevention activities.

We recognize that there is a continuum of risk of transmitting pathogens via routine player treatments. This risk is lowest and minimal during activities such as taping of intact skin and highest when there is direct hand-to-skin contact with abraded, cut, or nonintact skin.

Tips and Advice: Make Hand Hygiene Easy to Access

- We recommend adding alcohol-based hand hygiene dispensers in the following specific strategic locations:
  - Entrances and "pinch points" through which people routinely pass
    - Entry to the general facility
    - Entry to the training room
    - Entry to the examination procedure room
    - Entry to the locker room
    - Entry to the hydrotherapy room
    - Entry to the cafeteria and other refreshment areas
  - Throughout the training room, including between treatment beds
  - Throughout the players' locker room
- Particularly emphasize player hand hygiene when entering and leaving the weight room. Some athletes have a higher prevalence of MRSA colonization of the hands.
- Alcohol-based hand hygiene products can be delivered as foams, gel, or liquids. There is no difference in effectiveness between these forms.
- Dispensers should be located in easily accessible and visible locations.

✓ Recommendation 3 Clean hands with soap and water instead of alcohol-based products when they are visibly soiled or heavily contaminated with dirt, debris, body fluids, or blood.

✓ Recommendation 4 Clean hands with soap and water instead of alcohol-based products after treating a player with a diarrheal illness.

Rationale: Alcohol-based hand hygiene products are not effective when hands are heavily soiled with dirt or other material such as oils or blood. Alcohol does not kill two important pathogens that cause highly transmissible diarrheal illness—norovirus and *Clostridioides difficile* (also known as "*C. diff*").

✓ Recommendation 5 Ensure moisturizing hand lotions or emollients are available to staff and players to prevent dry or cracked skin.

Rationale: Frequent use of alcohol-containing hand hygiene products can occasionally lead to dry and cracked skin. While most hand hygiene products also contain emollients to prevent drying of skin, frequent use may still result in some degree of drying and cracking of skin. Dry, cracked, or irritated skin is more likely to harbor pathogens such as MRSA. Thus, ensuring that lotion is available for use can help overcome this potential side effect of increased hand hygiene.

Dry, cracked, or irritated skin is more likely to harbor pathogens such as MRSA.

⊘ **Recommendation 6** Use hospital-grade soap from prefilled/packaged dispensers in the training, treatment, and examination/procedure rooms.

Rationale: As detailed above, a few situations require hand washing with soap and water rather than alcohol-based products. Medical treatment facilities typically use antibacterial soap dispensed from prefilled, replaceable dispensers.

We acknowledge that the use of antibacterial soap is controversial. There is no compelling evidence that antibacterial soaps prevent infection in the community better than plain soap and water.[14] Furthermore, triclosan, the active ingredient of most commercially available antibacterial liquid soaps, may disrupt reproductive or thyroid function in aquatic life and laboratory animals.[15,16] In fact, the FDA recently concluded that the majority of chemicals used in over-the-counter antiseptic soap, including triclosan, were "not generally recognized as safe and effective."[17] Thus, we currently do not recommend the use of soaps containing triclosan in training facilities. Instead, we recommend liquid soaps containing chloroxylenol, benzalkonium, or chlorhexidine in prefilled dispensers. Finally, refillable soap dispensers have a known risk of becoming contaminated with potential pathogens such as *Pseudomonas* and *Serratia*. Thus, we recommend using prefilled/packaged dispensers that can be replaced when the soap content becomes empty or low instead of "topping off" refillable dispensers.

Decrease Risk of Infection From Athletic Activities

PLAYER HYGIENE

As described above, medical personnel must diligently perform hand hygiene to decrease the indirect transmission of pathogens from player to player through transiently contaminated medical personnel hands. Player hygiene is equally important. Improved player hygiene leads to decreased risk of direct transmission from player to player and indirect transmission through decreased environmental contamination.

Athletes have unique risks compared to the general population. For example, rates of MRSA colonization among athletes are as high as rates of MRSA colonization among patients admitted to intensive care units. Investigators from Brown University published a meta-analysis of the worldwide literature on the prevalence of asymptomatic MRSA nasal and/or skin colonization in athletes.[18] They reviewed 382 prior studies of MRSA infections in athletes and selected 15 studies in which prospective screening cultures for MRSA colonization were performed in team athletes. The mean pooled prevalence of MRSA colonization was 8% among American athletes.

- MRSA colonization among athletes was six times higher than the rate of colonization in the community.
- Colonization rates were higher in collegiate athletes (13%) than in professional athletes and significantly higher in wrestlers (22%) as compared to football players (4%-8%) and basketball players (8%).
- The risk of subsequent MRSA infection was seven times higher for colonized athletes than noncolonized athletes.

These findings reinforce numerous recommendations made throughout this manual related to regular hand hygiene by players and staff, prompt care of cuts and other skin injuries, and attention to disinfection of training tables and medical equipment.

▶ **Best Practice** Shower after practice to decrease the risk of bacterial transmission from player to player and from player to environment.

⊘ **Recommendation 1** Mandate postpractice showers for all players.

Rationale: The highest risk of transmission of important pathogens such as MRSA from one player to another likely occurs during and immediately after practice. Approximately 1% to 3% of the general American population is colonized with MRSA,[19,20] but up to 10% to 20% of athletes are colonized.[18,21,22] Put another way, if a team roster includes 50 players, approximately 5 to 10 players may be silently colonized with MRSA. Thus, contact with MRSA is inevitable in team settings. MRSA exposure in the setting of skin abrasions and cuts acquired through routine athletic activities substantially increases the risk of subsequent infection.

Athletes are more likely to have MRSA on their skin than nonathletes.

✓ **Recommendation 2** Do not provide bar soap in showers.

✓ **Recommendation 3** Use soap dispensers that utilize prefilled/packaged liquid soap in the showers.

Rationale: Bar soap has been previously implicated as a potential source of MRSA transmission; sharing bar soap was associated with MRSA infections during an outbreak among football players and in an outbreak in a prison.[23] Thus, the easiest way to reduce the risk of sharing or using previously used bars of soap in the shower is to remove them. Nonrefillable soap dispensers (ie, dispensers that utilize prefilled/packaged liquid soap products) should be used instead of refillable dispensers.

▶ **Best Practice** Perform "source control" routinely during the season.

✓ **Recommendation 1** Instruct players to bathe with chlorhexidine gluconate (CHG) three times each week.

✓ **Recommendation 2** Add 2% or 4% CHG soap dispensers to team showers to promote routine source control.

Rationale: "Source control" is the routine application of a disinfectant to skin to reduce the number of pathogenic bacteria that live on the skin. Source control has not been studied in the athletic team environment. Our recommendations are based on the use of source control strategies in ICU patients and military recruits. The use of CHG for routine bathing of ICU patients has emerged as a key practice for preventing infections in the hospital. Daily bathing with CHG in the ICU reduces the infection burden by 37% compared to routine bathing.[24] Two studies in military recruits using three times weekly CHG cloths demonstrated a statistically significant reduction in acquisition of *Staphylococcus aureus* **and** MRSA (3.3% vs 6.5%) colonization.[25,26] Thus, while the use of CHG is typically targeted at reducing the risk of MRSA, it also reduces the risk from methicillin-susceptible *Staphylococcus aureus* (MSSA).

FDA Announcement About Chlorhexidine Gluconate

The FDA released a safety communication about chlorhexidine gluconate (CHG) in 2017 warning about potential but rare allergic reactions, likely related to increased use of CHG throughout health care. Thus, as with any chemical, it is important to monitor for and routinely inquire about a history of CHG allergy. A recent study analyzed over 25,000 patients admitted to ICUs who received daily bathing with CHG; seven patients had mild adverse events related to CHG, and no patients experienced serious adverse events. We believe the substantial benefit from CHG outweighs potential risks and continue to strongly advocate for CHG use in myriad infection prevention interventions.

The delivery of CHG includes logistical challenges. Ideally, source control would be performed using CHG-impregnated wipes. However, the process of using wipes requires distribution of wipes and reliance on players to use them properly. Thus, for routine source control, we recommend use of the liquid, detergent-based preparations containing 2% to 4% CHG. *For additional information about using CHG for source control and strategies for implementation, please see Appendix 1J. In the event that a cluster of infections occurs, we recommend changing from liquid to wipes, as outlined in Chapter 5.*

Other products can potentially be used to reduce the number of pathogens on the skin. These products have limitations related to logistics and/or lack of clinical data. For example, daily dilute bleach baths (15-minute soak in ¼ cup bleach per tub) are highly effective at reducing colonization with MRSA; some centers recommend bleach baths as part of a decolonization strategy.[27] This strategy is not practical for widespread use in the team environment. However, this strategy has been made more practical by the development of bleach-containing body washes. Small trials involving 28 to 50 children with moderate to severe atopic dermatitis demonstrated that use of a bleach-containing body wash three times weekly led to decreases in the amount and severity of atopic dermatitis symptoms and *S. aureus* colonization.[28] Finally, some companies have begun using silver antiseptics for body washes. One formulation coupled with aloe, vitamin E, and allantoin was deemed "noninferior" to 4% CHG in a study involving effectiveness of inguinal fold disinfection in 81 health volunteers.[29]

⊙ **Best Practice** Develop and enforce a policy to guide hygienic use of common balms, lotions, and creams.

⊘ **Recommendation 1** Dispense balms, lotions, and creams via pumps whenever possible.

Rationale: A central theme throughout this manual is promoting the use of individual-use equipment and materials. The use of pumps to dispense balms, lotions, and creams, when available, achieves the spirit of this theme and greatly reduces the risk of contaminating these commonly used materials with unclean hands. In the event that a specific balm or cream cannot be dispensed via a pump (ie, due to viscosity), the following two recommendations should be followed.

⊘ **Recommendation 2** Ensure athletic trainers and players perform hand hygiene prior to accessing balms, lotions, and creams in communal tubs, even if gloves are being used.

⊘ **Recommendation 3** Ensure athletic trainers and players do not reenter communal tubs without performing hand hygiene prior to reentry.

Rationale: For materials that can only be provided in communal tubs, contamination of the materials can be greatly reduced by performing hand hygiene and wearing gloves prior to entry. Other strategies for obtaining materials, such as the use of wooden tongue depressors, may serve as an alternative to using hands. Importantly, some healthcare workers believe that wearing gloves is equivalent to performing hand hygiene. **This assumption is incorrect.** In fact, hands frequently become contaminated with important pathogens (eg, MRSA) present on gloves as gloves are removed.[30] Thus, hand hygiene must be performed after removing gloves.

Wearing gloves? Sorry, you still need to wash your hands.

Overall, the risk of transmission of important pathogens from one player or athletic trainer to another via contaminated balms, lotions, or creams is low, particularly when these materials are applied to intact skin. Thus, we acknowledge that the effort to closely follow and police the above recommendations and policy may be difficult to achieve. If or when one or more cases of MRSA is detected in the training facility, however, we believe the effort to enforce these policies must be expended.

CUT CARE

▶ **Best Practice** Establish a protocol for the routine care of simple abrasions, cuts, and lacerations.

Healthy, intact skin is the body's primary defense against infection.

✓ **Recommendation 1** Develop and use a written and comprehensive policy for "cut care."

Rationale: Although simple abrasions and other breaks in the integrity of the normal cutaneous barrier are usually uncomplicated, such injuries are also a common antecedent in players who develop skin and soft-tissue infections. Thus, we advise the use of a standard protocol that includes specific details about wound cleaning, the use of antibacterial ointments, and wound dressings.

A sample "Cut Care Protocol" is provided in **Appendix 1C.**

✓ **Recommendation 2** Use CHG for standard wound cleaning.

Rationale: Although soap and water are adequate cleaning agents, we recommend the general use of an antiseptic agent for standard wound care. Specifically, we advise using 4% CHG (Hibiclens or Betasept wash) for standard wound care.

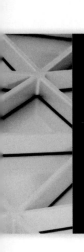

Why Use Chlorhexidine Gluconate for Wound Care?

- Chlorhexidine gluconate (CHG) products have in vitro bactericidal activity against methicillin-resistant and methicillin-susceptible staphylococci, streptococci, and most bacteria that colonize normal skin.[31]
- They are well tolerated and safe.
- Unlike Betadine/iodophors, CHG's activity is not diminished by the presence of organic debris or material such as blood.
- CHG produces a prolonged antibacterial effect after application.
- CHG "sticks" are now available for use and should replace Betadine sticks in all settings.
- While bacterial resistance has been demonstrated to chlorhexidine,[32] this occurs only rarely and its clinical significance in everyday practice is currently insignificant.

Iodophor-containing topical agents such as povidone-iodine (Betadine) are also effective topical agents. In head-to-head comparison studies, however, **CHG has been shown to have superior antibacterial activity** and less inactivation by organic debris or body fluids such as blood.[33] For this reason, we advise CHG-containing agents prior to most surgical procedures and for all wound care.

We are not aware of any data demonstrating superiority of topical agents containing quaternary ammonium such as benzathonium chloride (eg, dermal skin cleanser). Some quaternary ammonium compounds also contain surfactants that facilitate cleansing dirt and debris from the skin. However, in laboratory tests, topical quaternary ammonium components are bacteriostatic. We prefer agents that are bactericidal and known to rapidly kill pathogenic bacteria on contact. In addition, contamination of quaternary ammonium compounds by organisms such as *Pseudomonas aeruginosa* is a rare but well-recognized phenomenon and risk. This contamination is especially likely to occur when large-volume containers are used to store stock solutions that are dispensed into smaller containers.

Topical solutions (including povidone-iodine and chlorhexidine) that contain alcohol have the best and fastest antibacterial effects. However, we advise **against** using alcohol-containing solutions for routine care of cuts and abrasions for the following reasons:

- These solutions cause burning when applied to nonintact skin.
- These solutions predictably cause drying of the skin.

We advise against the use of iodophors such as povidone-iodine (Betadine) for routine care of cuts and abrasions for the following reasons:

- Although iodophors are generally safe and well tolerated, these compounds are more likely to cause contact dermatitis than other commonly used skin antiseptics.
- Iodophor solutions are prone to becoming contaminated (especially with *P. aeruginosa*) when stock solutions are stored in large bottles. Contaminated Betadine solutions have been associated with numerous outbreaks of healthcare-associated infections, particularly when used prior to injections or other invasive procedures. Note, this risk is eliminated when single-unit doses of iodophors are used (eg, individually wrapped, premoistened swabs).

☑ **Recommendation 3** Apply mupirocin or silver-containing ointments to cuts and scrapes as part of standard care.

Rationale: Many athletic trainers and medical professionals routinely apply antibacterial ointments prior to the placement of a clean, dry dressing. These agents are safe and effective. Although topical antibacterial ointments are probably not required for every cut or abrasion, we recommend their use for most skin injuries, especially if extensive, deep, or otherwise a concern. Choices for topical therapy include the following:

- Mupirocin
- Silver sulfadiazine creams and silver nanoparticle creams
- Bacitracin
- Bacitracin/polymyxin B or bacitracin, neomycin, and polymyxin B

Of the four therapeutic options listed above, we prefer mupirocin for the following reasons:

- It has established activity against MRSA, other strains of *S. aureus*, and common skin pathogens such as streptococci.
- It is safe and has few, if any, significant side effects.
- MRSA is the predominant pathogen causing skin and soft-tissue infection in the United States[34]; thus, using an agent with proven activity against MRSA for primary prevention is logical.
- Although emergence of antimicrobial resistance is a concern when mupirocin is used, the likelihood that regular use of mupirocin *as topical therapy* will result in the emergence of resistance in a small closed population such as an athletic team is unlikely.

Silver-containing creams and ointments can be used in place of mupirocin but are typically more costly. While older silver sulfadiazine creams frequently became dry, crusty, and difficult to use, these issues have been obviated by new nanoparticle formulations of silver ointment.

Bacitracin topical activity is inferior to mupirocin against MRSA and other common bacterial pathogens.[35]

Bacitracin, bacitracin/polymyxin B, neomycin, double-antibiotic, and triple-antibiotic creams are often used for topical therapy. However, we prefer mupirocin over these other agents for the following reasons:

- Bacitracin topical activity is inferior to mupirocin against MRSA and other common bacterial pathogens.[35]
- Bacitracin, neomycin, and polymyxin B and bacitracin/polymyxin B ointments are not effective against MRSA and can lead to allergic reactions that may be confused with an infection.

✓ **Recommendation 4** Use hydrocolloid dressings if simple bandages are insufficient.

Rationale: We recognize that there are no reliable published data to guide the choice of dressings for wounds or large areas of skin damage. Thus, the choice and type of dressing to apply to skin injuries is primarily a matter of clinical judgment and local preference. Although Band-Aid and other "breathable" bandages are fine for small and minor skin injuries, hydrocolloid dressings such as DuoDERM are preferable to gauze for deeper and more extensive skin injuries. Hydrocolloid dressings protect injured skin from drying and can be left in place for longer periods of time. Finally, these products are easy and painless to remove. Hydrocolloidal dressings containing CHG are also available, but few and limited data are currently available to assess their superiority compared to standard hydrocolloid dressings.

We are aware of increasingly advanced wound dressings, such as "electroceutical" wound dressings that generate a low-level electrical field in the bandage when wound exudate is present. For example, silver-zinc redox-coupled electroceutical wound dressings can disrupt *Pseudomonas* biofilm formation in laboratory conditions[36] and can reduce costs in chronic wound patients when coupled with negative-pressure wound therapy.[37] To date, however, we are unable to determine if these dressings offer advantages over standard dressings and disinfection strategies described above.

✓ **Recommendation 5** Ensure all materials required for effective wound therapy are readily available and easily accessible via a "wound care cart."

Rationale: A central theme throughout our manual is to "make it easy to do the right thing" through strategic placement of materials and organization of strategies (eg, hand hygiene or influenza vaccines). Wound care can be made easier through the use of a well-organized "wound care cart" or designated wound care area that provides easy access to all necessary materials and equipment.

HYDROTHERAPY

▶ **Best Practice** Develop, use, and enforce a policy for appropriate use of the hydrotherapy room.

✓ **Recommendation 1** Prevent players with open wounds from entering pools unless the wounds are covered with an impermeable dressing.

✓ **Recommendation 2** Require players to shower prior to using the hydrotherapy pools.

✓ **Recommendation 3** Prevent players with known MRSA infections from entering the pools until the infection is completely resolved.

✅ **Recommendation 4** If a player with an uncovered open wound uses the hydrotherapy pool, do not allow another player to use the pool until it has been drained, dried, and disinfected.

Rationale: Whirlpools have been implicated in previous outbreaks of MRSA among athletes. For example, one MRSA outbreak of 10 college football players (2 of whom required hospitalization) was linked to a whirlpool.[38] Players who used the whirlpools during or after players with MRSA infections entered the water had a 12-fold higher risk of MRSA infection. Pool environments can also spread other pathogens like *Pseudomonas, Cryptosporidium,* and *Legionella.*

Open sores or breaks in the skin can become infected by bathing in contaminated pool water. The Centers for Disease Control and Prevention (CDC) recommends that individuals with an open wound avoid going into swimming pools.[39] However, we understand that hydrotherapy can be essential for athlete rehabilitation. Therefore, athletes with open wounds who require hydrotherapy should always cover open wounds with impermeable dressings. If a player with an uncovered open wound uses a hydrotherapy pool, we recommend draining, drying, and disinfecting the pool. Subsequent players may be at risk for infection.

Other body fluids can also contaminate pools. The CDC recommends adjusting free chlorine levels following known stool or vomit contamination[40] Pool volumes, however, may be significantly different in public pools than in a small hydrotherapy pool. We recommend draining, drying, and disinfecting the pool in the unlikely and rare event of contamination from body fluids such as vomit or stool.

Over half of swimming pools contain fecal bacteria.[41] Such contamination not only spreads bacteria but also can interfere with disinfection chemicals.[40] Showers remove perianal fecal material, sweat, excess skin cells, and dirt before bathers enter the pool. Thus, showering before entering a hydrotherapy pool reduces the risk of contamination and helps maintain the cleanliness of the pools. In fact, showers prior to pool entry are required by some state and local regulations.

✅ **Recommendation 5** Ensure clean, laundered towels are available for individual use.

Remind Players—Never Share Towels

Rationale: Sharing towels places athletes at higher risk of developing MRSA and other infections. In one study, football players who shared towels were over eight times more likely to develop MRSA than those who did not.[42] Thus, as yet another example of "make it easy to do the right thing," clean laundered towels must be readily available for use by players exiting the hydrotherapy pools.

✅ **Recommendation 6** Place a sign in the hydrotherapy room to remind players of the hydrotherapy room policy.

See Chapter 6 and section on Maintenance of Hydrotherapy Rooms for additional recommendations.

Rationale: We realize it is not feasible or practical for teams to strictly monitor compliance with some of the preceding recommendations. However, signage, education, and frequent reminders about the preceding risks and recommendations may help improve compliance. In addition, players often consider requirements such as showering prior to using the hydrotherapy room to be a nuisance. Placing signs in the hydrotherapy rooms will help to serve as a reminder of the policy, will increase the culture of safety of the training room, and enforce the commitment to infection prevention practices. *Please see the e-book version of this book for an example of a sign that can be used in the hydrotherapy room.*

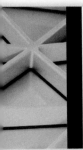

Above and Beyond: Hydrotherapy Room

✅ **Recommendation** Install a shower in the hydrotherapy room, if possible.

Rationale: This recommendation may not be feasible in all facilities, but we strongly encourage this strategy, when possible, to improve compliance with the policy to shower prior to hydrotherapy pool entry. Installation of a shower in the hydrotherapy room accompanied by appropriate signage and education is another example of our theme "make it easy to do what's right."

Diagnosis and Treatment of Infections and Transmissible Pathogens

Infections can and do occur regularly in athletes. In most cases, prompt identification and treatment of infections will decrease the risk of adverse events, including loss of playing time and, just as importantly, transmission to other athletes. While *Chapter 1 provides basic information about many of the infections that commonly occur in athletes*, this section provides specific information related to diagnosis and treatment of infections caused by pathogens that easily spread within a locker room, including tips and content for use in standardized diagnosis and treatment protocols.

The guidance included in this section is intended to provide basic and general strategies for diagnosis of common skin and soft-tissue infections, diarrheal illness, and respiratory illness. In all cases, treatment should be performed by a qualified clinician and individualized to the specific patient and scenario.

BACTERIAL SKIN AND SOFT-TISSUE INFECTIONS

▶ **Best Practice** Develop and use a standard protocol for diagnosis and treatment of skin and soft-tissue infections.

Although special clinical findings and circumstance may require unique or nonstandard treatment approaches, most common soft-tissue infections in athletes can and should be treated using the options outlined in a standardized protocol. Standard protocols also can prevent errors in management.

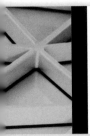

Key Components for a Protocol for Treatment of Skin and Soft-Tissue Infections

- Most likely bacterial pathogens
- Common antibiotic choices and routes of administration
- Weight-based dosing
- Alternatives for common drug allergies
- Options for de-escalation when culture results return.

✅ **Recommendation 1** Choose an antibiotic with activity against MRSA for empiric treatment of purulent skin infections.

Rationale: Infections of the skin can be divided into two clinical categories: purulent and non-purulent.[43] Sixty to seventy percent of purulent skin infections (eg, abscess, boil, carbuncle, or furuncle) are caused by MRSA.[34] It is impossible to distinguish purulent skin and soft-tissue infections due to MRSA from those due to other gram-positive bacteria, including strains of *S. aureus* that are susceptible to methicillin.

As a general rule, purulent infections are due to MRSA until proven otherwise.

As a result, we recommend starting one of the two following regimens (**Figure 4.1**; **Table 4.1**):

1. Trimethoprim/sulfamethoxazole double strength (DS) one to two tablets orally two times per day

OR

2. Linezolid 600 mg orally two times per day

There are important advantages and disadvantages to each of these approaches. Individual teams and team physicians will need to choose which of these two approaches to include in the individual policy used on each team based on the following issues:

1. Weight-based dosing
   a. Trimethoprim/sulfamethoxazole—Players who weigh >100 kg (220 pounds) require increased doses of Bactrim, which should be directed by the team physician.
   b. Linezolid—No weight-based dosing required.

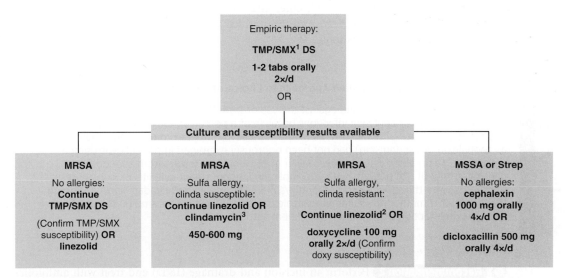

[1] TMP/SMX, trimethoprim/sulfamethoxazole (Bactrim). Players who weigh > 100 kg (220 pounds) may require increased doses of Bactrim, which should be directed by the team physician.

[2] Tedizolid can be used instead of linezolid. Tedizolid should be dosed at 200 mg orally once daily.

[3] While the recommended dose for clindamycin is 450-600 mg, many athletes may require 600 mg due to size.

Figure 4.1 Treatment algorithm for skin and soft-tissue infections.

Table 4.1 Antibiotic Recommendations for Purulent Skin/Soft-Tissue Infection

Empiric Antibiotics	First line: Trimethoprim/sulfamethoxazole (TMP/SMX), Linezolid
	Alternative: Doxycycline, clindamycin
Known pathogen	**Direct therapy based on pathogen and susceptibilities**
MRSA	Above, then based on susceptibilities
MSSA	Cephalexin, dicloxacillin
Streptococcus sp.	Penicillin, dicloxacillin, cephalexin

2. Streptococcal coverage
   a. Bactrim has activity against streptococci, but it is not the first choice for therapy for serious Group A *Streptococcus* infections.
   b. Linezolid has excellent activity against streptococci.
3. Cost
   a. Bactrim is very cheap.
   b. Linezolid is now also inexpensive as it is available in generic formulation.
4. Allergy
   a. Patients with glucose-6-phosphate dehydrogenase (G6PD) deficiency should not receive trimethoprim/sulfamethoxazole.
      i. The American Association of Family Practitioners recommends that neonates should be screened for G6PD deficiency when family history, appearance of neonatal jaundice, or ethnic or geographic origin suggests the possibility of G6PD deficiency.[44] Of note, African descent is associated with increased risk; thus, most African-American athletes should undergo screening as part of routine evaluation.

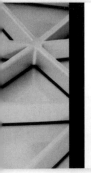

Tips and Advice: Use a Simplified Approach to Choice of Empiric Antibiotic Treatment

Previously, many experts argued against the use of trimethoprim/sulfamethoxazole (Bactrim) for nonpurulent skin infections because of a perceived decrease of efficacy against streptococci. Until recently, its relative efficacy compared to other oral agents (such as cephalexin or clindamycin) had not been rigorously examined in patients with simple cellulitis and skin abscesses. However, Miller et al. published results from a randomized controlled trial of 524 patients with uncomplicated, nonpurulent cellulitis or skin abscesses.[45] Cure rates were the same for trimethoprim/sulfamethoxazole and clindamycin, confirming the idea that trimethoprim/sulfamethoxazole can be safely used for empiric therapy for *any* type of skin infection treated in the outpatient setting.

✓ **Recommendation 2** Perform an incision and drainage (I&D) and treat with antibiotics for all purulent skin infections.

Rationale: Prior to the emergence of community-associated MRSA, it was widely believed that I&D without subsequent antibiotic therapy was the standard and accepted therapy for small (<5 cm) abscesses. MRSA is now, however, the most common cause of skin infections associated with visible pus. Thus, we and many other physicians believe that **all** pus-containing skin lesions should be treated with I&D **and** antibiotics. While simple I&D may be sufficient to cure some infections, the combination of I&D and effective antibiotics decreases the need for further drainage procedures and risk of recurrence after initially effective treatment.[46]

Two large trials further support this recommendation. The first of these studies included 1220 patients who presented to one of five participating emergency departments in the United States with a skin abscess greater than 2 cm in size. Enrolled patients (mean age 35 years) were randomized to I&D plus trimethoprim-sulfamethoxazole for 7 days or I&D plus placebo for 7 days. Eighty-one percent of 630 patients randomized to treatment with I&D and trimethoprim-sulfamethoxazole were cured compared to 74% of patients randomized to only I&D treatment ($P = .005$).[47] Moreover, rates of subsequent surgical drainage, new skin infections, and household member infections were lower in the trimethoprim-sulfamethoxazole arm. Subjects who received trimethoprim-sulfamethoxazole, however, had higher rates of GI side effects.

The second study enrolled 786 patients with a "simple" skin abscess less than 5 cm in size; each patient was randomized to one of three treatment arms: I&D plus trimethoprim-sulfamethoxazole for 10 days, I&D plus clindamycin for 10 days, or I&D plus placebo for 10 days.[48] The cure rates for both of the antibiotic treatment arms were significantly higher than the cure rate for the placebo arm (82%, 83%, and 69%, respectively). Rates of relapse were lower in the clindamycin arm, but rates of adverse events were also two times higher with clindamycin.

A similar percentage (roughly 50%) of patients in both studies had cultures that grew MRSA prior to treatment.

For most minor boils and abscesses, incision and drainage can be performed at the training facility, but complicated skin and skin-structure infections may require debridement in operating rooms.

✓ Recommendation 3 Obtain a culture from purulent skin infections to determine the infecting organism.

Rationale: Although empiric treatment of skin infections without concurrent collection of samples for making a microbiological diagnosis is commonly done in community practice, we advise against this practice when purulence is observed in an athlete. While the majority of purulent skin infections are caused by MRSA, other pathogens can also cause purulent infections that mimic those caused by MRSA. This observation is clinically important, as pathogens such as streptococci and MSSA can be easily treated with antibiotics that are safer than those required to treat MRSA.

Why Obtain a Culture From a Purulent Skin Infection?

1. A positive culture often leads to a definitive diagnosis that, in turn, can direct the most effective and safest treatment for an individual player. Ultimately, a positive culture with susceptibilities is the only way to determine if the selected antibiotic is active against the pathogen.

2. A positive culture may lead to confirmation that antibiotics prescribed empirically were indeed effective and optimal.

3. A positive culture may provide the necessary information to initiate contingency protocols that are designed to decrease the risk of additional cases in team members if epidemiologically important organisms such as MRSA are identified.

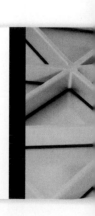

⊘ Recommendation 4 Change the antibiotic to specifically treat the infecting organism identified on culture and sensitivity of purulent skin infections.

Rationale: Initial antimicrobial therapy is typically chosen to "cover all the bases." As noted above, we believe trimethoprim/sulfamethoxazole (Bactrim, DS) can serve this purpose for the majority of skin and soft-tissue infections. Broad, empiric antimicrobial therapy will often require changes to narrow activity to the organism identified on culture (**Figure 4.1**). This approach is a standard and highly recommended practice as part of "antimicrobial stewardship."

- If the culture reveals MRSA and if the player is not allergic to sulfa-containing medicines, continue or switch to trimethoprim/sulfamethoxazole (Bactrim, DS), one to two tablets two times per day for 5 days or until the infection is gone (*confirm Bactrim susceptibility on culture result*).
  - If the player is sulfa-allergic AND if the isolate is clindamycin-susceptible, continue or switch to
    - linezolid 600 mg orally two times per day for 5 days or until the infection is gone OR
    - doxycycline 100 mg orally two times per day OR
    - clindamycin 450 to 600 mg orally three times per day, but it carries a higher risk of *C. difficile* colitis
  - If the player is sulfa-allergic AND if the organism is clindamycin-resistant, continue or switch to linezolid or doxycycline as outlined above.
- If the culture reveals *S. aureus* that is methicillin-sensitive (MSSA), treat with cephalexin 500 to 1000 mg orally four times per day or dicloxacillin 500 mg orally four times per day for 5 days or until the infection is gone.
  - Players who weigh >100 kg (220 pounds) can be safely given 1 g of cephalexin orally four times a day. Amoxicillin/clavulanate 875 mg orally two times per day is an acceptable alternative to cephalexin and dicloxacillin.
- If the culture reveals Group A streptococci (*Streptococcus pyogenes*) treat with Pen Vee K or Pen VK 1000 mg orally four times per day or Amoxicillin 500 mg orally three times per day for 5 days or until the infection is gone.

⊘ Recommendation 5 Store materials for the proper collection of diagnostic specimens on-site at the athletic training facility.

Rationale: If access to immediate medical evaluation and care is not conveniently and readily available, then storage of culture swabs in the athletic training facility is advised to facilitate diagnosis of common skin infections. Storage and use of culture swabs at the athletic training facility ensures that the specimen can be obtained and sent for analysis *immediately* upon diagnosis.

⊘ Recommendation 6 Include information regarding which laboratory receives the culture specimens and who receives the results in the treatment protocol.

Rationale: The receiving microbiology laboratory should be able to report positive results (to a designated person or telephone number) within 24 to 48 hours. Reporting exclusively via mail as opposed to telephone or e-mail should be discouraged, as receipt of test results and implementation of optimal treatment might be delayed.

⊘ Recommendation 7 Choose an antibiotic with activity against streptococci and MSSA for treatment of nonpurulent skin infections.

Rationale: Nonpurulent skin and soft-tissue infections such as cellulitis and erysipelas are unlikely to be due to MRSA.[43] Instead, streptococci are the primary cause of nonpurulent skin and soft-tissue infections. Given the absence of pus, no cultures are required for this type of infection (and thus therapy cannot be targeted against organisms identified on culture results).

For nonpurulent skin and soft-tissue infections, we recommend treatment with cephalexin 500 to 1000 mg orally four times a day or dicloxacillin 500 mg orally four times a day for 5 to 7 days or until the infection is gone. If the infection does not improve after 2 to 3 days of therapy, we recommend culturing the wound (if pus has developed in the interim) and broadening antibiotics to cover MRSA (see above recommendations).

⊘ **Recommendation 8** Immediately refer players with signs and symptoms of sepsis to the team physician and/or emergency room.

Rationale: Players with severe skin infections and/or concomitant signs and symptoms of sepsis (ie, fever, chills, tachycardia, or hypotension) should be seen by a clinician as soon as possible to determine if IV antibiotics or emergent incision and drainage are required.

VIRAL SKIN AND SOFT-TISSUE INFECTIONS

Viral infections may occasionally mimic bacterial skin infections, leading to unnecessary antibiotic therapy. In particular, it is important for team medical personnel to be aware of and be able to recognize two of these infections: herpes infection and hand, foot, and mouth disease (HFMD). Both infections typically have cutaneous manifestations in addition to systemic symptoms. Both are highly contagious; thus, failure to quickly diagnose these infections can lead to subsequent exposure and transmission to teammates and other athletes.

⊙ **Best Practice** Routinely evaluate athletes for manifestations of herpes virus to decrease transmission.

⊘ **Recommendation 1** Perform routine skin checks for manifestations of herpes infection.

⊘ **Recommendation 2** Withhold athletes from practice and competition with other athletes if active herpes lesions are present.

Rationale: Herpes is a very common viral infection. More than 50% of people have been exposed to herpes by the time they reach adulthood. Oral herpes or "cold sores" are the most common manifestation of herpes infections. Athletes who participate in contact sports, particularly wrestling, are at increased risk of herpes infections involving the skin and eyes. Contamination likely occurs by inoculation of skin abrasions by infected saliva.

Herpes gladiatorum typically occurs on the face, neck, and arms of athletes. Because the erythematous fluid-filled vesicular lesions often progress to an erythematous ulceration, the infection is often mistaken for folliculitis or impetigo. Herpetic whitlow typically occurs on fingers and hands, but otherwise has a similar appearance.

Numerous outbreaks of herpes infections in wrestlers have been documented. In one well-documented example, more than 50 wrestlers from 23 different teams were ultimately diagnosed with symptomatic herpes gladiatorum following a statewide tournament. Wrestling was stopped in the state of Minnesota for 8 days in order to stop the outbreak.[49]

In general, herpes infections do not routinely require treatment. However, groups such as the National Athletic Trainers' Association suggest that athletes with herpes gladiatorum must be on antiviral treatment for at least 5 days with no new lesions in 3 days before they can return to play.[50] When treatment is necessary, valacyclovir 1000 mg given two times a day for 7 to 10 days is recommended.

> ▶ **Best Practice** Routinely evaluate athletes for manifestations of HFMD.

> ✓ **Recommendation 1** Provide supportive treatment for players with symptoms of HFMD.

> ✓ **Recommendation 2** Perform a thorough cleaning of the facility if a player is diagnosed with HFMD, with particular emphasis on areas that hands encounter (eg, weights, balls, meeting room chairs, and arm rests).

Rationale: As outlined in *Chapter 1*, HFMD is typically a mild viral infection that occurs in children in the summer and fall; it can be caused by several viruses but is typically caused by Coxsackievirus or enterovirus. Rash on the hands (often vesicular on the palms or soles) and lesions in the mouth (mild ulcers) are often visible on physical examination. HFMD in adults is also typically a mild illness with widely varying presentation; most patients will believe they have a "cold." Some adults may not have the same type of rash or skin lesions seen on children with HFMD; in contrast, a rash may be the only symptoms present in other adults. HFMD is spread by oral ingestion of contaminated feces, following direct exposure to saliva or vesicular fluid (that then enters into the mouth), or following indirect exposure via a contaminated environment.

> ✓ **Recommendation 3** Exclude athletes with HFMD from team activities until afebrile and vesiculopapular lesions can be covered.

Rationale: The benefit of isolation for HFMD is controversial. An extensive outbreak occurred on the east coast of the United States in 2016, particularly impacting high-school students in New Jersey and Connecticut.[51] During this outbreak, health departments in these states issued warnings for athletes and parents. Numerous sporting events were canceled or postponed. In the daycare setting, however, removal of children with HFMD does not decrease transmission, as children shed virus before, during, and after symptoms. Nevertheless, isolation and removal from team activities coupled with more intensive environmental disinfection likely decrease risk of subsequent spread.

DIARRHEAL ILLNESS

Diarrhea can be caused by numerous viruses and bacteria, though the vast majority of sporadic and community-onset cases are viral.[52]

> ▶ **Best Practice** Develop and use a standard protocol for diagnosis and treatment of diarrheal illness.

> ✓ **Recommendation 1** Utilize signs and symptoms to make an empirical diagnosis of the cause of diarrhea in an ill athlete.

> ✓ **Recommendation 2** Have a high suspicion of norovirus if a player is vomiting and has diarrhea.

> ✓ **Recommendation 3** Promptly treat symptoms (ie, fluid loss) of diarrheal illness.

Rationale: Because most cases of diarrhea are viral and because most cases of diarrhea are minor, self-limiting short-duration illnesses, culturing stool specimens is not normally necessary or beneficial.

Norovirus is the most common cause of outbreaks of acute gastroenteritis in the United States. It is responsible for an estimated 21 million annual cases of diarrhea in Americans each year. Outbreaks spread rapidly from person to person.

Norovirus infections range in severity from mild to severe; diarrhea from norovirus is typically accompanied by vomiting. Fever is present in approximately half of infected adults with norovirus. Patients often have headache, myalgia, and malaise, but they rarely appear acutely ill. Treatment is typically limited to supportive treatment such as fluids. Antibiotics are not required for norovirus.

Please see **Appendix 1G** *for an example policy for diagnosis and treatment of diarrheal illness.*

✅ **Recommendation 4** Educate players to promptly notify team personnel when they have vomiting and/or diarrhea.

Rationale: Epidemics or sustained outbreaks of norovirus infection are a common and recurrent problem because norovirus is exceptionally contagious. The incubation period of norovirus infection is short (24-48 hours). Transmission occurs from person to person (via the fecal to oral route) and via aerosols, food, or contact with contaminated environmental surfaces. Infected patients shed astonishing quantities of viral particles. For example, diarrheal specimens from infected patients may contain up to 770 *trillion* viral particles per gram of stool. Because as few as 18 viral particles may produce infection in a healthy person, it is not surprising that outbreaks of infection with this virus are common.

Vomit from infected patients is also highly infectious. Individuals who are in the same room as a person vomiting due to norovirus infection are usually exposed to significant quantities of aerosolized norovirus particles. Norovirus particles can also be aerosolized from simply flushing a toilet. Once aerosolized, viral particles may contaminate surfaces and objects that can subsequently lead to transmission via hands or contact with inanimate objects (fomites).

To make matters worse, norovirus persists on environmental surfaces for prolonged periods. Such contamination is resistant to cleaning with common disinfectants (such as alcohol-containing gels or quaternary-ammonium–containing compounds; *see Chapter 6*).

Outbreaks of norovirus infection have occurred among athletes. For example, an outbreak of norovirus infections occurred in 1999 because of transmission *during* a football game between Duke University and Florida State University. The original source of the infection was deduced to be turkey sandwiches in box lunches served to members of the Duke team approximately 50 hours before the game. Fifty-four (50%) of 108 Duke team personnel became ill immediately before and during the game (43 were infected via contaminated food; the remainder developed secondary infections). Eleven Florida State players developed norovirus infections after the game. Transmission to these players was thought to have occurred during the game (via contact with jerseys of their opponents that had been soiled by vomit and/or feces). Aerosol transmission via retching and close direct contact during the game was also thought to have occurred. Molecular studies demonstrated the norovirus strain responsible for illness in both teams was identical.[53]

Similarly, 21 players and 3 team staff from 13 NBA teams developed gastroenteritis predominately due to norovirus infections from November 10 to December 20, 2010. Transmission between players on the same team occurred. Similarly, team-to-opposing team transmission occurred during at least two games.

Large outbreaks have occurred on cruise ships and college campuses, in nursing homes and hospitals, and among patrons of restaurants with food handlers who have norovirus infections.[54,55] In one case report, an outbreak was traced to an odd cause—a package of sealed packaged cookies, the outside of which became contaminated while stored in an open plastic grocery bag in a bathroom where an index case of norovirus had vomited.[56] While these settings are notable, the most probable source of transmission among athletes is through endemic spread from infected children or siblings. Adults with young children, particularly children in daycare settings, are most likely to be exposed to norovirus during endemic spread of the virus each winter.

⊘ **Recommendation 5** Refer players with severe or persistent diarrhea to team or primary care physicians for evaluation.

Rationale: Prompt notification and removal from team activities are key interventions to prevent an outbreak of diarrheal illness among players. *See Chapter 5 for additional strategies for prevention of diarrheal outbreaks.* A physician should promptly evaluate players with severe or persistent diarrhea. Signs of severe diarrhea may include fever >38.5°C, bloody diarrhea, profuse diarrhea leading to hypovolemia (six or more unformed stools in a 24-hour period), severe abdominal pain, or diarrhea in the setting of recent antibiotic use.[57,58] If a player has severe diarrhea or persistent (>72 hours) nonsevere diarrhea, we suggest performing a stool test for fecal leukocytes and routine stool culture. If the player has recently received antibiotic therapy, we suggest sending a test for *C. difficile* infection.

RESPIRATORY ILLNESS

From "colds" to "the flu," viral respiratory illnesses are common at all ages. Almost all viral respiratory illnesses are transmittable from one person to the next. In contrast, the majority of bacterial respiratory illnesses are not easily transmitted. An important exception that team medical personnel must recognize is "whooping cough" (caused by the bacterium *Bordatella pertussis*).

▶ **Best Practice** Develop a protocol for diagnosis and treatment of respiratory or influenza-like illness.

⊘ **Recommendation 1** Obtain diagnostic tests for influenza from players with influenza-like illness when typical symptoms of influenza occur during "flu season."

Rationale: Influenza is classically associated with the acute onset of fever, chills, muscle pains, headache, cough, loss of appetite, and generalized feelings of weakness. This pattern of illness is highly predictive of influenza in the setting of a documented outbreak or high community prevalence. However, these symptoms are **not** a reliable way to diagnose sporadic cases of influenza in the absence of an outbreak, as numerous other common viral pathogens can cause an illness indistinguishable from influenza. Also, the severity of influenza can vary substantially between individuals infected with the same strain of influenza, leading to a false assumption that a simple uncomplicated viral illness is present.

Testing provides two important benefits to overall team health. First, players may then be provided anti-influenza medications such as oseltamivir (Tamiflu) 75 mg two times per day by mouth for 5 days to decrease the duration of symptoms. Use of this medication for treatment of influenza may shorten the duration of symptoms by 1 to 2 days. A second treatment option, baloxavir (Xofluza) was approved by the FDA in 2018 for treatment of influenza; a single dose of 40 mg (if <80 kg) or 80 mg (if >80 kg) is given at the time of diagnosis. Second, knowledge that a player has influenza can allow medical staff to initiate a tiered response protocol *as described in Chapter 5*.

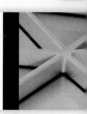

Tips and Advice: Diagnosis of Influenza-like Illness

Testing is best achieved by referring the player to the team physicians, as specific testing strategies may differ by site.

However, be sure polymerase chain reaction (PCR)-based molecular tests are used at the office to ensure more reliable results.

✓ **Recommendation 2** Use PCR-based molecular tests to diagnose influenza, not rapid antigen tests.

Rationale: Most influenza testing is completed through one of two methods: rapid antigen testing or molecular assays such as reverse transcriptase (RT)-PCR. Rapid antigen tests, which are commonly used in outpatient locations because they can be completed in the clinic within 15 minutes without specialized equipment, are, unfortunately, not sensitive or specific. Various studies have shown the sensitivity (which measures the ability to detect a case when it is present) ranges from 50% to 60%. The specificity of such tests in nonoutbreak settings is similarly low (averaging 53%-54%) in several large studies. In other words, these tests are actually not much better than a coin toss in determining that a patient does or does not have influenza. In contrast, RT-PCR assays are highly sensitive and specific. A recently published meta-analysis and systematic review of 162 studies concluded that pooled sensitivity of RT PCR testing for detecting influenza A was 92% compared to rapid antigen test sensitivity of 54%.[59]

✓ **Recommendation 3** Do not routinely obtain cultures for bacterial pathogens in players with influenza-like illness or the "common cold."

✓ **Recommendation 4** Do not routinely treat players with influenza-like illness or the "common cold" with antibiotics.

Rationale: Although the use of nasal cultures may identify a small subset of patients with bacterial infections (*Haemophilus influenzae*, *Moraxella catarrhalis*, or *Streptococcus pneumoniae*) who might respond to antimicrobials, the practice of routinely obtaining bacterial cultures in such patients is **not** recommended. Bacterial culture results take several days to return. More importantly, many, if not most, positive cultures in individuals with upper respiratory infection are due to coincidental colonization in persons with viral illnesses.

The potential benefit of nasal cultures was examined in a double-blind, placebo-controlled trial involving 314 patients who presented with common cold symptoms. Subjects were randomly assigned to 5 days of treatment with amoxicillin-clavulanate (375 mg, three times per day) or placebo.[60] Of 300 patients who had nasal aspirates performed, 72 had negative bacterial cultures, 167 had cultures that were positive only for bacteria not responsible for respiratory infections, and 61 had cultures positive for *H. influenzae*, *M. catarrhalis*, or *S. pneumoniae*. Antibiotic therapy benefited only those in the last group; the cure rate in this subset of patients increased from 4% (in placebo-treated patients) to 27%, and symptoms scores improved.

In summary, we **do not** recommend performing nasal cultures in any patient with symptoms suggestive of the common cold. Similarly, the vast majority of patients with acute sinusitis have viral illnesses that do not require cultures or antibiotic therapy even if they have copious purulent-appearing nasal or postnasal drainage.

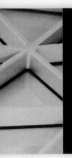

It is not necessary to culture nasal secretions in patients with the common cold for these reasons:

- The majority of cultures of nasal discharge taken from patients with colds are negative or reveal nonpathogenic bacteria.
- Results of cultures are not immediately available to guide treatment.
- A positive culture is not diagnostic of bacterial infection.
- The presence of yellow or green nasal secretions is common in many viral infections and is not a reliable way to determine if a bacterial infection is present.

⊘ Recommendation 5 Refer players with influenza-like illness and signs and symptoms of secondary bacterial infection to primary care or team physicians.

Rationale: Symptoms of acute rhinosinusitis and secondary bacterial infection include nasal congestion and obstruction, maxillary tooth discomfort, and facial pain or pressure that is worse when bending forward. Other signs and symptoms include fever, fatigue, cough, ear pressure or fullness, headache, and halitosis. Most secondary bacterial infections occur more than 10 days after onset of symptoms. Thus, if antibiotic therapy is used at all, it should typically be reserved for players with symptoms that persist **AND** worsen after 10 days.

▶ Best Practice Develop and use a standard protocol for diagnosis and treatment of pertussis ("whooping cough").

⊘ Recommendation 1 Diagnose pertussis with culture, PCR, or serology testing, depending on duration of symptoms.

Rationale: Pertussis, or "whooping cough," is highly contagious and can easily cause outbreaks in sports teams. For example, a high-school football team in Arkansas experienced an outbreak of pertussis involving 77 players, despite the fact that most players had received pertussis vaccination as children.[61]

See Chapter 1 for information regarding the three stages of pertussis: catarrhal, paroxysmal, and convalescent.

Diagnosing pertussis in adults requires a high index of suspicion. Early diagnosis is important as it can prevent the spread of infection, particularly in vulnerable populations (eg, infants and young children). In addition, antibiotic treatment may shorten the duration of symptoms. The clinical case definition advocated by the CDC and the World Health Organization (WHO) is a cough illness lasting 2 weeks with one of the following symptoms: paroxysms of coughing, inspiratory whoop, or posttussive emesis.[62,63]

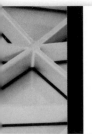

Confirmed cases of pertussis are defined as[64]:

- Patients with an acute cough illness of any duration and culture positive from nasopharyngeal secretions.
- Patients who meet the clinical case definition with laboratory confirmation by PCR from nasopharyngeal secretions.
- Patients who meet the clinical case definition and are epidemiologically linked to a case confirmed by either culture or PCR.

In the absence of an outbreak, the choice of diagnostic tests depends upon the duration of cough.[65-67] Perform both culture and PCR for patients with less than 4 weeks of cough. Both tests should be performed since the accuracy of PCR as a stand-alone diagnostic test is not well established. Perform serologic testing alone for patients with 4 weeks or more of cough.

Obtaining a specimen from the posterior nasopharynx is uncomfortable. Suboptimal specimen collection is common. In fact, proper specimen collection will typically induce cough or sneeze. The CDC has developed publicly available videos to guide clinicians with proper specimen collection (***https://www.cdc.gov/pertussis/clinical/diagnostic-testing/specimen-collection.html***).

⊘ **Recommendation 2** Use a calcium alginate or Dacron culture swab to diagnose pertussis.

Rationale: Cotton or rayon swabs contain fatty acids that are toxic to the organism that causes pertussis and should not be used. Calcium alginate swabs can be used for serology testing but not for PCR assays. Thus, Dacron swabs are optimal.

⊘ **Recommendation 3** Treat confirmed cases of pertussis with azithromycin.

Rationale: The treatment of choice for confirmed cases of pertussis is azithromycin 500 mg (day 1) followed by 250 mg each day for days 2 through 5 (ie, a "Z-pak").[68]

⊘ **Recommendation 4** Provide postexposure prophylaxis with azithromycin to players exposed to a confirmed case of pertussis.

Rationale: Players in close contact with another player with pertussis are at substantial increased risk of becoming infected. "Close contact" is defined as (1) face-to-face exposure within 3 feet of a symptomatic person, (2) direct contact with respiratory, oral, or nasal secretions from a symptomatic person, or (3) sharing the same confined space in close proximity with a symptomatic patient for ≥1 hour.[68] As with treatment of infection, treat personnel or players who have had "close contact" with a player infected with pertussis with azithromycin (500 mg on day 1 and 250 mg on days 2 through 5) for postexposure prophylaxis.

Initiation of postexposure prophylaxis within 21 days of exposure to the index case can prevent the development of symptoms in exposed asymptomatic contacts.

ATHLETE'S FOOT (TINEA PEDIS)

▶ **Best Practice** Diagnose and treat tenia pedis ("athlete's foot") to prevent bacterial skin infections.

⊘ **Recommendation 1** Diagnose tinea pedis using clinical signs and symptoms.

⊘ **Recommendation 2** Treat players with tinea pedis with topical or oral antifungal therapy.

Rationale: Tinea pedis in athletes is typically contracted through exposure to arthrospores shed on training facility floors by infected individuals. The majority of cases of tinea pedis are chronic. If untreated, infection may persist indefinitely.

Tinea pedis can be easily diagnosed by the presence of interdigital skin erythema, fissures, scaling, and/or pruritus (**Figure 4.2**). Treatment typically consists of a topical antifungal cream for 4 weeks.[69] Numerous antifungal creams are available for use; most are available over the counter. Treatment with allylamines like terbinafine leads to slightly higher cure rates than topical treatment with azole drugs such as itraconazole or fluconazole.[69] Players with extensive disease and/or players who have failed topical treatment may require oral therapy such as terbinafine 250 mg PO per day for 2 weeks, itraconazole 200 mg PO two times per day for 1 week, or fluconazole 150 mg PO one time weekly for 6 weeks.[70]

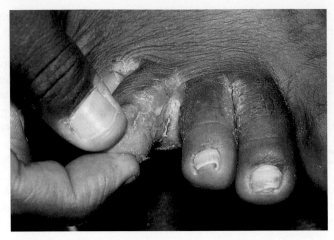

Figure 4.2 Athlete's foot (tinea pedis). (Reprinted with permission from Goodheart HP. *Goodheart's Photoguide of Common Skin Disorders*. 2nd ed. Philadelphia: Lippincott Williams & Wilkins; 2003.)

Treatment of tinea pedis is important for two reasons. First, it reduces the shedding and environmental burden of arthrospores that may in turn lead to infection in other players. Second, tinea pedis is a known and significant risk factor for primary and recurrent leg cellulitis,[71] particularly among individuals with high BMIs.[72] In general, players should wear shower shoes or sandals to avoid exposure to athrospores. Players known to have tinea pedis should wear shower shoes or sandals to reduce the risk of spread to other players.

Decrease Risk of Infection During Invasive Procedures

Athletes regularly require invasive procedures as part of treatment. The most common procedure in all of medical care—injections—is also the most common procedure for athletes. In some cases, athletes require surgical procedures. Any and every invasive procedure—from placing an IV to major surgery—includes some risk of infection. The information provided in this section is intended to help team medical personnel reduce the risk of infection associated with these invasive procedures.

SAFE INJECTION PRACTICES

▶ **Best Practice** Use safe injection practices at all times.

✓ **Recommendation 1** Medical staff must consistently and carefully utilize safe injection practices.

Rationale: Injections are used for the prevention, diagnosis, and treatment of various illnesses and are the most common interventions in health care. Unsafe injection practices put patients and healthcare providers at risk of infectious and noninfectious adverse events. Safe injection practices are part of Standard Precautions and are aimed at ensuring a basic level of safety for patients and providers.

Injections are the most common interventions in health care.

Safe injection practices must be used during all activities in which an athlete's skin is penetrated with a needle. Therefore, these practices are important for procedures other than injection, including joint aspiration with or without injection of corticosteroids, placement of

IVs, the use of insulin syringes, and the use of glucometers. Safe injection practices are particularly important in ambulatory care and in the sports medicine setting, given the high volume of procedures performed.

Adherence to safe injection practices can effectively prevent the transmission of viral pathogens such as hepatitis B virus (HBV), hepatitis C virus (HCV), and HIV and bacteria such as *S. aureus*. Thus, all healthcare providers must be familiar with safe injection techniques. In fact, many institutions mandate annual certification regarding safe injection practices to ensure competency and knowledge base.

Failure to adhere to safe injection practices has led to well-publicized outbreaks, patient suffering, severe legal ramifications, and even imprisonment. More than 150,000 patients in the United States have been potentially exposed to bloodborne pathogens such as HBV, HCV, and HIV due to unsafe injection practices. For example, the CDC investigated an endoscopy clinic in southern Nevada in 2007 and discovered that up to 63,000 patients were potentially exposed to HBV, HCV, and HIV due to unsafe injection practices. A total of 115 patients contracted hepatitis C as a result of clinic staff reusing syringes to draw up medications from single-use vials for use among multiple patients. As a result, the clinic closed, and the medical providers were stripped of their licenses and sentenced to life-in-prison due to gross negligence.[73]

In 2009, the CDC published a review of outbreaks of hepatitis that occurred from 1998 to 2008 in outpatient settings such as doctor's offices, outpatient clinics, dialysis centers, and nursing homes. The review identified 33 hepatitis outbreaks resulting from deficient safe injection practices such as reuse of syringes and use of single vial medications for multiple patients.[74]

These outbreaks related to unsafe injection practices indicate that some healthcare personnel are unaware of, do not understand, or do not adhere to basic principles of infection prevention and aseptic technique. A survey of US healthcare workers who provide medication through injection found that 1% to 3% reused the same needle and/or syringe on multiple patients.[75] Specific deficiencies identified in recent outbreaks included a lack of oversight of personnel and failure to follow up on reported breaches in infection prevention practices in ambulatory settings. Therefore, principles of infection prevention and aseptic technique need to be reinforced and incorporated into institutional polices that are monitored for adherence to ensure that all healthcare personnel understand and adhere to recommended practices.

✅ **Recommendation 2** Use aseptic technique to avoid contamination of sterile injection equipment.

✅ **Recommendation 3** Do not administer medications from a syringe to multiple players, even if the needle or cannula on the syringe is changed.

✅ **Recommendation 4** Use fluid infusion and administration sets (ie, intravenous bags, tubing, and connectors) for one player only and dispose appropriately after use.

✅ **Recommendation 5** Open the packaging of sterile needles/cannulas/syringes immediately before use (not ahead of time).

✅ **Recommendation 6** Dispose of needles in a sharps container.

✅ **Recommendation 7** Store vials in accordance with the manufacturer's recommendations. Discard if sterility is compromised or questionable.

✅ **Recommendation 8** Place signage in your medical treatment rooms to remind clinicians: "one needle, one syringe, one vial, one time."

Never reuse needles, cannulas, or syringes.

Rationale: Aseptic technique reduces the risk of contamination of sterile injection equipment.[75,76] Needles, cannulas, and syringes are sterile, single-use items; they **MUST NEVER** be reused for another patient or to access a medication or solution that might be used for a subsequent patient. In other words, consider a syringe or needle/cannula contaminated once it has been used to enter or connect to a patient's intravenous infusion bag or administration set.

The best illustration of the dangers of the above practice can be seen in the 2008 southern Nevada outbreak of hepatitis C that was traced to an endoscopy clinic. In that outbreak, an anesthetist was directly observed reusing syringes and medication vials. After administering propofol to one patient, the needle was changed, but the same syringe was used to access the same vial of propofol. These open vials were also used on subsequent patients. These inappropriate practices led to the transmission of HCV and the notification of ~63,000 persons (the largest ever in US history) by public health officials.[73]

Most state health agencies require specific disposal of sharps and biohazardous waste. Thus, we recommend contracting with a professional company to dispose of sharps containers in order to ensure biohazardous materials are disposed of properly. This approach also reduces the risk of needle sticks among athletic training staff. Finally, ensure that sharps containers are available in all areas where needles are used.

▶ **Best Practice** Do not use multiuse or multidose medication vials.

✓ **Recommendation 1** Use single-use vials for all injections and discard after use.

✓ **Recommendation 2** Do not administer medications from single-dose vials or ampules to multiple players or combine leftover contents for later use.

Rationale: Safe injection practices can be summarized by the phrase **"One Needle, One Syringe, Only One Time."** This approach is endorsed by the CDC and professional societies and has led to the "One and Only Campaign." This campaign and website (***http://www. oneandonlycampaign.com***) provide useful information and resources to patients and providers that promote safe injection practices.[77] In fact, when providers deviate from these safe practices, patients are placed at risk of infections and adverse outcomes. Since 2007, at least 19 outbreaks have been tied to the misuse of single use medications (7 involving bloodborne pathogens and 12 others involved bacterial infections).[75] *Posters to promote "One Needle, One Syringe, Only One Time" are provided in the e-book version of this book.*

✓ **Recommendation 3** Do not keep multidose vials in the immediate player treatment area.

✓ **Recommendation 4** If the medication (eg, lidocaine) is only available in multidose vials, use the vial as a single-dose vial and discard even if it contains residual medication.

✓ **Recommendation 5** Never use bags or bottles of intravenous solution as a common source of supply for multiple patients.

✓ **Recommendation 6** Discard vials immediately after use or prior to manufacturer's expiration date.

Rationale: Bags of saline and other intravenous solutions frequently become contaminated when needles and syringes are used to obtain fluid for irrigation or flushing of IV lines. Such unsafe practices have led to transmission of bloodborne pathogens. For example, this practice led to the transmission of HCV to 89 patients in a hematology/oncology clinic in Nebraska. A nurse was observed reusing disposable syringes to withdraw saline from common 500 mL bags. Saline for a single IV bag was subsequently used to flush IV lines or heparin locks in up to 25 to 50 patients per day. Patients affected by this outbreak even reported seeing blood in the saline bags. The state of Nebraska revoked the professional licenses of the oncologist and the nurses who were involved in this outbreak. Patients also filed litigation claims against the medical professional, the nurse, and the hospital involved in this outbreak.[78]

Regulations banning the use of multidose vials do not exist. Ideally, multidose vials should be dedicated for use in an individual patient. Multidose vials can, however, be used to provide doses to multiple patients. The correct use of these vials requires the multidose vial can only be accessed in a **dedicated medication preparation area**, away from immediate patient treatment areas.[64] In our experience, no training facility has a dedicated medication preparation area; thus, all multidose vials should be used as single-dose vials and discarded after use.

All vials used for injections must be stored in specific conditions recommended by the manufacturer of the vial (eg, 40°F refrigerator). Any vials that are discovered to be "left out" of their normal storage location should be immediately discarded. Similarly, vials should be discarded if there are any questions or concerns regarding their sterility or prior use.

PREVENT SURGICAL SITE INFECTIONS

▶ **Best Practice** Adhere to standard and widely accepted guidelines for the prevention of surgical site infections (SSIs).

✓ **Recommendation 1** Provide guidelines and evidence-based practices to reduce the risk of SSI to team or personal orthopedic surgeons.

Rationale: Injuries are common and often unavoidable for athletes. Some of the serious injuries that occur during practices and games require surgical intervention. The majority of surgical procedures performed on athletes are orthopedic. Most surgical procedures have low risks of postoperative infection (eg, arthroscopic knee surgery, ligament repair, or tendon repairs). Despite these low risks, postoperative SSIs may occur in a small proportion of players, particularly when metal or hardware is implanted. Indeed, SSIs in several high-profile athletes have resulted in adverse consequences for individual players and their teams. Occasionally, postoperative infections can end careers.

On average, 1% to 3% of surgical procedures performed in the United States result in an SSI. These SSIs range in severity from nuisance infections that require little intervention to devastating invasive infections that require admission to the hospital, IV antibiotics, and a return to the operating room. In the general population, orthopedic procedures have lower risk of SSI compared with other major procedure categories. For example, the rate of *S. aureus* SSI following orthopedic procedures in a study of more than 90,000 procedures was 0.27%.[79] Nevertheless, when one SSI occurs, a player's playing status is jeopardized and, in some cases, his or her career may be adversely affected.

Four societies have published guidelines for prevention of SSI. We summarize and emphasize several of the most important interventions below and include a recommendation based on the high prevalence of MRSA colonization among athletes as previously described.

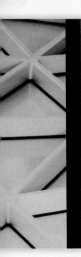

Guidelines to prevent SSI have recently been published by four major societies: the World Health Organization (WHO), the American College of Surgeons (ACS)/Surgical Infection Society (SIS), the Infectious Disease Society of America (IDSA)/Society for Healthcare Epidemiology of America (SHEA), and the Healthcare Infection Control Practices Advisory Committee (HICPAC) of the CDC.

These guidelines can all be viewed and accessed online:

1. **HICPAC/CDC** (https://jamanetwork.com/journals/jamasurgery/fullarticle/2623725)—Centers for Disease Control and Prevention Guideline for the Prevention of SSI, 2017.
2. **WHO** (http://www.who.int/gpsc/ssi-prevention-guidelines/en/)—Global guidelines on the prevention of surgical site infection, published in 2016.
3. **ACS/SIS** (http://online.liebertpub.com/doi/10.1089/sur.2016.214)—Surgical Site Infection Guidelines, 2016 Update.
4. **SHEA/IDSA** (http://www.jstor.org/stable/10.1086/676022)—Strategies to Prevent Surgical Site Infection in Acute Care Hospitals: 2014 Update.

✅ Recommendation 2 Adjust dosing of perioperative antimicrobial prophylaxis based on the player's weight.

Rationale: Antimicrobial prophylaxis is a fundamental strategy for the prevention of SSI.[80] Dosing of many antibiotics used for preoperative prophylaxis, including cefazolin, the most commonly used antibiotic for antimicrobial prophylaxis, needs to be adjusted based on weight.

Cefazolin should be dosed as follows:

- Players who weigh less than 120 kg (260 pounds), should receive 2 g cefazolin within 60 minutes prior to surgical incision.
- Players who weigh more than 120 kg (260 pounds), should receive 3 g cefazolin within 60 minutes prior to surgical incision.

✅ Recommendation 3 Control blood glucose (<180 mg/dL) during the immediate postoperative period.

Rationale: Many athletes are at high risk of metabolic syndrome, diabetes mellitus, and postoperative increases in blood glucose due to body size. High blood glucose increases the risk of SSI by two- to fourfold.[81,82] Importantly, blood glucose can rise in the postoperative period even if a player does not have diabetes. As a result, all patients undergoing major surgical procedures should have their plasma glucose closely monitored in the immediate postoperative period.

✅ Recommendation 4 Use CHG- and alcohol-containing skin preps in the operating room.

Rationale: All surgical skin preps should include alcohol. Persistent and cumulative antisepsis is improved by combining alcohol with CHG or povidone-iodine. We believe CHG has advantages over povidone-iodine in the absence of alcohol for three reasons. First, CHG has a longer duration of residual antibacterial activity on the skin. Second, CHG has superior antibacterial effects in the presence of blood or serum. Third, CHG does not require complete drying to produce an antibacterial effect, unlike povidone-iodine.[33,83] In fact, randomized controlled trials[84] and systematic reviews conclude that CHG is superior to povidone-iodine for preoperative skin antisepsis.[85]

✅ Recommendation 5 Perform *S. aureus* decolonization for all players undergoing an elective surgical procedure.

Rationale: As previously discussed, athletes are at higher risk of colonization with *S. aureus* than the general population. Colonization with *S. aureus* (either MSSA or MRSA) is a risk factor for SSI. As a result, we believe specific interventions to reduce this risk should be employed for athletes undergoing elective procedures.

Three potential strategies could be used to address this risk: (1) screen players for colonization and perform decolonization among patients with positive screening cultures, (2) provide vancomycin as antimicrobial prophylaxis for all players undergoing a procedure, or (3) provide decolonization for all players (and do not screen). Screening is an imperfect approach, as up to 25% of patients with MRSA colonization may be missed because of colonization outside of the nares. If a screening strategy is employed, ensure that the player is screened for both MRSA and MSSA. Widespread use of vancomycin is not advised, as it may lead to adverse drug events and resistance. Instead, vancomycin should only be used for players with known MRSA colonization or a history of infection. No studies have compared the effectiveness of these strategies, but we advise the use of decolonization for any player undergoing a surgical procedure, regardless of screening status. In fact, we believe this approach would obviate the need for screening.

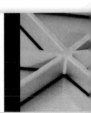

Decolonization can be achieved through this simple regimen:
- Apply mupirocin ointment to both nares two times each day for 5 days.
- Bathe with CHG each day using Hibiclens (4% CHG) as soap in the shower for up to 5 days. If the procedure is scheduled to occur within 5 days, then continue the use of CHG after the procedure.

✓ **Recommendation 6** For players who are known to be colonized with MRSA, add vancomycin to cefazolin for perioperative antimicrobial prophylaxis.

Rationale: Players colonized with MRSA are at increased risk of subsequent MRSA infection if they undergo surgical procedures.[86] Cefazolin does not have activity against MRSA. Although vancomycin has activity against MRSA, unlike cefazolin, it does not provide coverage for important gram-negative pathogens such as *Escherichia coli* (the fourth most common cause of SSI).[87] In addition, vancomycin has less activity than cefazolin against MSSA, now the most common cause of SSI.[88,89] Thus, we recommend **adding** vancomycin to cefazolin for preoperative prophylaxis in players known to be colonized with MRSA in order to ensure that the perioperative prophylaxis regimen has activity against both MRSA and important gram-negative bacteria. Vancomycin should be dosed as 15 mg/kg and administered within 2 hours prior to surgical incision.[80]

REFERENCES

1. Weiser TG, Haynes AB, Dziekan G, et al. Effect of a 19-item surgical safety checklist during urgent operations in a global patient population. *Ann Surg.* 2010;251(5):976-980.

2. Shekelle PG, Wachter RM, Pronovost PJ, et al. Making health care safer II: an updated critical analysis of the evidence for patient safety practices. *Evid Rep Technol Assess (Full Rep).* 2013;(211):1-945.

3. Septimus E, Yokoe DS, Weinstein RA, Perl TM, Maragakis LL, Berenholtz SM. Maintaining the momentum of change: the role of the 2014 updates

to the compendium in preventing healthcare-associated infections. *Infect Control Hosp Epidemiol.* 2014;35(5):460-463.

4. Pronovost P, Needham D, Berenholtz S, et al. An intervention to decrease catheter-related bloodstream infections in the ICU. *N Engl J Med.* 2006;355(26):2725-2732.

5. Wick EC, Hobson DB, Bennett JL, et al. Implementation of a surgical comprehensive unit-based safety program to reduce surgical site infections. *J Am Coll Surg.* 2012;215(2):193-200.

6. Mittal V, Hall M, Morse R, et al. Impact of Inpatient Bronchiolitis Clinical Practice Guideline Implementation on Testing and Treatment. *J Pediatr.* 2014;165(3):570-576.e3.

7. Kahanov L, Gilmore EJ, Eberman LE, Roberts J, Semerjian T, Baldwin L. Certified athletic trainers' knowledge of methicillin-resistant *Staphylococcus aureus* and common disinfectants. *J Athl Train.* 2011;46(4):415-423.

8. Boyce JM, Pittet D. Guideline for hand hygiene in health-care settings. Recommendations of the Healthcare Infection Control Practices Advisory Committee and the HICPAC/SHEA/APIC/IDSA Hand Hygiene Task Force. Society for Healthcare Epidemiology of America/Association for Professionals in Infection Control/Infectious Diseases Society of America. *MMWR Recomm Rep.* 2002;51(RR-16):1-45, quiz CE41-44.

9. Thomas Y, Boquete-Suter P, Koch D, Pittet D, Kaiser L. Survival of influenza virus on human fingers. *Clin Microbiol Infect.* 2014;20(1):O58-O64.

10. Pittet D, Allegranzi B, Sax H, et al. Evidence-based model for hand transmission during patient care and the role of improved practices. *Lancet Infect Dis.* 2006;6(10):641-652.

11. Allegranzi B, Pittet D. Role of hand hygiene in healthcare-associated infection prevention. *J Hosp Infect.* 2009;73(4):305-315.

12. WHO guidelines on hand hygiene in health care. 2009. http://whqlibdoc.who.int/publications/2009/9789241597906_eng.pdf. Accessed July 1, 2019.

13. Picheansathian W. A systematic review on the effectiveness of alcohol-based solutions for hand hygiene. *Int J Nurs Pract.* 2004;10(1):3-9.

14. Aiello AE, Larson EL, Levy SB. Consumer antibacterial soaps: effective or just risky? *Clin Infect Dis.* 2007;45 suppl 2:S137-S147.

15. Hwang J, Suh SS, Chang M, et al. Effects of triclosan on reproductive prarmeters and embryonic development of sea urchin, *Strongylocentrotus nudus. Ecotoxicol Environ Saf.* 2014;100:148-152.

16. Crofton KM, Paul KB, Devito MJ, Hedge JM. Short-term in vivo exposure to the water contaminant triclosan: evidence for disruption of thyroxine. *Environ Toxicol Pharmacol.* 2007;24(2):194-197.

17. FDA issues proposed rule to determine safety and effectiveness of antibacterial soaps. 2013. http://www.fda.gov/NewsEvents/Newsroom/PressAnnouncements/ucm378542.htm. Accessed March 1, 2019.

18. Karanika S, Kinamon T, Grigoras C, Mylonakis E. Colonization With Methicillin-resistant *Staphylococcus aureus* and Risk for Infection Among Asymptomatic Athletes: A Systematic Review and Metaanalysis. *Clin Infect Dis.* 2016;63(2):195-204.

19. Kuehnert MJ, Kruszon-Moran D, Hill HA, et al. Prevalence of *Staphylococcus aureus* nasal colonization in the United States, 2001-2002. *J Infect Dis.* 2006;193(2):172-179.

20. Salgado CD, Farr BM, Calfee DP. Community-acquired methicillin-resistant *Staphylococcus aureus:* a meta-analysis of prevalence and risk factors. *Clin Infect Dis.* 2003;36(2):131-139.

21. Creech CB, Saye E, McKenna BD, et al. One-year surveillance of methicillin-resistant *Staphylococcus aureus* nasal colonization and skin and soft tissue infections in collegiate athletes. *Arch Pediatr Adolesc Med.* 2010;164(7):615-620.

22. Oller AR, Province L, Curless B. *Staphylococcus aureus* recovery from environmental and human locations in 2 collegiate athletic teams. *J Athl Train.* 2010;45(3):222-229.

23. Nguyen DM, Mascola L, Brancoft E. Recurring methicillin-resistant *Staphylococcus aureus* infections in a football team. *Emerg Infect Dis.* 2005;11(4):526-532.

24. Huang SS, Septimus E, Kleinman K, et al. Targeted versus universal decolonization to prevent ICU infection. *N Engl J Med.* 2013;368(24):2255-2265.

25. Whitman TJ, Schlett CD, Grandits GA, et al. Chlorhexidine gluconate reduces transmission of methicillin-resistant *Staphylococcus aureus* USA300 among Marine recruits. *Infect Control Hosp Epidemiol.* 2012;33(8):809-816.

26. Morrison SM, Blaesing CR, Millar EV, et al. Evaluation of methicillin-resistant *Staphylococcus aureus* skin and soft-tissue infection prevention strategies at a military training center. *Infect Control Hosp Epidemiol.* 2013;34(8):841-843.

27. Fritz SA, Camins BC, Eisenstein KA, et al. Effectiveness of measures to eradicate *Staphylococcus aureus* carriage in patients with community-associated skin and soft-tissue infections: a randomized trial. *Infect Control Hosp Epidemiol.* 2011;32(9):872-880.

28. Ryan C, Shaw RE, Cockerell CJ, Hand S, Ghali FE. Novel sodium hypochlorite cleanser shows clinical response and excellent acceptability in the treatment of atopic dermatitis. *Pediatr Dermatol.* 2013;30(3):308-315.

29. Paulson DS, Topp R, Boykin RE, Schultz G, Yang Q. Efficacy and safety of a novel skin cleansing formulation versus chlorhexidine gluconate. *Am J Infect Control.* 2018;46(11):1262-1265.

30. Tenorio AR, Badri SM, Sahgal NB, et al. Effectiveness of gloves in the prevention of hand carriage of vancomycin-resistant enterococcus species by health care workers after patient care. *Clin Infect Dis.* 2001;32(5):826-829.

31. McDonnell G, Russell AD. Antiseptics and disinfectants: activity, action, and resistance. *Clin Microbiol Rev.* 1999;12(1):147-179.

32. Cookson BD, Bolton MC, Platt JH. Chlorhexidine resistance in methicillin-resistant *Staphylococcus aureus* or just an elevated MIC? An in vitro and in vivo assessment. *Antimicrob Agents Chemother.* 1991;35(10):1997-2002.

33. Larson E. Guideline for use of topical antimicrobial agents. *Am J Infect Control.* 1988;16(6):253-266.

34. Moran GJ, Krishnadasan A, Gorwitz RJ, et al. Methicillin-resistant *S. aureus* infections among patients in the emergency department. *N Engl J Med.* 2006;355(7):666-674.

35. Soto NE, Vaghjimal A, Stahl-Avicolli A, Protic JR, Lutwick LI, Chapnick EK. Bacitracin versus mupirocin for *Staphylococcus aureus* nasal colonization. *Infect Control Hosp Epidemiol.* 1999;20(5): 351-353.

36. Banerjee J, Das Ghatak P, Roy S, et al. Silver-zinc redox-coupled electroceutical wound dressing disrupts bacterial biofilm. *PLoS one.* 2015;10(3):e0119531.

37. Ghatak PD, Schlanger R, Ganesh K, et al. A wireless electroceutical dressing lowers cost of negative pressure wound therapy. *Adv Wound Care (New Rochelle).* 2015;4(5):302-311.

38. Begier EM, Frenette K, Barrett NL, et al. A high-morbidity outbreak of methicillin-resistant *Staphylococcus aureus* among players on a college football team, facilitated by cosmetic body shaving and turf burns. *Clin Infect Dis.* 2004;39(10):1446-1453.

39. Sehulster L, Chinn RY. Guidelines for environmental infection control in health-care facilities. Recommendations of CDC and the Healthcare Infection Control Practices Advisory Committee (HICPAC). *MMWR Recomm Rep* 2003;52(RR-10):1-42.

40. The Model Aquatic Health Code - The Code - Release for Final Public Comment. 2014. http://www.cdc.gov/healthywater/pdf/swimming/pools/mahc/mahc-complete-draft-CODE-for-2nd-round-of-comments.pdf. Accessed July 30, 2014.

41. Centers for Disease Control and Prevention. Microbes in pool filter backwash as evidence of the need for improved swimmer hygiene - metro-Atlanta, Georgia, 2012. *MMWR Morb Mortal Wkly Rep.* 2013;62(19):385-388.

42. Centers for Disease Control and Prevention. Methicillin-resistant *Staphylococcus aureus* among players on a high school football team–New York City, 2007. *MMWR Morb Mortal Wkly Rep.* 2009;58(3):52-55.

43. Stevens DL, Bisno AL, Chambers HF, et al. Practice guidelines for the diagnosis and management of skin and soft tissue infections: 2014 update by the Infectious Diseases Society of America. *Clin Infect Dis.* 2014;59(2):e10-e52.

44. Frank JE. Diagnosis and management of G6PD deficiency. *Am Fam Physician.* 2005;72(7):1277-1282.

45. Miller LG, Daum RS, Creech CB, et al. Clindamycin versus trimethoprim-sulfamethoxazole for uncomplicated skin infections. *N Engl J Med.* 2015;372(12):1093-1103.

46. Ruhe JJ, Smith N, Bradsher RW, Menon A. Community-onset methicillin-resistant *Staphylococcus aureus* skin and soft-tissue infections: impact of antimicrobial therapy on outcome. *Clin Infect Dis.* 2007;44(6):777-784.

47. Talan DA, Mower WR, Krishnadasan A, et al. Trimethoprim-sulfamethoxazole versus placebo for uncomplicated skin abscess. *N Engl J Med.* 2016;374(9):823-832.

48. Daum RS, Miller LG, Immergluck L, et al. A placebo-controlled trial of antibiotics for smaller skin abscesses. *N Engl J Med.* 2017;376(26):2545-2555.

49. Anderson BJ. Managing herpes gladiatorum outbreaks in competitive wrestling: the 2007 Minnesota experience. *Curr Sports Med Rep.* 2008;7(6):323-327.

50. Zinder SM, Basler RS, Foley J, Scarlata C, Vasily DB. National athletic trainers' association position statement: skin diseases. *J Athl Train.* 2010;45(4):411-428.

51. Three more schools infected by 'unprecedented' hand-foot-and-mouth disease outbreak. 2016. http://highschoolsports.nj.com/news/article/-3132375131977714380/unprecedented-hand-foot-and-mouth-disease-outbreak-reported-at-shore-conference-school/. Accessed June 1, 2019.

52. Jones TF, Bulens SN, Gettner S, et al. Use of stool collection kits delivered to patients can improve confirmation of etiology in foodborne disease outbreaks. *Clin Infect Dis.* 2004;39(10):1454-1459.

53. Becker KM, Moe CL, Southwick KL, MacCormack JN. Transmission of Norwalk virus during football game. *N Engl J Med.* 2000;343(17):1223-1227.

54. Wikswo ME, Cortes J, Hall AJ, et al. Disease transmission and passenger behaviors during a high morbidity Norovirus outbreak on a cruise ship, January 2009. *Clin Infect Dis.* 2011;52(9):1116-1122.

55. Centers for Disease Control and Prevention. Norovirus outbreaks on three college campuses - California, Michigan, and Wisconsin, 2008. *MMWR Morb Mortal Wkly Rep.* 2009;58(39):1095-1100.

56. Repp KK, Keene WE. A point-source norovirus outbreak caused by exposure to fomites. *J Infect Dis.* 2012;205(11):1639-1641.

57. DuPont HL. Guidelines on acute infectious diarrhea in adults. The Practice Parameters Committee of the American College of Gastroenterology. *Am J Gastroenterol.* 1997;92(11):1962-1975.

58. Guerrant RL, Van Gilder T, Steiner TS, et al. Practice guidelines for the management of infectious diarrhea. *Clin Infect Dis.* 2001;32(3):331-351.

59. Merckx J, Wali R, Schiller I, et al. Diagnostic accuracy of novel and traditional rapid tests for influenza infection compared with reverse transcriptase polymerase chain reaction: a systematic review and meta-analysis. *Ann Intern Med.* 2017;167(6):394-409.

60. Kaiser L, Lew D, Hirschel B, et al. Effects of antibiotic treatment in the subset of common-cold patients who have bacteria in nasopharyngeal secretions. *Lancet.* 1996;347(9014):1507-1510.

61. Centers for Disease Control and Prevention. Updated recommendations for use of tetanus toxoid, reduced diphtheria toxoid and acellular pertussis vaccine (Tdap) in pregnant women and persons

who have or anticipate having close contact with an infant aged <12 months – Advisory Committee on Immunization Practices (ACIP), 2011. *MMWR Morb Mortal Wkly Rep*. 2011;60(41):1424-1426.

62. Immunization Surveillance, Assessment, and Monitoring. 2014. http://www.who.int/immunization/monitoring_surveillance/en/. Accessed May 23, 2014.

63. Pertussis (Whooping Cough) – Surveillance & Reporting. 2014. http://www.cdc.gov/pertussis/surv-reporting.html. Accessed June 3, 2014.

64. Centers for Disease Control and Prevention. Questions about multi-dose vials. 2019. https://www.cdc.gov/injectionsafety/providers/provider_faqs_multivials.html. Accessed August 22, 2019.

65. Pertussis (Whooping Cough) – Diagnosis Confirmation. 2013. http://www.cdc.gov/pertussis/clinical/diagnostic-testing/diagnosis-confirmation.html. Accessed May 1, 2014.

66. Hewlett EL, Edwards KM. Clinical practice. Pertussis–not just for kids. *N Engl J Med*. 2005;352(12):1215-1222.

67. von Konig CH, Halperin S, Riffelmann M, Guiso N. Pertussis of adults and infants. *Lancet Infect Dis*. 2002;2(12):744-750.

68. Tiwari T, Murphy TV, Moran J. Recommended antimicrobial agents for the treatment and postexposure prophylaxis of pertussis: 2005 CDC guidelines. *MMWR Recomm Rep*. 2005;54(RR-14):1-16.

69. Crawford F, Hollis S. Topical treatments for fungal infections of the skin and nails of the foot. *Cochrane Database Syst Rev*. 2007;(3):CD001434.

70. Gupta AK, Cooper EA. Update in antifungal therapy of dermatophytosis. *Mycopathologia*. 2008;166(5-6):353-367.

71. Bisno AL, Stevens DL. Streptococcal infections of skin and soft tissues. *N Engl J Med*. 1996;334(4):240-245.

72. McNamara DR, Tleyjeh IM, Berbari EF, et al. A predictive model of recurrent lower extremity cellulitis in a population-based cohort. *Arch Intern Med*. 2007;167(7):709-715.

73. Fischer GE, Schaefer MK, Labus BJ, et al. Hepatitis C virus infections from unsafe injection practices at an endoscopy clinic in Las Vegas, Nevada, 2007-2008. *Clin Infect Dis*. 2010;51(3):267-273.

74. Thompson ND, Perz JF, Moorman AC, Holmberg SD. Nonhospital health care-associated hepatitis B and C virus transmission: United States, 1998-2008. *Ann Intern Med*. 2009;150(1):33-39.

75. Centers for Disease Control and Prevention. *Protect Patients Against Preventable Harm from Improper Use of Single–Dose/Single–Use Vials*; 2012. http://www.cdc.gov/injectionsafety/CDCposition-SingleUseVial.html. Accessed July 30, 2014.

76. Archer W. Methicillin-susceptible *Staphylococcus aureus* infections after intra-articular injections. 47th Annual Meeting of Infectious Diseases Society of America; October 29-November 1, 2009, 2009; Philadelphia, PA.

77. OneandOnlyCampaign.Org. One and Only Campaign. 2014. http://www.oneandonlycampaign.org/.

78. Macedo de Oliveira A, White KL, Leschinsky DP, et al. An outbreak of hepatitis C virus infections among outpatients at a hematology/oncology clinic. *Ann Intern Med*. 2005;142(11):898-902.

79. Anderson DJ, Arduino JM, Reed SD, et al. Variation in the type and frequency of postoperative invasive *Staphylococcus aureus* infections according to type of surgical procedure. *Infect Control Hosp Epidemiol*. 2010;31(7):701-709.

80. Bratzler DW, Dellinger EP, Olsen KM, et al. Clinical practice guidelines for antimicrobial prophylaxis in surgery. *Am J Health Syst Pharm*. 2013;70(3):195-283.

81. Dronge AS, Perkal MF, Kancir S, Concato J, Aslan M, Rosenthal RA. Long-term glycemic control and postoperative infectious complications. *Arch Surg*. 2006;141(4):375-380; discussion 380.

82. Olsen MA, Nepple JJ, Riew KD, et al. Risk factors for surgical site infection following orthopaedic spinal operations. *J Bone Joint Surg Am*. 2008;90(1):62-69.

83. Aly R, Maibach HI. Comparative antibacterial efficacy of a 2-minute surgical scrub with chlorhexidine gluconate, povidone-iodine, and chloroxylenol sponge-brushes. *Am J Infect Control*. 1988;16(4):173-177.

84. Tuuli MG, Liu J, Stout MJ, et al. A randomized trial comparing skin antiseptic agents at cesarean delivery. *N Engl J Med*. 2016;374(7):647-655.

85. Dumville JC, McFarlane E, Edwards P, Lipp A, Holmes A, Liu Z. Preoperative skin antiseptics for preventing surgical wound infections after clean surgery. *Cochrane Database Syst Rev*. 2015;(4):CD003949.

86. Perl TM, Cullen JJ, Wenzel RP, et al. Intranasal mupirocin to prevent postoperative *Staphylococcus aureus* infections. *N Engl J Med*. 2002;346(24):1871-1877.

87. Anderson DJ, Sexton DJ, Kanafani ZA, Auten G, Kaye KS. Severe surgical site infection in community hospitals: epidemiology, key procedures, and the changing prevalence of methicillin-resistant *Staphylococcus aureus*. *Infect Control Hosp Epidemiol*. 2007;28(9):1047-1053.

88. Berrios-Torres SI, Yi SH, Bratzler DW, et al. Activity of commonly used antimicrobial prophylaxis regimens against pathogens causing coronary artery bypass graft and arthroplasty surgical site infections in the United States, 2006-2009. *Infect Control Hosp Epidemiol*. 2014;35(3):231-239.

89. Bull AL, Worth LJ, Richards MJ. Impact of vancomycin surgical antibiotic prophylaxis on the development of methicillin-sensitive *Staphylococcus aureus* surgical site infections: report from Australian Surveillance Data (VICNISS). *Ann Surg*. 2012;256(6):1089-1092.

5

Reducing Transmission of Pathogens Between Athletes

Samuel Hume | Daniel J. Sexton

Introduction

Multiple athletes in close quarters is a key risk factor for transmission of pathogens. Simply put, more close interactions with other athletes lead to more movement of pathogens such as bacteria and viruses. These pathogens can be transmitted directly from one player to another in close quarters such as a locker room or training facility. However, transmission through direct contact is not the only way that pathogens can spread (**Table 5.1**). Pathogens can move from player to player through a contaminated environment, droplets in the air after a cough or sneeze, contaminated food, or, rarely, through exposure to blood.

Various interventions to decrease the risk of transmission and the risk of infection are outlined throughout this book. In this chapter, we first outline key concepts on pathogen transmission among athletes. We then summarize general principles to prevent transmission. Some of these principles should sound familiar by this point. As this chapter focuses specifically on reducing transmission of pathogens between athletes, we emphasize the importance of vaccination strategies and outbreak mitigation.

Concepts of Microbial Spread

Microbes may be transmitted in numerous ways that are particular to the type of organism (**Figure 5.1**). Each method of transmission requires different prevention strategies.

Direct and Indirect Contact

Common bacteria such as staphylococci (including methicillin-resistant *Staphylococcus aureus* [MRSA]) and respiratory viruses such as influenza primarily are transmitted between persons through either direct contact such as when shaking hands, grappling, or tackling or indirectly through contamination of environmental surfaces and objects such as shared gym equipment. In order for pathogens to spread via environmental surfaces,

Table 5.1 Transmission of Pathogens Between Athletes

Mode of Transmission	Pathogens	Examples of Transmission	Methods of Prevention
Contact—direct	• **Staphylococcus aureus (including MRSA)** • Group A streptococci • **Influenza** • **Respiratory viruses and the "common cold"** • Herpes simplex • Tinea (Tinea capitis, T. corporis, T. pedis) • Pubic lice (pediculosis pubis) • Norovirus • Molluscum contagiosum • Warts (human papillomavirus) • Scabies (Sarcoptes scabiei)	• Hand shaking • Direct player contact on field	• Hand hygiene • Showering after practice
Contact—indirect (via fomites/ environment)	• **S. aureus** (including MRSA) • **Norovirus** • **Influenza**	• Sharing towels • Gym equipment • Shared razors	• Minimize shared items • Disinfect equipment between users
Droplet	• **Influenza** • Mumps • **Respiratory viruses and the "common cold"** • Whooping cough (pertussis) • Neisseria meningitis • Group A streptococci	• Sitting next to a symptomatic player on a team bus or flight	• Vaccination • Masks • Exclusion of symptomatic and exposed players
Airborne droplet nuclei	• Measles • Tuberculosis • Chicken pox (varicella)	• Shared bus, hotel, or meeting room with the infected player	• Vaccination • Masks • Exclusion of symptomatic and exposed players
Foodborne/ enteric	• **Norovirus** • Salmonella • Campylobacter • Hepatitis A • Giardia • Cryptosporidiosis • Bacillus cereus • Leptospirosis	• Eating a contaminated packed meal while travelling • Exposure to fecally contaminated equipment	• Exclusion of symptomatic players • Avoiding undercooked or contaminated meat/surfaces
Bloodborne	• Hepatitis B • Hepatitis C • HIV	• Failure to use safe injection practices (eg, using contaminated multidose vial for joint injection)	• Safe injection practices: • Single-use vials • Sharps container • Self-retracting needles

Note: some pathogens **in bold** can be transmitted through multiple modes.

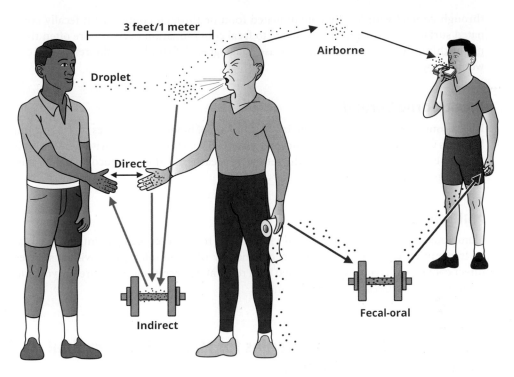

Figure 5.1 Methods for microbe transmission between athletes.

they must survive long enough to remain viable when the next person touches the surface. Unfortunately, most pathogens summarized in **Table 5.1** can live for hours or longer on environmental surfaces.

Respiratory Droplet Spread

Other organisms, such as the mumps virus, spread via droplets of saliva or respiratory tract secretions induced by sneezing, coughing, or speaking. Droplets can travel up to 3 feet (1 m) from the source to people or to environmental surfaces.

Airborne Droplet Nuclei Spread

Smaller infective particles called droplet nuclei that result from coughing can remain airborne for prolonged periods. Thus, these particles may lead to infection in individuals who are well beyond the 3 feet (1 m) that droplets travel. Essentially, these droplet nuclei can permeate an entire room and often remain suspended in the air for hours. These particles can even lead to transmission and infection of people who enter the vicinity hours later. Examples include the measles virus and tuberculosis.

Enteric Spread (Fecal-to-Oral Spread)

Certain bacteria such as *Salmonella* and viral pathogens such as norovirus and hepatitis A virus can be transmitted via contaminated food or water. For example, *Salmonella* may be transmitted by contaminated raw or undercooked chicken or eggs. Hepatitis A is transmitted through the ingestion of fecally contaminated food or water. Norovirus can be spread through contact with fecally contaminated food or through contact with fecally contaminated surfaces. Unfortunately, exposure to fecal contamination occurs more often than one might think. As an old infectious disease adage goes, "if stool were fluorescent, the world would glow."

Bloodborne Spread

Direct contact with blood may result in transmission of bloodborne viruses such as hepatitis B, hepatitis C, and human immunodeficiency virus (HIV). Direct contact with blood with intact skin poses no risk, but contact in the setting of breaches in skin or mucous membranes can lead to risk of transmission.

Multiple Routes

Numerous organisms are transmitted via multiple routes. For example, influenza virus may be transmitted via droplet spread to people nearby when an infected individual sneezes, via direct contact with hands contaminated with respiratory secretions, or indirectly via touching contaminated surfaces such as door handles.

General Principles—Strategies for Minimizing Microbial Spread Between Athletes

Colonization, Subclinical Infection, and Infection (Table 5.2)

As described in **Chapter 4**, athletes can be either colonized or infected with certain microbes. Colonization implies the host does not have any symptoms or ill effects attributable to the organism. Infection means that the host is suffering ill effects from the organism, and the patient is symptomatic. During the early phases of infection, a pathogen may be present and starting to grow or incubate but is not yet causing symptoms. This phenomenon is labeled as a "subclinical infection." In general, this label implies that the process is *about* to lead to symptoms of infection. The term "subclinical infection" is also used to describe an infection that leads to mild symptoms.

Bacterial and viral pathogens can be transmitted to others regardless if causing colonization, subclinical infection, or infection. As an example, hepatitis A virus can be transmitted in the latter half of the incubation period prior to the onset of symptoms. Similarly, athletes whose skin is colonized with MRSA can transmit the bacteria to others. In fact, people colonized with MRSA may lead to more environmental contamination than people undergoing treatment for an MRSA infection.[1]

Table 5.2 Organisms Don't Always Cause Symptoms

	Organism Present?	Organism Increasing in Number?	Organism Causing Symptoms?	Transmission of Organism Possible?
Colonization	Yes	No	No	Yes
Subclinical infection	Yes	Yes	No	Yes
Infection	Yes	Yes	Yes	Yes

On one hand, people with infection must follow infection prevention cornerstone concept #1: **people with infection should be isolated from uninfected people.** Don't come to work if you're sick or you will infect your coworkers. For athletes, don't participate in team activities if you're sick or you will infect teammates and team staff. On the other hand, people without symptoms of infection can transmit pathogens when they are colonized or during a subclinical phase of infection. This fact leads to infection prevention cornerstone concepts for the prevention of transmission between athletes #2—*standard precautions*, #3—*hygiene*, and #4—*vaccination*.

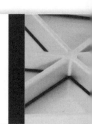

Cornerstone Principles of Infection Prevention

1. Isolate
2. Standard ("universal") precautions
3. Hygiene
4. Vaccination

Standard Precautions

Standard precautions, also known as "universal precautions," are used in healthcare facilities in all situations in which healthcare workers come into contact with patients. As we've noted throughout this book, athletic training facilities are healthcare facilities; thus, standard precautions should be used at all times. While healthcare providers are routinely trained in the use of standard precautions, we believe it is equally important for athletes to use standard precautions to the greatest extent possible.

The elements of standard precautions include hand hygiene; the use of gloves, gowns, and eyewear where contact with bodily fluid can be reasonably expected; cough etiquette; and safe injection and needle disposal practices. *The importance of hand hygiene and safe injection practices is discussed in detail in Chapter 4.* Cough or respiratory etiquette involves covering the mouth and nose during coughing, promptly disposing of facial tissues contaminated with respiratory secretions, and performing hand hygiene after contact with respiratory secretions. These precautions are central to the reduction of transmission of infections within healthcare settings and contained environments where people come into close contact such as within sporting facilities, military barracks, and cruise ships. In general terms, standard precautions for athletes include cough etiquette; frequent use of hand hygiene before and after training sessions and at times when the group comes together for team meetings and to eat and travel; and segregation of personal care products such as soap, razors, towels, and drink bottles.

Both formal and informal team policies can endorse a culture of safety and reinforce each individual's contribution to both personal and team health. Below are a series of practical and (where possible) evidence-based recommendations that enhance infection prevention between athletes and within teams.

HYGIENE

Strategies to promote and improve hand and body hygiene are core components of infection prevention. Improving hygiene reduces risk of infection for the individual and for others. *Hygienic practices such as hand hygiene, postpractice showering, and source control are discussed in detail in Chapter 4.*

*Hygienic practices such as hand hygiene, postpractice showering, and source control are discussed in detail in **Chapter 4.***

VACCINATION

Vaccination is a cornerstone of infection prevention efforts. Several highly transmissible and potentially serious infections can be reliably prevented among athletes and players using safe and effective vaccines. Vaccination provides temporary or lifelong immunity against specific infections and is a mainstay of infection prevention practices. Immunity is effective and long-lasting for some infections such as hepatitis A and B, while it provides incomplete or short protection for other infections such as influenza. Vaccination prevents infections through two mechanisms. First, vaccinated individuals have increased protection. Second, community or herd immunity reduces transmission risk when a high enough proportion of a population has been immunized. Thus, vaccination in the population setting actually protects unimmunized individuals.

While standard childhood vaccination schedules provide protection into adolescence and early adulthood, some persons may have inadvertently or deliberately missed critical vaccinations, or immunity may have waned with time leaving individuals at risk for infection. Reviewing vaccination history, testing for protective antibodies, and then undertaking catch up or revaccination is a reasonable strategy to prevent infections within teams—both for the individual athlete and for the entire team. While standard childhood and adult catch-up immunization schedules are subject to both national and local variability, vaccination should be considered against the pathogens listed in **Table 5.3**.

Valuable methods for minimizing the impact of vaccine-preventable illnesses on athlete health include (1) developing a reliable system to assess the vaccination status of athletes and support staff and (2) implementing strategies to ensure both standard and selected additional vaccinations have been provided.

▶ **Best Practice** Develop a written policy for vaccine-preventable infectious diseases among players and team personnel.

✓ **Recommendation 1** Develop a policy about immunizations for vaccine-preventable diseases (influenza, pertussis, meningococcus, measles, mumps, and chicken pox) in players and team personnel.

Rationale: Several highly transmissible and potentially serious infections can be easily prevented among athletes using safe vaccines: influenza, *Bordetella pertussis* (pertussis or "whooping cough"), meningococcal meningitis, measles, mumps, and chicken pox. ***An example of a policy for vaccine-preventable diseases is included in Appendix 1D***. Vaccine Information Sheets (VISs) for influenza vaccine, tetanus-diphtheria-acellular pertussis (Tdap) vaccine, meningococcal vaccine, measles-mumps-rubella (MMR) vaccine, and chicken pox vaccine are provided by the Advisory Committee on Immunization Practices (ACIP) and should be reviewed prior to vaccine administration (https://www.cdc.gov/vaccines/acip/index.html).

Table 5.3 Catch-up Vaccinations Recommended on a Population Level

Measles	Tetanus	Polio
Mumps	Pertussis	Human papillomavirus
Rubella	Hepatitis A and B	Influenza
Diphtheria	Meningococcus ACWY, B	Varicella

Vaccines are highly effective and safe.

Influenza

⊙ **Best Practice** Provide influenza vaccination to prevent influenza (the "flu").

⊘ **Recommendation 1** Provide influenza vaccination to all players and staff annually.

⊘ **Recommendation 2** Track compliance with influenza vaccination among players and staff.

Rationale: Influenza is a common and partially preventable respiratory infection that is readily transmitted from person to person. Influenza infection significantly reduces respiratory capacity and athletic performance even in players with relatively mild infections. A small but important percentage of young and otherwise healthy individuals who acquire influenza may develop severe infections that require hospitalization and, occasionally, intensive care.

Vaccination is the most effective method to prevent flu. Influenza vaccines have proven benefits that are important for athletes and teams. **Most importantly, players who receive influenza vaccines are less likely to have fever or influenza-like illness, are less likely to miss practice and games, and are less likely to spread influenza to teammates.**[2-4] It is important to recognize, however, that numerous viruses can cause "influenza-like illness"; thus, vaccination will not prevent all episodes of influenza-like illness. This fact should be emphasized when players or skeptics complain *"I received influenza vaccine, and I got the flu anyway."* **We are including specific educational materials regarding facts and myths about the benefits and safety of influenza vaccination in Appendix 1E.**

Vaccination is the most effective method to prevent flu.

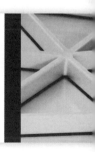

Common Myths About and Barriers to Flu Vaccine

1. I am healthy, and the flu isn't serious.
2. The vaccine doesn't work.
3. The vaccine causes the flu.
4. The vaccine causes side effects.
5. I live with someone with a weak immune system.

From a team perspective, vaccinated players who are exposed to influenza are less likely to spread the virus and are, thus, less likely to cause a locker room–wide outbreak that could potentially devastate a team. Thus, immunization has benefits for individual players **and** the team.

We continue to believe the best and most effective approach is to **require that all** players receive influenza vaccination. This approach is now widely used in most hospitals in the United States. We acknowledge, however, that this approach may not be feasible in some settings without union, parent, and/or player approvals. Compliance among athletes is typically low, between 20% and 30%. However, some programs have achieved much higher rates of compliance (even up to 90%) through highly visible and active campaigns.

Strategies for Improving Uptake of Influenza Vaccination Among Athletes

- Use influenza vaccination "blitzes," in which vaccination is provided by practitioners at the team facilities on specific days and times, so that influenza vaccination can be immediately provided onsite to whomever consents. However, don't limit access to these blitzes. Make sure it is clear the vaccination is available any time.
- Use influenza vaccination mobile "stations" that move frequently between strategic, high-traffic locations (eg, cafeteria, training room, outside locker room) so that individuals can be immunized during the course of their normal activities without an appointment or clinic visit.
- Provide educational materials to players at the beginning of influenza season describing the benefits of the vaccination and debunking the myths about the vaccine *(see Appendix 1E)*.
- Recruit player champions to promote the use of the vaccination. Champions are ideally team leaders who can "show the way" for younger players. If someone in your facility has been impacted by influenza (the player or family member), have that player share his or her story and help advocate for the vaccination.
- Focus on players with families, pregnant partners, and young children. Vaccination of the player provides protection against importing influenza into the team from his family **as well as** protecting his family against importation of the virus from the team. These players should have the biggest motivation for vaccination.
- Demonstrate receipt of the vaccination by team leaders and coaches (ie, lead by example).
- Post signs promoting influenza vaccination *(see the ebook version of this book for example signs)*.

Vaccination can be given intranasally or via intramuscular (IM) injection. In 2017, the ACIP recommended against the use of the intranasal formulation (a live attenuated vaccine) due to lack of efficacy against the common H1N1 influenza strain. However, the intranasal vaccine was reintroduced and approved by the ACIP for the 2018 season (and beyond) following a change in the H1N1 component.[5] We welcome the reintroduction of the intranasal vaccine, as it provides a method for overcoming one of the key excuses for not receiving a vaccine—the injection or "shot." Similarly, egg allergies are no longer sufficient to prevent receipt of the vaccine, as egg-free formulations now exist. Injections can be given using either trivalent (covers three types of flu) or quadrivalent (covers four types of flu) vaccine.

⊘ **Recommendation 4** Mandate that all athletic trainers and team medical staff receive annual influenza vaccination.

Rationale: Most US healthcare institutions now require that all healthcare workers receive annual influenza vaccination.[6] Requiring that team healthcare providers, including athletic trainers and team physicians, receive annual influenza vaccination leads to two benefits. First, it helps improve the "culture of safety" by providing an outward and visible demonstration of the importance of influenza prevention. Second, as athletic trainers have regular close contact with players, immunized athletic trainers are unlikely to spread influenza from one player to another during their routine work and activities.

Hepatitis A and Hepatitis B

⊙ **Best Practice** Provide vaccine to prevent hepatitis A and hepatitis B infections.

⊘ **Recommendation 1** Ensure athletes have been vaccinated against hepatitis A and B.

Rationale: Hepatitis A and hepatitis B are viral infections that can cause serious liver damage. Hepatitis A is an acute illness acquired by ingestion of contaminated food. Hepatitis B can be an acute and/or chronic disease that is acquired from exposure to contaminated blood (eg, a needle stick).

Hepatitis A vaccine became available in the United States in 1996 but was not widely used prior to 2006 when it became part of the standard vaccines administered to American children. However, many young adults did not receive this vaccination in childhood and thus remain vulnerable to acquiring hepatitis A.

In light of the above, it is not surprising that outbreaks of hepatitis A continue to occur even though the overall incidence of hepatitis A has declined. A large and persistent outbreak of hepatitis A began in San Diego in 2015 and continued into 2017.[7] Cases linked to this outbreak have occurred in multiple states including Arizona, Indiana, Michigan, Colorado, and Tennessee. The average age of 3421 cases reported in 2017 was 40 years; two-thirds of the affected individuals were men. Over 25,000 cases were reported between November 2016 and September 2019, contributing to 15,500 hospitalizations and 259 deaths.[8]

Due to these outbreaks, the United States Centers for Disease Control and Prevention (CDC) supports the use of hepatitis A vaccine after known or possible exposure to a single case of hepatitis A. Some experts have recommended vaccination in athletes involved in close-contact sports "because this disease typically leads to months of reduced physical performance and [because] hepatitis A can be easily transferred to teammates and opponents."[9] Another aspect of hepatitis A risk is international travel. For example, the CDC recommends that travelers to most Central American, South American, and Southeast Asian destinations receive vaccination against hepatitis A, as the virus can be acquired via contaminated food or water regardless of where you are eating or staying. Specific recommendations for specific destinations can be found at https://wwwnc.cdc.gov/travel/destinations/list.

Hepatitis B vaccine became part of routine childhood immunizations in the United States in 1991. Outbreaks are more likely to occur in locations where health care is provided. More specifically, these outbreaks occur because of poor, unsafe, and sometimes illegal activities during invasive medical procedures (eg, hemodialysis, surgical centers, injections) (https://www.cdc.gov/hepatitis/outbreaks/healthcarehepoutbreaktable.htm). The CDC reported 23 outbreaks of hepatitis B related to health care from 2008 through 2017; 18 occurred in long-term care facilities and 5 occurred in medical settings such as dental clinics, outpatient oncology clinic, surgical center, and two pain clinics. *See Chapter 4 for additional information about safe injection practices to prevent the risk of hepatitis B transmission.*

Hepatitis B is more contagious than hepatitis C or HIV. Transmission has occurred in contact sports, such as among members of a Japanese sumo wrestling club,[10] during American football,[11] and among cross-country runners in Sweden.[12]

⊘ **Recommendation 2** Vaccinate all athletic trainers and team medical personnel against hepatitis B.

⊘ **Recommendation 3** Document that all athletic trainers and team medical personnel have been vaccinated against hepatitis B.

Rationale: The risk of transmission due to high-risk exposures to blood infected with hepatitis B is approximately 33% (one in three). Vaccination is highly effective in reducing this risk to near zero, is long-lasting, and is safe.[13] In fact, healthcare facilities that do not offer the hepatitis B vaccine to employees have been sued for negligence.[14] Therefore, most medical facilities require hepatitis B vaccination as a requirement for employment.

Based on previous discussions with athletic trainers, we believe the vast majority of athletic trainers and team physicians are already vaccinated against hepatitis B. In the event that athletic trainers or team physicians have not been vaccinated against hepatitis B, we recommend they receive the vaccination series. We also recommend documenting the vaccination status for each athletic trainer and physician. This requirement is especially important for new staff members.

Pertussis

▶ **Best Practice** Provide vaccine to prevent pertussis infection ("whooping cough").

✓ **Recommendation 1** Ensure all athletes have completed recommended DTaP series.

Rationale: Pertussis is widely and erroneously believed to be a rare disease of infants and children. In fact, pertussis is common. An estimated 2 million Americans acquire pertussis each year. Pertussis causes an illness that typically manifests as cough (often prolonged) with or without fever. During the second phase of illness, cough due to pertussis can be so severe that it leads to vomiting (ie, paroxysms of cough leading to posttussive vomiting). Among children, the illness often causes a characteristic "whooping" sound or "whooping cough."

Vaccination is the key strategy to prevent infection with pertussis. The ACIP currently recommends that children in the United States receive five doses of the diphtheria-tetanus-pertussis (DTaP) vaccine: 2 months, 4 months, 6 months, 15 to 18 months, and 4 to 6 years old.[15]

✓ **Recommendation 2** Ensure athletes have received at least one dose of Tdap.

✓ **Recommendation 3** Provide the Tdap vaccine in place of standard tetanus when indicated.

Rationale: The ACIP recommends that children in the United States receive one dose of Tdap vaccine at age 11 or 12 years.[16] "Acellular" refers to the fact that the immune response is triggered by immunogenic proteins, toxins, and other cellular components and is not due to an intact bacterium. **As such, pertussis vaccine cannot and does not cause pertussis.** As this recommendation is relatively recent, most adult athletes will not have received a dose. As a result, adult athletes should receive a dose of Tdap. If the athlete is unsure if he or she has received Tdap, the CDC recommends providing a booster. Furthermore, if a player requires a tetanus booster due to an injury that requires sutures, the Tdap can be given instead of the standard tetanus booster.

The fact that immunization for pertussis in childhood does not produce durable immunity in adults is widely underappreciated. While infants have more severe infections, adolescents and adults actually account for >60% of cases in the vaccination era.[17]

Because immunity induced by pertussis vaccine characteristically declines with time, adults who were vaccinated during childhood can and do become infected with *B. pertussis*. For example, 40% of previously immunized adults contract pertussis after exposure to infected children.[18] Though unlikely to cause death, adults with pertussis often have prolonged, significant illnesses. Pertussis infection regularly results in unnecessary doctor visits, unnecessary use of antibiotics, and most importantly from a team perspective, increased absenteeism from work.[19] Several studies have demonstrated that the majority of adults with pertussis missed between 7 to 10 days of work[20]; 10% to 16% of adults with pertussis missed more than a month of work.[21-24]

Pertussis is highly contagious. It can spread rapidly, and it frequently causes outbreaks or clusters of infection in populations in close quarters such as sports teams.[25] While an infection of a single player may be easy to deal with, having a teamwide outbreak can be devastating.

Childhood pertussis immunization does not produce durable immunity in adults.

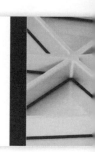

We believe athletes can and should be given the Tdap vaccination in the following scenarios:
- Tdap can be given to any player who has not previously received it. The ACIP previously recommended a wait period of 2 years since the prior Td (regular tetanus and diphtheria toxin booster), but this restriction has been removed.
- Td boosters are currently recommended for adults every 10 years.
  - If an individual player is now due for his or her next Td booster or if a Td booster is needed as a component of wound management, simply replace the Td booster with Tdap.

Meningococcus

▶ **Best Practice** Prevent meningococcal disease by administering meningococcal vaccine.

✓ **Recommendation 1** Provide meningococcal vaccine to players who previously have not been immunized.

Rationale: The ACIP currently recommends that all children receive one of two quadrivalent meningococcal vaccines between the ages of 11 and 18 years. If given at the age of 11 or 12 years, a booster is recommended at approximately 16 years of age. In fact, most US universities require proof of receipt within 5 years prior to matriculation.

We recommend that team medical staff assess the prior receipt of meningococcal vaccine in new players. In particular, players from other countries (eg, Australia) may not have received meningococcal vaccine. Vaccine should be offered to team members who have not received this vaccine.

The meningococcal vaccine is effective and safe. In addition, it is safe to reimmunize players who are not certain if they have or have not previously received this vaccine. This policy and the high effectiveness of meningococcal vaccines led to a 21% decrease in the incidence of meningitis in developed countries from 1993 to 2011.[26]

Measles and Mumps

▶ **Best Practice** Prevent measles and mumps by administering MMR vaccine.

✓ **Recommendation 1** Provide MMR vaccine to players who previously have not been immunized.

Rationale: Infections like measles and mumps ravaged populations and children prior to the development of the MMR vaccine in the 1950s. The impact of the vaccine on childhood health has been labeled as one of the 10 greatest medical accomplishments of the past 100 years. The ACIP currently recommends that children in the United States receive two doses of MMR: one dose between 12 and 15 months and a second dose between 4 and 6 years of age.[27] Two doses of MMR is 88% effective at preventing mumps and 97% effective at preventing measles.

Measles was declared eradicated from the United States in 2000. Unfortunately, the incidence of measles has increased over the past decade. In fact, numerous measles outbreaks have occurred in recent years. For example, 24 separate measles outbreaks occurred in the United

States in 2014, including one large outbreak involving 383 people. Another outbreak in 2014 involving 125 cases was linked to visitors to a California amusement park. Forty-five percent of patients in this outbreak were unvaccinated, and an additional 43% had unknown vaccination status. The remaining 12% contracted measles despite one, two, or even three prior doses of measles vaccine.

Measles transmission and outbreaks have occurred in the sporting context as well. An outbreak of measles occurred at an international youth baseball tournament when an infectious player from Japan resided in a shared compound with other athletes.[28] The CDC recommends documentation of vaccination status for participants and support staff by organizers of large gatherings.

Finally, 2019 was the worst year for measles in the United States since "eradicated" in 2000. Over 1200 cases, including 128 hospitalizations, were reported—more in 6 months than any year in previous decade, with three separate outbreaks that started in late 2018.[29]

The number of cases of mumps increased significantly in recent years as a direct consequence of declining vaccination rates. The number of annually reported cases of mumps in the United States increased 27-fold from 229 in 2012 to 6109 in 2017.[30] The highest proportion of these cases occurred in the >30 years age group. In fact, 2016 and 2017 had the highest number of reported cases in a decade.[31] Proper vaccination (two doses) is only 88% effective at preventing cases. Thus, older individuals remain vulnerable even with well-documented vaccination status.

ACIP now recommends an additional dose of MMR for (1) students who lack documentation of prior receipt of two doses of MMR at the time of entry into college; (2) healthcare and day care workers who are at increased risk of exposure who similarly lack documentation; or (3) any individual exposed during an outbreak. Athletes that are currently or have previously attended college in the United States have probably (but not definitively) received one or more doses of MMR. For these athletes, we recommend seeking documentation of two doses or, if documentation is unavailable, administering a booster of MMR to ensure adequate immunity, as per ACIP recommendations.

In the event that a player did not attend a college in the United States, we recommend immunizing the player with a booster of MMR vaccine to improve "herd immunity" and decrease the risk of a measles or mumps outbreak in the team.

Chicken Pox ("Varicella")

⊙ **Best Practice** Prevent chicken pox by administering the varicella ("chicken pox") vaccine.

✓ **Recommendation** Ensure all athletes have received the varicella vaccination or have a clear, documented prior history of chicken pox.

Rationale: After introduction of the chicken pox vaccine in 1995, the CDC recommended that all children receive one dose of vaccine at 12 months of age and a second dose prior to age 6 years. Since then, infection rates have declined remarkably in the United States. However, sporadic outbreaks of chicken pox continue to occur, primarily because many young adults who are now in their late 20s to early 30s were not immunized as infants or subsequently. Because of widespread "herd immunity," these susceptible individuals may have avoided acquiring natural infection with chicken pox, yet they remain at risk if they are directly exposed to a case of chicken pox. Thus, the risk of chicken pox exists in college and professional adult athletes. For example, five San Diego State football players developed chicken pox in August 2017.[32] The first player to develop symptoms had never developed chicken pox nor received chicken pox vaccine during his childhood. SDSU officials had difficulty determining the risk of further infection for teammates and staff because San Diego State did not require documentation of prior chicken pox disease or vaccination prior to college admission. Practices were canceled to allow time for locker room disinfection, and infected team members were removed from play during their illness.

Immunization Status

⊙ **Best Practice** Ensure vaccination status is known, documented, and easily accessible for all of the below vaccine-preventable pathogens.

⊘ **Recommendation 1** Determine vaccine status through documentation or, if necessary, screening.

⊘ **Recommendation 2** If a player is found not to have immunity to a vaccine-preventable infection, offer a booster to improve immunity.

Rationale: Any and all of the infections described in this section can cause infection and outbreaks in players and teams. Vaccines remain the primary strategy to prevent these infections, but the prevention strategy is not 100% effective. In general, the team environment is associated with increased risk of infection transmission and outbreaks. As a result, we recommend that the vaccination status for all of the below pathogens be documented and easily accessible, including influenza, pertussis, meningococcus, mumps, hepatitis A, hepatitis B, measles, and chicken pox (varicella).

Obtain athletes' vaccination status for influenza, pertussis, meningococcus, mumps, hepatitis A, hepatitis B, measles, and chicken pox (varicella).

This information is critical to stop or to mediate an outbreak from occurring, as it will provide the team physicians with critical information about players' risks if one or more of these vaccine-preventable infections occur. Ideally, these data are documented in the electronic health record (EHR). If documentation in the EHR is not feasible, each team should document vaccine status locally.

While vaccination is the best intervention to prevent infections such as measles, mumps, and chicken pox, the strategy is imperfect. As outlined in the discussions of various outbreaks above, infections can occur despite prior vaccination. Conway et al recently summarized the vaccination status of 98 professional athletes in the NBA and MLB; screened the players for immunity to measles, mumps, rubella, and chicken pox; and compared their results to data published from the NHANES cohort for adults aged 20 to 29 years.[33] In general, the prevalence of immunity was lower among athletes compared to age-matched controls; approximately one-third of the athletes had insufficient immunity to one or more viruses. Neither birth in the United States nor attendance at a US college was associated with increased immunity. Though the analysis was a small cross-sectional analysis, we believe these data emphasize two important points. First, these data underscore the concern that athletes are at increased risk of infection from vaccine-preventable infections. Second, record keeping and requirements at US colleges may be insufficient to determine immune status. As a result, it is reasonable to offer screening for immune status against measles, mumps, and varicella to new college and professional athletes, particularly if vaccine status is otherwise unknown or unclear. If a player is found to have decreased or no immunity to one of the vaccine-preventable infections outlined above, discuss the issue with the player and offer a booster to improve immunity and decrease risk of infection.

Outbreak Investigations and Mitigation

Many pathogens can spread between athletes, leading to transmission of infection and clusters or outbreaks in a team. Recommendations throughout this textbook are designed to decrease this risk. However, the risk of infection and transmission is never zero. As a result, team medical personnel must be well aware of strategies for identification of transmission, clusters, and/ or outbreaks. As with most topics, management of outbreaks first starts with an understanding of basic definitions and concepts, including strategies for detection and early recognition. We end this section with specific tier-based recommendations to manage outbreaks related to common infections among athletes.

Definitions: An outbreak is defined as an occurrence of infectious disease in excess of its normal incidence in a specific population such as a hospital ward, a school, or an athletic team. The term "outbreak" typically implies that transmission between individuals has occurred. Epidemic has a similar definition as outbreak, but epidemic is the generally preferred term when an excess number of cases over the normal incidence occurs in a large geographic area.

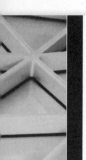

What's the Difference Between a "Cluster" of Infections, an Outbreak, and an Epidemic?

- Cluster—an unusual aggregation of infections grouped in space and time at a frequency greater than normal.
- Outbreak—infectious disease in excess of its normal incidence in a specific population due to transmission between individuals.
- Epidemic—an outbreak in a large geographic area.
   In general, outbreaks represent a small proportion of clusters, and epidemics are a small proportion of outbreaks (**Figure 5.2**).

In contrast, cluster is generally used to describe an unusual aggregation (either real or perceived) of infections or healthcare events that are grouped in space and time at a frequency that is greater than normal (even though the normal incidence of such events may not be known or knowable). For example, a perceived increase in the occurrence of colds, sore throats, or skin rashes in members of an athletic team may be more appropriately defined as a cluster rather than an outbreak. Often such clusters are hard to investigate and manage, as a perception of an increase in incidence is difficult to confirm statistically or clinically. Because conditions such as colds, sore throats, and skin rashes commonly have multiple different and unrelated causes, widespread perception that there is an outbreak can lead to confusion and, in some cases, to unnecessary investigations, interventional measures, and unwarranted media attention.

Clusters of healthcare events occasionally lead to the detection of a true outbreak or even an epidemic. For example, Legionnaires' disease was identified after investigation of a cluster of cases of unexplained pneumonia in people staying in a single Philadelphia hotel.[34] HIV was identified following an investigation of a single cluster of an unusual opportunistic infection (*Pneumocystis jiroveci* pneumonia) in Los Angeles, paving the way for the subsequent worldwide epidemic.[35]

Detection and Management of Clusters or Outbreaks

Clusters or outbreaks of infectious diseases in athletic teams can be sudden or gradual in onset. For example, outbreaks of norovirus infection, food poisoning, and respiratory infections such as influenza tend to be sudden in onset, immediately obvious, and involve

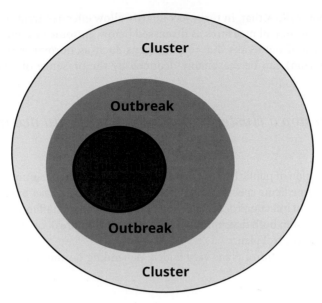

Figure 5.2 Relationship of clusters, outbreaks, and epidemics.

a substantial portion of a team. In contrast, outbreaks of MRSA or herpetic skin infections (herpes gladiatorum) are frequently gradual in onset. Initially, it may be difficult or even impossible to determine if the observed cases are simply sporadic and unrelated occurrences or if transmission is occurring between team members. An outbreak cannot be defined by the occurrence of a specific number of cases. For example, even one case of measles in an athletic team would be considered an outbreak as the normal incidence of measles in the United States should be zero. In the case of infections such as meningococcal meningitis, a single case, although not truly a cluster, may appropriately be approached and managed as a cluster.

Pathogens with a known propensity to cause outbreaks include bacteria such as *Staphylococcus aureus* and *Streptococcus pyogenes* (also known as Group A strep); viruses such as norovirus, enterovirus, herpes simplex, and influenza; mycobacteria such as *Mycobacterium tuberculosis*; fungal organisms such as the organisms that cause tinea pedis; and even arthropods such as head lice.

EARLY RECOGNITION OF A CASE

Outbreak detection can be easy and straightforward or extremely difficult. In general, the first step in control and mitigation of any outbreak is to make a diagnosis. *Steps for diagnosing common infections in athletes are discussed in Chapter 4.* For example, the occurrence of respiratory illnesses among multiple team members could be due to multiple unrelated respiratory viruses or a single highly communicable pathogen such as influenza virus. Thus, diagnostic testing for influenza virus should be an early step in the investigation of a cluster of respiratory infections during the winter months. An accurate diagnosis can directly lead to effective therapy and antiviral prophylaxis of exposed but not yet clinically ill team members. The presence of documented cases of influenza virus infection in the community greatly increases the likelihood that a cluster will occur in an athletic team. Similarly, accurate diagnosis of skin and soft-tissue infections can lead to the detection of pathogens such as MRSA that, in turn, secondarily allow effective treatments and stepwise implementation of control measures as discussed below. In some circumstances, the likely or probable cause of outbreaks due to pathogens such as norovirus or Herpes simplex (herpes gladiatorum) can be reasonably deduced by the presence of characteristic signs and symptoms.

First step to stop a cluster or outbreak—make an accurate diagnosis.

Early notification of public health officials or trained medical personnel such as infectious diseases or sports medicine specialists should be considered on a case-by-case basis when an outbreak or cluster of infections occurs in team players or athletic staff in a single facility. These individuals can assist in both determining the cause of the outbreak or cluster and developing a management and control plan.

Management and control plans vary widely depending on the size and likely or known cause of an outbreak.

OUTBREAK MITIGATION

Designing mitigation measures to prevent further microbial spread is relatively easy in some outbreaks, whereas mitigation can be exceedingly difficult in others (eg, in outbreaks in which cases in the community "spill over" into team members).

Temporary removal (ie, isolation or "quarantine") and treatment of ill individuals is critical to stop any cluster or outbreak. Removal alone may be sufficient to terminate direct person-to-person transmission in some clusters or outbreaks (such as those with active herpetic skin or mucous membrane lesions from a wrestling team). In contrast, norovirus outbreaks require measures to interrupt direct transmission via person-to-person contact **and** indirect transmission via secondary environmental contamination. Thus, removal of acute ill team members coupled with extensive and careful environmental cleaning with bleach and hand hygiene are required to interrupt and then terminate norovirus transmission.

A preexisting, well-constructed, and medically sound plan to manage a case or cluster of infections in team members can prevent confusion and errors made by "ad hoc" decisions that are not fully informed. Preexisting written contingency policies should be designed to allow "stepwise" implementation of control measures. Tier-based contingency policies for managing clusters of common pathogens in athletes are discussed below. ***Templates for these policies are provided in Appendix 1F.***

The foundation for these policies is related to alterations in risk and the cost:benefit equation of added risk reduction. As described several times throughout this book, athletes are inherently at risk for transmission of bacterial and viral pathogens. Standard recommendations throughout this manual are considered best strategies when risk is at baseline. Put another way, some additional activities *could* be implemented to reduce risk even further, but these additional activities may include great logistical challenges and/or lead to the elimination of activities, procedures, or products that have value for the players. However, when risk is elevated above baseline (eg, when one or more cases of a transmissible infection occurs in the facility), then the cost:benefit equation may shift so the reduced risk provided by the additional activities outweighs the energy required to overcome the logistical challenges and "cost" for the player.

Methicillin-resistant *Staphylococcus aureus*

▶ **Best Practice** Use a tiered contingency protocol to guide appropriate responses when a case or cluster of MRSA infections occurs in team personnel.

Tier 1 recommendations include all of the standard recommendations for infection prevention provided in this manual. In other words, tier 1 recommendations should be followed even in the absence of any cases of MRSA. Tier 2 interventions should be implemented when a single case of MRSA occurs in a team facility. Tier 3 interventions should be implemented when two or more cases of MRSA occur in close temporal proximity in a team facility. Each tier includes new recommendations, but all recommendations from the prior tier should still be followed.

Tier 2 Interventions—Recommendations When One Player Has an MRSA Infection

▶ **Best Practice** Reduce the risk of new or ongoing colonization with MRSA after one player has been diagnosed with an MRSA infection.

✓ **Recommendation 1** Decolonize the player(s) diagnosed with MRSA.

Rationale: Decolonization strategies are moderately effective at temporarily reducing the burden of MRSA on the skin. Approximately 60% of people who undergo a topical decolonization strategy remain decolonized 30 days later.[36] We recommend topical decolonization after completion of antibiotics as follows:

- Apply mupirocin ointment to both nares two times each day for 5 days.
- Shower with chlorhexidine gluconate (CHG) each day using a 4% CHG-containing soap in the shower for 5 days.

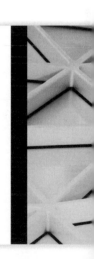

Tips and Advice: Decolonization

- Use a dual cotton-tip applicator to apply mupirocin ointment to one nostril. Turn the applicator over and use the other end to apply to the other nostril. This approach avoids contamination of the mupirocin bottle.
- Begin regimen on the same day the player *finishes* antibiotic treatment for the infection. Patients receiving antibiotics for infection are less likely to shed MRSA into the environment than patients with MRSA colonization (and not receiving antibiotics)[37]; thus, the end of antibiotic treatment is the optimal time to decolonize an individual infected patient.
- We recommend decolonizing the player diagnosed with MRSA even if screening cultures are negative, as screening does not identify 100% of colonization and antibiotic therapy will decrease the yield of the test even further. Essentially, if you have an infection with MRSA, you are considered colonized with MRSA at that time.

✓ **Recommendation 2** Use CHG-containing wipes to perform intensive "source control" for 14 days when a case or cluster of MRSA infections has been identified in team personnel.

Rationale: Two percent CHG-impregnated cloths are more effective and have a lower risk of side effects than liquid CHG preparations.[38] These cloths are commercially available in alcohol-free prepackaged unit doses sufficient for bathing a single person. Four to ten 7.5 × 7.5-inch cloths are needed to bathe a single, standard-sized (70 kg) adult. More cloths will likely be needed for larger athletes. *We have provided a sample protocol to guide use of CHG-containing cloths for source control in Appendix 1J.*

Perform intensive source control for 14 days.

We recommend using disposable prepackaged 2% CHG-impregnated cloths for the following reasons:

- They have a track record of success[39,40]
- They are available as a prepackaged product with a consistent and effective concentration of CHG
- They are disposable
- They are safe—allergic side effects are extremely rare and minor
- Packets are relatively inexpensive and portable
- They result in rapid and long-lasting (>24 hours) killing of MRSA on skin surfaces[41]

No rinsing is needed after application as CHG dries on the skin. If used after showering, wipes should be used after the skin is dry and cool. Warmers can be used to heat CHG-impregnated cloths prior to application.

There are no reliable data regarding ideal time of day for CHG administration for non-hospitalized individuals. We recommend applying prepackaged body wipes to athletes **after** the postpractice shower. CHG should not be applied to the face; we recommend instructing athletes to apply wipes to all skin surfaces below the chin.

(▶) **Best Practice** Increase education and strictly enforce infection prevention policies to prevent further transmission when a case or cluster of MRSA infections has been identified in team personnel.

(✓) **Recommendation 1** Increase educational efforts when a case or cluster of MRSA infections is identified.

Rationale: Educate and alert players that an MRSA infection has occurred in the team facility and that, by definition, they are now also at higher risk for infection. This information also provides full disclosure to players who are logically concerned about their health. Such notification may also provide a stimulus for improved personal hygienic practices among players. Notification also overcomes the occasional problem of the perception of secrecy regarding MRSA. Players should be educated about the newly recommended control strategies. We also recommend a "no exception" approach to enforcement of infection prevention recommendations among team members (see below). Finally, we recommend that medical personnel specifically remind players to present to training staff with **any** skin abrasion, cuts, or infection.

Enforcing "no exception" policies may require the assignment of monitors to observe practices.

Players must also be educated that MRSA transmission can (and often does) occur at home and among family members. In fact, one of the most important risk factors for the spread of MRSA in the community is living in the same home with someone who has an MRSA skin infection.[42] Thus, athletes who have family members—particularly children—with boils, pimples, infected cuts, or minor skin infections should urge their family and household members with actual or suspected skin infections to seek medical care in order to get a correct diagnosis and prompt treatment. Other measures to prevent the spread of MRSA at home include:

- Handwashing with soap and water or hand hygiene with an alcohol-containing hand rub before and after wound dressings are changed.

- The infected person should keep their wounds or draining skin lesions covered at all times.
- Family members should avoid handling soiled bandages.
- Family members should not share hand or bath towels, clothes, or other common personal hygiene objects such as razors, toothbrushes, or eating utensils.
- Special cultures (eg, nasal swabs) are NOT recommended when a single or multiple family members have an infection due to MRSA. However, when more than one family member is infected, we advise the empirical use of topical nasal mupirocin and chlorhexidine showers as described in the recommendation for decolonization. If MRSA infections continue to recur, consultation with a local infectious diseases specialist is recommended.
- Any skin lesion that **drains pus** (even a minor cut) should be cultured and treated, especially if one of more family members currently has or has recently had an infection due to MRSA. This intervention is important, as it is impossible to clinically distinguish an MRSA infection from a staphylococcal infection due to methicillin-sensitive strain of S. *aureus.*

All family members should shower with 2% to 4% CHG soap daily until all family members are well and free of infection. Family members should then continue these daily applications of CHG for 5 additional days.

⊘ **Recommendation 2** Enforce "no exception" policies for handwashing, postpractice showering, and use of the hydrotherapy room when a case or cluster of MRSA infections has been identified

⊘ **Recommendation 3** Strictly enforce a policy banning use of communal tubs of balm, lotion, or cream when a case or cluster of MRSA infections has been identified unless hand hygiene is performed.

Rationale: Ensure that standard recommendations in tier 1 are followed. For example, ensure that all players and staff wash their hands upon entering and exiting the training facility. All athletic trainers must wash hands between player treatments. All athletic trainers and players also must wash hands between uses of communal tubs or containers used for balms and ointments. Similarly, it is important for teams to insist that all players shower following practices and prior to further use of the training facility. Finally, ensure that players with skin infections do not use the pools in the hydrotherapy room. In other words, do not allow players with skin infections in the whirlpools even if the wound is covered with a hydrocolloid bandage when a case or cluster of MRSA infections is known or suspected in team members. Enforcement of "no exception" policies may require the designation of monitors to observe the above scenarios and provide corrective education as needed. If a player with an infection must use the hydrotherapy room, use individual whirlpools, and ensure the whirlpool is drained and properly cleaned after use, as described in *Chapter 6*.

⊘ **Recommendation 4** Ban sharing of personal equipment, including towels and water bottles, when a case or cluster of MRSA infections has been identified.

Rationale: Sharing of personal equipment, including towels and water bottles during a game or practice, is part of the culture of most teams but is also a risk factor for acquiring MRSA.[43,44] Thus, players must be educated that sharing of these types of equipment should not occur after a single case of MRSA has been identified. Athletic trainers and other staff must help players enforce this policy. To improve the likelihood that this ban is successful, players should be given individual towels for use during the day. Similarly, individual water bottles can be provided or players can use individual cups to obtain water from larger coolers.

Provide individual towels and water bottles for practice.

Tier 3 Interventions—Recommendations When Two or More Players Have an MRSA Infection

⊙ **Best Practice** Reduce the risk of new or ongoing colonization with MRSA after two or more players have been diagnosed with an MRSA infection.

⊘ **Recommendation 1** Ensure that equipment throughout the training facility is thoroughly cleaned a minimum of one time per day and that such cleaning is carefully documented or monitored when a case or cluster of MRSA infections has been identified.

Rationale: While skin-to-skin contact is the most likely method for transmission of MRSA, MRSA can be spread via inanimate objects such as training equipment. Thus, thorough and regular cleaning of the training facility is an important step to reduce the risk of MRSA transmission. Not only should equipment and rooms be cleaned, but cleaning should also be documented. We recommend that supervisory personnel responsible for facility cleaning assume responsibility for reviewing these cleaning logs on a daily basis.

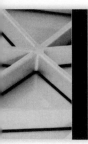

Tips and Advice

- Provide adequate numbers of bottles of disinfectant sprays throughout training facility and encourage all players and/or staff to spray and wipe down equipment after they use equipment in the weight room, *AND/OR*
- Place disposable pop-up dispensers of disinfectant cleaning wipes (eg, bleach or quaternary ammonium) in convenient areas such as weight rooms to make it easy for players to wipe down equipment after each use.

⊙ **Best Practice** Ban shaving below the neck when a case or cluster of MRSA infections has been identified in team personnel.

⊘ **Recommendation 1** Enforce a policy prohibiting cosmetic shaving below the neck when a case or cluster of MRSA infections is identified in an individual team.

Rationale: As described previously, body or cosmetic shaving is a well-known risk factor for MRSA infection as it leads to microscopic skin abrasions that increase the risk of MRSA infection.[45] While we recognize that this behavior cannot be prevented outside of the training facility, we strongly encourage that players be urged to stop this practice when a cluster of MRSA has been identified in the facility to reduce the risk of additional infections.

MRSA

If more than one team member develops a boil or other type of skin or soft-tissue infection due to MRSA, enact the highest tier prevention strategies for MRSA:

1. Increase player and staff education about common signs and symptoms of MRSA to encourage early evaluation and treatment by medical personnel.
2. Enforce "no exception" policies for handwashing, postpractice showering and use of hydrotherapy facilities.
3. Strictly enforce a policy banning the communal use of single tube or containers of balm, lotion, or creams unless hand hygiene and gloves are used for application.
4. Ban sharing of personal equipment such as towels and water bottles.
5. Enhance current protocols for cleaning equipment, training tables, and common use areas.
6. In addition to prompt treatment of all known or suspected cases, decolonize players who are known to be infected with MRSA.
7. Use chlorhexidine-containing soaps for all showering until the outbreak is deemed to be over.
8. Ban body shaving (ie, shaving below the neck).

Diarrheal Illness/Norovirus

⊙ **Best Practice** Use a tiered contingency protocol to guide appropriate responses when a case or cluster of diarrheal illness occurs in team personnel.

⊘ **Recommendation 1** Develop a tiered contingency protocol to guide responses when diarrheal illness is detected in team personnel.

Rationale: We prefer a tiered approach to guide responses to a case or cluster of diarrheal infection. Tier 1 recommendations include all of the standard recommendations for infection prevention provided in this manual. In other words, tier 1 recommendations should be followed even in the absence of any cases of diarrhea. Tier 2 interventions can be implemented when a single case of diarrhea **not** related to food poisoning occurs in a team facility. Tier 3 interventions can be implemented when two or more cases of diarrhea occur in close temporal proximity in a team facility. The following best practices and recommendations are predicated on the fact that the majority of cases of diarrhea are caused by highly transmissible viruses such as norovirus. Each tier includes new recommendations, but all recommendations from the prior tier should still be followed. *A sample tiered contingency protocol to decrease the risk of diarrheal transmission is provided in Appendix 1G.*

Tier 2 Interventions—Recommendations When One Player Has an Acute-Onset Diarrheal Illness

⊙ **Best Practice** Isolate any player(s) with acute-onset of diarrheal illness to avoid contact with other players.

⊘ **Recommendation 1** Immediately send any player(s) with diarrheal illness home as soon as symptoms are recognized.

Players with diarrhea must be sent home ASAP.

Rationale: Diarrheal illness is defined as three or more loose or liquid stools in a 24-hour period.[46] We strongly recommend that any player with a diarrheal illness be sent home, away from the training facility, as quickly as possible. This recommendation stems from the fact that the majority of diarrheal illnesses are caused by highly contagious viruses such as norovirus. Of note, not all acute-onset diarrheal illness is due to viral illness. Some diarrheal illness may be caused by food poisoning. Nonetheless, a standard and well-proven intervention to decrease transmission is to remove (ie, isolate) the contagious person from uninfected personnel until symptoms resolve or an alternative, nontransmissible cause is determined.

Norovirus is typically a self-limited illness with symptom duration of approximately 2 days; norovirus infections can cause significant illness that impacts player performance. Furthermore, if ill players are not removed from other players and staff, this virus can cause outbreaks, impacting many team members simultaneously. For example, significant norovirus outbreaks have occurred on athletic teams, and transmission between players has been demonstrated when the only contact between some affected players occurred on the playing field.[47] We think the benefit of preventing a teamwide diarrheal outbreak outweighs the downside of one to two missed days of practice for affected players who, if allowed to practice and train with the team, will not be at full strength.

▶ **Best Practice** Adjust infection prevention practices to prevent spread of illness when a case of acute-onset diarrheal infections has been identified.

✓ **Recommendation 1** Wear gloves for all contact with players with diarrheal illness.

✓ **Recommendation 2** Enforce a strict policy of hand hygiene using soap and water among players and athletic trainers when a case or cluster of diarrheal illness has been identified.

✓ **Recommendation 3** Educate team personnel that hand hygiene requires soap and water, not alcohol-based products because some viruses (eg, norovirus) are not inactivated by alcohol.

Rationale: "Contact precautions," the practice of wearing gloves and disposable gowns when interacting with patients with potentially transmissible infections, is standard of care when treating patients with norovirus in acute care hospitals in the United States.[48] Because the use of gowns is not practical in outpatient settings, we recommend wearing gloves when treating any player with a diarrheal illness. Gloves should be removed immediately after contacting the infected player. Hand hygiene with soap and water should be performed immediately **after** removing gloves because hand contamination during glove removal is common and significant. This practice will reduce the risk of secondary and indirect transmission via hand and environmental contamination in the facility.

Wearing gloves? You still need to wash your hands after you remove them.

As mentioned above, alcohol foam is ineffective against norovirus. Soap does not kill norovirus either, but the practice of lathering and emulsifying hands followed by rinsing effectively removes norovirus from hands. A meta-analysis of seven studies looking at the effect of handwashing with soap and water showed that the rate of transmission of diarrheal illness decreased by 47% when hand hygiene with soap and water was used.[49]

▶ **Best Practice** Use cleaning products that effectively kill norovirus when a case of diarrheal illness has been identified in team personnel.

✓ **Recommendation 1** Use a hypochlorite-, phenol-, or hydrogen peroxide–containing disinfectant to clean surfaces in direct contact or close proximity to a player(s) with acute-onset diarrheal illness.

✓ **Recommendation 2** Use a hypochlorite-, phenol-, or hydrogen peroxide–containing solution to clean all surfaces when a cluster of diarrheal illness has been identified in team personnel.

✓ **Recommendation 3** Use a hypochlorite-, phenol-, or hydrogen peroxide–containing solution to clean all surfaces until the cluster has resolved.

Rationale: Quaternary ammonium–containing solutions ("quats") are **not** effective against norovirus. In contrast, bleach, phenol, or hydrogen peroxide **is** effective.[50] Toilets are a major source of contamination from norovirus. Approximately 78% of toilets, including the seat, handles, and the area surrounding the toilet, may be contaminated following use by a patient with diarrheal illness.[51] As a result, we recommend cleaning all toilets and bathrooms with one of the above effective agents after a single player has been diagnosed with acute-onset diarrheal illness. If a Kaivac system is used to clean the facility's bathrooms, ensure the appropriate disinfectant is used in this system as well. In addition, we recommend using the same cleaning agents to clean surfaces in the training facility that are known or assumed to be contaminated from contact by the player or players with diarrheal illness.

Quats don't work against norovirus. Double-check to make sure your disinfectant is active against norovirus.

▶ **Best Practice** Educate players about the risk of acquiring diarrheal illness and changes to infection prevention practices when a case or cluster of acute-onset diarrheal illness has been identified.

✓ **Recommendation 1** Provide education to all players and team personnel when a case or cluster of diarrheal illness is identified in team personnel.

✓ **Recommendation 2** Strictly enforce a policy of no food or food containers in the locker room, bathroom, or in the treatment areas when a cluster of diarrheal illness is identified in team personnel.

Rationale: All of the recommendations in this section will require direct education of players and team personnel. More specifically, we suggest providing education regarding the following:

- Use soap and water for hand hygiene when norovirus infection is suspected. Such hygienic measures should be continued for at least 72 hours after symptoms resolve in individuals with acute illnesses compatible with norovirus infections.
- Restriction of activities of all acutely ill individuals. Players who are acutely ill or who have been ill in the preceding 24 to 36 hours should not practice or play.
- Recognition when their family members, in particular young children, have symptoms. Players who have family members with gastroenteritis can introduce norovirus into the facility.

We also advise team medical personnel to educate their players and staff to report all instances of acute illness that include vomiting and diarrhea so that the enhanced hygienic measures can be employed before a widespread outbreak occurs. Medical staff may wish to place signs outlining this basic control measure on bulletin boards and at the entrance of training facilities.

Tier 3 Interventions—Recommendations When Two or More Players Have Acute-Onset Diarrheal Illness

⊙ **Best Practice** Use more intrusive interventions to decrease risk of ongoing transmission.

⊘ **Recommendation 1** Ban food from the bathroom and treatment areas of the athletic training facility.

⊘ **Recommendation 2** Implement stricter hand hygiene and environmental disinfection requirements.

Rationale: Outbreaks of norovirus have been closely linked to food and food contaminated in the bathroom environment and in any area where vomiting occurs.[52] Thus, we suggest banning any food or food containers from the bathroom area and treatment areas when a cluster of diarrheal illness has been identified. This intervention decreases the chance food will come into contact with contaminated equipment or infected athletes.

As the number of personnel with infection increases, the risk of environmental contamination increases. Thus, when a cluster of diarrheal illness has been identified, we suggest changing the cleaning strategy throughout the facility. In such circumstances, environmental cleaning with an agent known to be effective against norovirus should be continued until the cluster has resolved (ie, until no further personnel have diarrheal symptoms >72 hours). Similarly, appropriate hand hygiene (with soap and water) must be used throughout the facility. In some instances, alcohol hand hygiene products can be removed from the facility and replaced with standard soap until no player has had symptoms of acute illness for 72 hours.

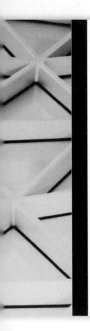

Diarrheal Illness

If more than one team member develops a diarrheal illness, enact the highest tier of infection prevention recommendations for norovirus:

1. Isolate (send home) any player(s) with acute-onset diarrheal illness to avoid contact with other personnel (until symptoms have resolved).
2. Wear gloves for all contact with players with diarrheal illness.
3. Enforce a policy of strict handwashing using soap and water among players and team personnel such as athletic trainers. Educate these individuals that use of alcohol-containing hand cleaning agents is NOT sufficient in this situation.
4. Use cleaning products that are effective against norovirus until the outbreak or cluster has resolved completely. Effective cleaning products in such a circumstance include hypochlorite- (bleach), phenol-, or hyrogen peroxide-containing product.
5. Educate players and staff about the reasons for and the importance of adherence to the above measures. Also educate players of the need to promptly report the onset of any new symptoms or signs.
6. Enforce a strict policy of no food or food containers in the training facility if a cluster of diarrhea illness occurs. Maintain this ban until the cluster or outbreak has completely resolved.

Influenza-like Illness

⊙ **Best Practice** Use a tiered contingency response protocol to guide appropriate responses when a case or cluster of respiratory or influenza-like illness occurs in team personnel.

⊘ **Recommendation 1** Develop a tiered contingency response protocol to guide appropriate responses when respiratory or influenza-like illness is detected in team personnel.

Rationale: We prefer using a tiered approach in response to an individual case or a true cluster of influenza-like or viral respiratory illness. *A sample protocol is provided in Appendix 1H.* Tier 1 recommendations include all of the standard recommendations for infection prevention provided in this manual. Tier 2 interventions can be implemented when a single case of flu-like illness occurs in a team facility. In addition to standard recommendations provided in tier 1, players should be educated and prompted to use "cough etiquette" when players or staff develop typical signs and symptoms of a respiratory tract infection.

Higher level (tier 3) recommendations for managing clusters of respiratory illness in players and/or staff must be individualized based on the likely or known diagnosis, the time of year, the presence or absence of a known outbreak of respiratory infection in the community, and the severity of observed illness. In general, we advise teams to seek input about management of such clusters from local or regional experts in infectious diseases and epidemiology. However, the following general guidelines can be utilized in assessing and managing such outbreaks:

- Make an etiologic or probable diagnosis whenever possible. Such efforts may include cultures for influenza or pertussis when appropriate.
- Symptomatic and ill individuals should be encouraged to avoid direct contact with healthy individuals whenever possible. In general, it is best to remove (ie, isolate) symptomatic/ill individuals from the training facility until the acute phase of their illness is over.
- Do not use antimicrobial therapy when the likely pathogen is viral.
- Decisions about return to full team activities should be made on a case-by-case basis by physicians.
  - In general, players with viral respiratory illness can return to training when they have been afebrile for >24 hours.
- Decisions about the utility and type of prophylaxis (eg, for influenza or pertussis) or the implementation of a teamwide vaccine program should be made by team physicians with input from infectious disease experts/epidemiologists or the local health department. Prophylaxis or vaccine use may need to be extended to household contacts of players or staff in selected cases.

Cough etiquette is simple: ill individuals should cover their mouths with a tissue or a body part when they cough, and they should promptly clean their hands when they are contaminated with respiratory secretions.

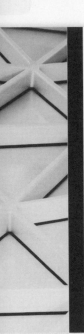

Respiratory Illness

If more than one team member develops a respiratory or flu-like illness, enact the highest tier of infection prevention recommendations for influenza:

1. Isolate any player(s) with acute flu-like illness to avoid contact with other personnel (until symptoms have resolved).
2. Obtain diagnostic tests to confirm or exclude influenza in players with flu-like symptoms during "flu season" or when documented influenza infections are known to be present in the community. This testing should consist of molecular-based tests such as PCR rather than rapid antigen tests (which lack sufficient specificity and sensitivity).
3. Do not obtain bacterial cultures in players with typical flu-like symptoms. Do not empirically give antibacterial therapy to these individuals or give antibiotics to players with typical symptoms of the common cold, sinusitis, or uncomplicated bronchitis.
4. Enforce a policy of strict handwashing using soap and water or hand cleaning with an alcohol-based agent among players and team personnel such as athletic trainers.
5. Educate players and staff about the importance of cough etiquette and the reasons for and the importance of adherence to the above measures (eg, that both droplet and hand-to-hand transmission of respiratory virus commonly occurs). Also educate players of the need to promptly report the onset of any new symptoms or signs consistent with a flu-like illness.

Hand, Foot, and Mouth Disease

▶ **Best Practice** Use a protocol to guide appropriate responses when a case or cluster of hand, foot, and mouth disease (HFMD) occurs in team personnel.

✓ **Recommendation 1** Develop a protocol to guide appropriate responses when HFMD is detected in team personnel.

Rationale: We prefer a tiered approach to guide responses when a case or cluster of HFMD occurs. Tier 1 recommendations include all of the standard recommendations for infection prevention provided in this manual. In other words, tier 1 recommendations should be followed even in the absence of any cases of HFMD. Tier 2 interventions can be implemented when a single case of HFMD occurs in a team facility. Tier 2 includes new recommendations, but all recommendations from the prior tier should still be followed. *A sample tiered contingency protocol to decrease the risk of HFMD transmission is provided in Appendix 1I.*

Outbreaks of HFMD can and do occur regularly. Most published reports of outbreaks are from settings outside of the United States, but the incidence of HFMD in the United States is on the rise. For example, an outbreak of HFMD due to coxsackievirus A6 occurred in 53 basic military trainees in 2015.[53] The patients infected during this outbreak were all young, and almost all were found to have a widespread vesiculopapular rash. Infected trainees wore masks and were isolated. No patients required hospitalization. A more extensive outbreak occurred on the east coast of the United States in 2016, particularly impacting high school students in New Jersey and Connecticut.[31] During this outbreak, numerous sporting events were canceled or postponed. Finally, we are aware of a small outbreak of HFMD that occurred in a professional football team. Impacted players were in the same practice group (eg, quarterback, center, and wide receiver). Transmission may have occurred via a contaminated football and frequent licking of hands or fingers for grip.

In light of the above routes of transmission, we recommend the following when one or more cases of HFMD are identified in the training facility:

1. Perform a thorough cleaning of the facility with particular emphasis on areas that hands encounter (eg, weights, training equipment, meeting room chairs and arm rests).
2. Implement "no exception" policy for hand hygiene.
3. Discard gloves used by players.

The benefit of isolation is controversial. In the day care setting, removal of children with HFMD does not decrease transmission, as children can shed virus before, during, and after symptoms. We suggest isolating infected players in general, but if the player cannot be removed from team activities, he or she may continue as long as afebrile and any vesiculopapular lesions can be covered.

Return to Play Guidelines for Athletes With Infectious Diseases

A frequent question among athletes with an infection is: "when can I come back to practice?"

Groups such as the National Athletic Trainers Association (NATA) have published guidance for return to play for some infections.[54] These recommendations are reviewed and expanded in this section. In addition, these recommendations should be considered as general guidance. Return to play decisions for individual players should be made by team physicians.

Skin and Soft-Tissue Infections

In general, athletes with skin infections such as cellulitis, impetigo, or abscesses due to MRSA or group Λ streptococci (*S. pyogenes*) should refrain from competition and team training activities until they have

1. started antibiotic therapy **and**
2. have had no new skin lesions for at least 48 hours **and**
3. resolution of moist, weeping, or draining purulent lesions as manifested by the presence of dry scabs.

Players with dry and crusted skin lesion may return to competition if these lesions are covered with an occlusive dressing.

Athletes with herpetic lesions (due to herpes simplex) should be excluded from practice and competition until systemic symptoms have resolved AND until resolution (drying and crusting) of all moist, oozing, or wet acute lesions of the skin and mucous membranes.

Athletes with chicken pox (varicella) should be excluded from team activities until all moist or wet skin and mucous membrane lesions have dried and crusted and there have been no acute new lesions for at least 48 hours.

Athletes such as swimmers, wrestlers, hockey players, and others involved in contact sports who have lesions consistent with molluscum contagiosum on exposed skin should avoid competition and team practices involving skin contact until the lesions have been curetted and removed. Lesions in nonexposed skin surfaces should be covered with tape or an appropriate occlusive dressing until they can be definitively treated with curettage.

Respiratory Infections

Players with pertussis should be excluded from direct close contact with team members until they have received at least 5 days of effective antibiotic therapy (usually with azithromycin) or until at least 3 weeks after the onset of cough.

Influenza

Players and team staff with influenza should not return to work until at least 24 hours after the resolution of fever (while not on antipyretics). If the infected individual still has cough, utilize cough etiquette and consider a face mask if close contact with team members is unavoidable.[55]

Diarrheal Illnesses

Athletes with norovirus infections should be excluded from all team activities until symptoms have resolved for at least 48 hours. Swimmers with diarrheal illness due to giardia or cryptosporidiosis should be excluded from training or competitive activities while ill and for 2 weeks after illness has resolved.

REFERENCES

1. Knelson LP, Williams DA, Gergen MF, et al. A comparison of environmental contamination by patients infected or colonized with methicillin-resistant *Staphylococcus aureus* or vancomycin-resistant enterococci: a multicenter study. *Infect Control Hosp Epidemiol.* 2014;35(7):872-875.

2. Nichol KL, Mendelman PM, Mallon KP, et al. Effectiveness of live, attenuated intranasal influenza virus vaccine in healthy, working adults: a randomized controlled trial. *J Am Med Assoc.* 1999;282(2):137-144.

3. Wilde JA, McMillan JA, Serwint J, Butta J, O'Riordan MA, Steinhoff MC. Effectiveness of influenza vaccine in health care professionals: a randomized trial. *J Am Med Assoc.* 1999;281(10):908-913.

4. Bridges CB, Thompson WW, Meltzer MI, et al. Effectiveness and cost-benefit of influenza vaccination of healthy working adults: a randomized controlled trial. *J Am Med Assoc.* 2000;284(13):1655-1663.

5. Grohskopf LA, Sokolow LZ, Broder KR, Walter EB, Fry AM, Jernigan DB. Prevention and control of seasonal influenza with vaccines: recommendations of the Advisory Committee on Immunization Practices-United States, 2018-19 influenza season. *MMWR Recomm Rep.* 2018;67(3):1-20.

6. Perl TM, Talbot TR. Universal influenza vaccination among healthcare personnel: yes we should. *Open Forum Infect Dis.* 2019;6(4):ofz096.

7. Foster MA, Hofmeister MG, Kupronis BA, et al. Increase in hepatitis A virus infections - United States, 2013-2018. *MMWR Morb Mortal Wkly Rep.* 2019;68(18):413-415.

8. Centers for Disease Control and Prevention. *Widespread Person-To-Person Outbreaks of Hepatitis A Across the United States;* 2019. Available at https://www.cdc.gov/hepatitis/outbreaks/2017March-HepatitisA.htm. Accessed September 13, 2019.

9. Gartner BC, Meyer T. Vaccination in elite athletes. *Sports Med.* 2014;44(10):1361-1376.

10. Kashiwagi S, Hayashi J, Ikematsu H, Nishigori S, Ishihara K, Kaji M. An outbreak of hepatitis B in members of a high school sumo wrestling club. *J Am Med Assoc.* 1982;248(2):213-214.

11. Tobe K, Matsuura K, Ogura T, et al. Horizontal transmission of hepatitis B virus among players of an American football team. *Arch Intern Med.* 2000;160(16):2541-2545.

12. Ringertz O, Zetterberg B. Serum hepatitis among Swedish track finders. An epidemiologic study. *N Engl J Med.* 1967;276(10):540-546.

13. Fitzsimons D, Francois G, Hall A, et al. Long-term efficacy of hepatitis B vaccine, booster policy, and impact of hepatitis B virus mutants. *Vaccine.* 2005;23(32):4158-4166.

14. Baker CH, Brennan JM. Keeping health-care workers healthy. Legal aspects of hepatitis B immunization programs. *N Engl J Med.* 1984;311(10):684-688.

15. Centers for Disease Control and Prevention. *Vaccine Information Statement - DTaP (Diphtheria, Tetanus, Pertussis) Vaccine: What You Need to Know;* 2019. Available at https://www.cdc.gov/vaccines/hcp/vis/vis-statements/dtap.pdf. Accessed September 15, 2019.

16. Centers for Disease Control and Prevention. *Tdap (Tetanus, Diphtheria, Pertussis) Vaccine Information Statement;* 2019. Available at https://www.cdc.gov/vaccines/hcp/vis/vis-statements/tdap.html. Accessed September 15, 2019.

17. Burgess MA, McIntyre PB, Heath TC. Pertussis re-emerging: who is responsible? *Aust N Z J Public Health*. 1998;22(1):9-10.

18. Storsaeter J, Hallander HO, Gustafsson L, Olin P. Low levels of anti-pertussis antibodies plus lack of history of pertussis correlate with susceptibility after household exposure to *Bordetella pertussis. Vaccine*. 2003;21:3542-3549.

19. Forsyth K. Pertussis, still a formidable foe. *Clin Infect Dis*. 2007;45(11):1487-1491.

20. Kretsinger K, Broder KR, Cortese MM, et al. Preventing tetanus, diphtheria, and pertussis among adults: use of tetanus toxoid, reduced diphtheria toxoid and acellular pertussis vaccine recommendations of the Advisory Committee on Immunization Practices (ACIP) and recommendation of ACIP, supported by the Healthcare Infection Control Practices Advisory Committee (HICPAC), for use of Tdap among health-care personnel. *MMWR Recomm Rep*. 2006;55(RR-17):1-37.

21. De Serres G, Shadmani R, Duval B, et al. Morbidity of pertussis in adolescents and adults. *J Infect Dis*. 2000;182(1):174-179.

22. Lee GM, Lett S, Schauer S, et al. Societal costs and morbidity of pertussis in adolescents and adults. *Clin Infect Dis*. 2004;39(11):1572-1580.

23. Thomas PF, McIntyre PB, Jalaludin BB. Survey of pertussis morbidity in adults in western Sydney. *Med J Aust*. 2000;173(2):74-76.

24. Trollfors B, Rabo E. Whooping cough in adults. *Br Med J*. 1981;283(6293):696-697.

25. Skrzypiec-Spring M, Krzywanski J, Karlikowska-Skwarnik M, et al. Pertussis outbreak in Polish shooters with adverse event analysis. *Biol Sport*. 2017;34(3):243-248.

26. Pellegrino P, Carnovale C, Perrone V, et al. Epidemiological analysis on two decades of hospitalisations for meningitis in the United States. *Eur J Clin Microbiol Infect Dis*. 2014;33(9): 1519-1524.

27. Centers for Disease Control and Prevention. *Vaccine Information Statement - MMR Vaccine (Measles, Mumps, and Rubella): What You Need to Know*. 2019. Available at https://www.cdc.gov/vaccines/hcp/vis/vis-statements/mmr.pdf. Accessed September 15, 2019.

28. Centers for Disease Control and Prevention. Multistate measles outbreak associated with an international youth sporting event–Pennsylvania, Michigan, and Texas, August-September 2007. *MMWR Morb Mortal Wkly Rep*. 2008;57(7):169-173.

29. Centers for Disease Control and Prevention. *Measles Cases and Outbreaks*; 2019. Available at https://www.cdc.gov/measles/cases-outbreaks.html. Accessed September 21, 2019.

30. Centers for Disease Control and Prevention. *Mumps Cases and Outbreaks*; 2019. Available at https://www.cdc.gov/mumps/outbreaks.html. Accessed September 21, 2019.

31. *Three More Schools Infected by 'unprecedented' Hand-Foot-And-Mouth Disease Outbreak*; 2016. Available at http://highschoolsports.nj.com/news/article/-3132375131977714380/unprecedented-hand-foot-and-mouth-disease-outbreak-reported-at-shore-conference-school/. Accessed June 1, 2019.

32. Golwalkar M, Pope B, Stauffer J, Snively A, Clemmons N. Mumps outbreaks at four universities - Indiana, 2016. *MMWR Morb Mortal Wkly Rep*. 2018;67(29):793-797.

33. Conway JJ, Toresdahl BG, Ling DI, Boniquit NT, Callahan LR, Kinderknecht JJ. Prevalence of inadequate immunity to measles, mumps, rubella, and varicella in MLB and NBA athletes. *Sports Health*. 2018;10(5):406-411.

34. Fraser DW, Tsai TR, Orenstein W, et al. Legionnaires' disease: description of an epidemic of pneumonia. *N Engl J Med*. 1977;297(22):1189-1197.

35. Centers for Disease C. Pneumocystis pneumonia–Los Angeles. *MMWR Morb Mortal Wkly Rep*. 1981;30(21):250-252.

36. Fritz SA, Camins BC, Eisenstein KA, et al. Effectiveness of measures to eradicate *Staphylococcus aureus* carriage in patients with community-associated skin and soft-tissue infections: a randomized trial. *Infect Control Hosp Epidemiol*. 2011;32(9):872-880.

37. Miller LG, Daum RS, Creech CB, et al. Clindamycin versus trimethoprim-sulfamethoxazole for uncomplicated skin infections. *N Engl J Med*. 2015;372(12):1093-1103.

38. Edmiston CE Jr, Seabrook GR, Johnson CP, Paulson DS, Beausoleil CM. Comparative of a new and innovative 2% chlorhexidine gluconate-impregnated cloth with 4% chlorhexidine gluconate as topical antiseptic for preparation of the skin prior to surgery. *Am J Infect Control*. 2007;35(2):89-96.

39. Huang SS, Septimus E, Kleinman K, et al. Targeted versus universal decolonization to prevent ICU infection. *N Engl J Med*. 2013;368(24):2255-2265.

40. O'Horo JC, Silva GL, Munoz-Price LS, Safdar N. The efficacy of daily bathing with chlorhexidine for reducing healthcare-associated bloodstream infections: a meta-analysis. *Infect Control Hosp Epidemiol*. 2012;33(3):257-267.

41. Block C, Robenshtok E, Simhon A, Shapiro M. Evaluation of chlorhexidine and povidone iodine activity against methicillin-resistant *Staphylococcus aureus* and vancomycin-resistant *Enterococcus faecalis* using a surface test. *J Hosp Infect*. 2000;46(2):147-152.

42. Moran GJ, Krishnadasan A, Gorwitz RJ, et al. Methicillin-resistant *S. aureus* infections among patients in the emergency department. *N Engl J Med*. 2006;355(7):666-674.

43. Kazakova SV, Hageman JC, Matava M, et al. A clone of methicillin-resistant *Staphylococcus aureus* among professional football players. *N Engl J Med*. 2005;352(5):468-475.

44. Oller AR, Province L, Curless B. *Staphylococcus aureus* recovery from environmental and human locations in 2 collegiate athletic teams. *J Athl Train.* 2010;45(3):222-229.

45. Hamilton HW, Hamilton KR, Lone FJ. Preoperative hair removal. *Can J Surg.* 1977;20(3):269-271, 274-265.

46. King CK, Glass R, Bresee JS, Duggan C. Managing acute gastroenteritis among children: oral rehydration, maintenance, and nutritional therapy. *MMWR Recomm Rep.* 2003;52(RR-16):1-16.

47. Abisheganaden JA, Avila PC, Kishiyama JL, et al. Effect of clarithromycin on experimental rhinovirus-16 colds: a randomized, double-blind, controlled trial. *Am J Med.* 2000;108(6):453-459.

48. *Management of Multidrug-Resistant Organisms in Healthcare Settings, 2006.* 2006. Available at http://www.cdc.gov/hicpac/pdf/MDRO/MDROGuideline2006.pdf. Accessed July 14, 2014.

49. Curtis V, Cairncross S. Effect of washing hands with soap on diarrhoea risk in the community: a systematic review. *Lancet Infect Dis.* 2003;3(5):275-281.

50. Centers for Disease Control and Prevention. Outbreaks of gastroenteritis associated with noroviruses on cruise ships–United States, 2002. *MMWR Morb Mortal Wkly Rep.* 2002;51(49):1112-1115.

51. Verani M, Bigazzi R, Carducci A. Viral contamination of aerosol and surfaces through toilet use in health care and other settings. *Am J Infect Control.* 2014;42(7):758-762.

52. Repp KK, Keene WE. A point-source norovirus outbreak caused by exposure to fomites. *J Infect Dis.* 2012;205(11):1639-1641.

53. Banta J, Lenz B, Pawlak M, et al. Notes from the field: outbreak of hand, foot, and mouth disease caused by Coxsackievirus A6 among basic military trainees - Texas, 2015. *MMWR Morb Mortal Wkly Rep.* 2016;65(26):678-680.

54. Zinder SM, Basler RS, Foley J, Scarlata C, Vasily DB. National athletic trainers' association position statement: skin diseases. *J Athl Train.* 2010;45(4):411-428.

55. Centers for Disease Control and Prevention. *Prevention Strategies for Seasonal Influenza in Healthcare Settings - Guidelines and Recommendations.* 2018. Available at https://www.cdc.gov/flu/professionals/infectioncontrol/healthcaresettings.htm. Accessed June 1, 2019.

6

Infection Risks From Shared Equipment

Christopher J. Hostler | Deverick J. Anderson

Introduction

Athletic equipment and facilities are a potential source of indirect disease transmission (**Figure 6.1**). As we've discussed throughout this book, athletes are commonly colonized with highly pathogenic organisms such as methicillin-resistant *Staphylococcus aureus* (MRSA). Interestingly, athletes tend to carry these organisms on their hands, rather than in more remote locations such as the groin or armpits, where hospitalized patients tend to be colonized.[1] Every time an athlete touches a surface, they deposit organisms onto that surface. This contamination can lead to disease transmission, as the next athlete or staff member to touch the same surface can acquire the previously deposited organisms and become colonized or infected.

Disease transmission through the environment occurs regularly in hospital settings. Patients in rooms previously occupied by other patients who have infections with important pathogens such as *Clostridioides difficile* and MRSA are at significantly greater risk of acquiring these pathogens during their hospital stay.[2,3] Healthcare providers routinely use "isolation precautions," which include the use of gowns and gloves, among other barrier precautions, to reduce the risk of transmission of these important pathogens from one patient to another. These transmission dynamics occur among athletes and the training environment as well.

Basic Premises of Cleaning and Disinfection

Given the type and intensity of care provided in athletic training facilities, athletic facilities and athletic equipment should be cleaned and disinfected using the same strategies and recommendations used to clean and disinfect healthcare facilities and medical equipment. Given similarities in colonization risk and environmental exposures between athletes and hospitalized

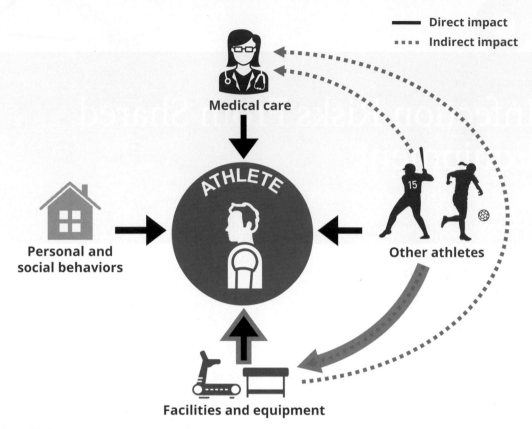

Figure 6.1 Equipment can serve as an indirect route of transmission between athletes.

patients, the need is all the greater. In that vein, we suggest following these basic best practices of cleaning and disinfection:

1. Use **EPA-registered cleaning and disinfection products** to perform routine disinfection of athletic facilities.
2. Apply disinfectant chemicals to surfaces for the appropriate amount of **contact time.**
3. Develop a standard cleaning and disinfection **protocol** that identifies who is responsible for routine cleaning, which products should be used on specific surfaces, and when cleaning should take place.

Tips and Advice

- Minimize the types and brands of disinfectant chemicals used in the facility. In our experience, numerous types of disinfectant chemicals are available for use at most training facilities, which can lead to confusion and misuse when disinfection is required. Pick one to be used throughout the facility.

- Make sure that cleaning and professional staff know that bleach-containing or hydrogen peroxide–containing solutions should be used for blood or body fluid spills and when clusters of infections due to norovirus occur.

- Storage of disinfectant solutions should occur in well-designed (safe and convenient) and consistent designated locations so that replacements can easily and conveniently be accessed.

⊙ **Best Practice** Use EPA-registered disinfection products to perform routine disinfection of athletic facilities.

⊘ **Recommendation 1** Use a quaternary ammonium–containing solution, a bleach-containing solution, or a hydrogen peroxide–containing solution for routine disinfection of surfaces in the training facility or when surfaces are visibly soiled.

Rationale: Training facilities should only use "hospital-grade" disinfectants registered by the Environmental Protection Agency (EPA) to "ensure chemical potency, materials compatibility, and safety." EPA-registered chemicals are recommended by the Centers for Disease Control and Prevention (CDC) for cleaning and disinfecting both routine surfaces and visibly soiled surfaces in healthcare facilities.[4]

A list of the EPA-registered disinfectants is available online through the EPA website (https://www.epa.gov/pesticide-registration/selected-epa-registered-disinfectants). Regardless of which product is used, we prefer the use of premixed bottles instead of concentrated disinfectants that require dilution in order to eliminate error related to mixing.

The most common EPA-registered disinfecting agents for surfaces in healthcare facilities include quaternary ammonium–containing solutions ("quats"), bleach-containing solutions, and hydrogen peroxide–containing solutions. All three products are effective against a wide variety of human pathogens. In fact, all three are equally effective against vegetative bacteria (including MRSA) and the vast majority of viruses. They do not, however, have equal effectiveness against two important causes of diarrhea: *C. difficile* spores and certain viruses such as norovirus. There are several advantages and disadvantages to each product.

Quats are the preferred disinfectant at most hospitals in the United States for routine disinfection of environmental surfaces because they are nontoxic to exposed skin, less corrosive to medical devices and equipment than other disinfectants, and cheap. These properties make quaternary ammonium compounds ideal for cleaning and disinfecting contaminated "high-touch" surfaces and equipment. Quats are ineffective, however, against some bacteria such as *C. difficile* and viruses such as norovirus.[5] In addition, the antimicrobial activity of quats can be reduced by dilution using "hard water" or by using cotton towels or gauze pads to apply these chemicals.[6]

Bleach-containing solutions are the second most commonly used EPA-registered disinfectant in hospitals. Bleach has several advantages over other disinfecting agents. Bleach-containing solutions have a broad spectrum of antimicrobial activity, they do not leave toxic residues on surfaces, and they are unaffected by water "hardness." In addition, bleach-containing solutions are inexpensive, fast-acting, and effectively remove dried organisms and biofilms from surfaces.[7] However, bleach-containing solutions also have disadvantages. Bleach-containing solutions can corrode metal surfaces, produce toxic chlorine gas when mixed with ammonia or acid, discolor fabrics, and irritate the mucous membranes of the eyes, mouth, and stomach when exposure is prolonged or intense. Bleach is also easily inactivated by organic materials.

EPA-registered disinfectant solutions containing hydrogen peroxide are less commonly used as a hospital disinfectant. Like bleach, most hydrogen peroxide–containing disinfectants have activity against *C. difficile* and norovirus. Hydrogen peroxide has one specific advantage over other disinfectants: it enhances the removal of organic matter and organisms from contaminated surfaces.[6] Hydrogen peroxide is also odorless, has a broad spectrum of antimicrobial activity, decomposes into water and oxygen, and is thus safe and nontoxic. However, use of currently available hydrogen peroxide–containing solutions can be irritating to the eye if splash exposure or other direct contact with the sclera or conjunctiva occurs. While hydrogen peroxide is generally more expensive than quaternary ammonium–containing and bleach-containing disinfectants, it represents the best combination of characteristics of EPA-registered disinfectants.

Quick Tips for Disinfection in the Athletic Training Environment

- Use an EPA-registered disinfectant
  - Apply with a microfiber cloth, especially if using a quaternary ammonium–containing disinfectant (a "quat")
- Ensure the disinfectant remains wet on the surface for the appropriate contact time—typically at least 1 minute
  - Don't apply and immediately wipe!
  - Even better, let disinfectants air dry
  - Liquid disinfectants are more reliable than foam disinfectants, which typically have longer contact times

✓ **Recommendation 2** Use microfiber cloths to disinfect surfaces if a quaternary ammonium–containing disinfectant is used.

Rationale: Microfiber cloths made with polyester and polyamide (nylon) threads are highly effective and should be used for all types of disinfection when a quaternary ammonium–containing solution is used. More specifically, we recommend using microfiber cloths for daily, routine disinfection of the facility and when equipment and treatment areas are disinfected between players. Microfibers are now widely used in clothing, shoes, accessories, upholstery and other textiles, industrial filters, and cleaning products.

Microfiber cloths have two specific properties that make them superior to cotton cloths in routine disinfection. First, microfiber cloths have phenomenal absorptive properties. A microfiber cloth can absorb up to six times its weight in water. Second, microfiber cloths have unique electrodynamic properties that allow them to lift and remove debris from a surface. Negatively charged dirt and dust are attracted to and retained by the positively charged microfibers until the microfiber cloth undergoes laundering.

Microfiber cloths effectively reduce the quantity of MRSA, *Escherichia coli*, and *C. difficile* by up to 99% from stainless steel, furniture laminate, and ceramic tile.[8] In contrast, cotton cloths remove only 30%.[9] Additionally, microfiber products more effectively deliver disinfectant solution to surfaces.[10] Cotton and gauze pads absorb and bind the active ingredients in quaternary ammonium–containing disinfectants and deliver less of the solution to a surface. Over time, a cotton cloth will release half of the amount of quaternary ammonium compound present in the original disinfectant.[11] In contrast, a microfiber cloth will release 85% of the amount of quaternary ammonium compound in the original disinfectant.

Microfiber cloths remove more bacteria than cotton towels.

✓ **Recommendation 3** Follow the manufacturer's instructions for use and laundering of microfiber cloths.

✓ **Recommendation 4** Replace microfiber cloths used for disinfection at least annually.

Rationale: Disinfection with and laundering of microfiber products require different techniques compared to standard cleaning materials. Traditional cotton mop pads, for example, are repeatedly placed in buckets with water and disinfectant and "wrung out" before each use. This "wringing out" process may occur up to 75 times during a typical work shift when a cotton mop is used, leading to contamination of the disinfectant solution.[12] In contrast, microfiber cloths and microfiber mop pads should be placed in a basin or bucket of disinfectant and removed one at a time for use. After use, the microfiber product is placed in a "used" bucket. In other words, microfiber cloths are designed to be used once and then laundered before subsequent use to prevent the transfer of microbes via contamination of disinfectants. A single standard-sized microfiber mop pad is sufficient to mop an average hospital room (~320 sq. ft); more mop pads are required for larger rooms such as the training room. Finally, it is also important to note that bleach degrades microfiber products. Thus, bleach-containing solutions should not be used with microfiber cloths and mops.

Though some microfiber cloths can be washed in regular washing machines, most microfiber cloths require a special laundering process that varies slightly depending on the brand of microfiber cloth. In particular, fabric softeners and bleach should not be used to launder these products. Similarly, water temperature should not exceed 160°F to avoid damaging the cloths. Microfiber mops can withstand over 300 standard laundering cycles in a washing machine, whereas the conventional cotton string mop withstands approximately 75 laundering cycles.[11] Refer to the manufacturer's recommendations regarding how many uses each microfiber product can withstand before losing its effectiveness.

Microfiber products should be replaced a minimum of once each year.

✅ **Recommendation 5** Use EPA-registered disinfectants on nonporous materials and launder porous materials.

✅ **Recommendation 6** Avoid use of porous materials that cannot be laundered (eg, wood, marble).

Rationale: Nonporous surfaces used throughout the facility (eg, vinyl, stainless steel, ceramic) should be disinfected with EPA-registered disinfectants, as outlined above. Occasionally, manufacturers may recommend that nonporous materials not undergo disinfection due to potential aesthetic concerns (eg, stainless steel adjacent to a shake station). We disagree with this approach, and strongly believe that all nonporous surfaces should undergo routine disinfection. All porous material used in the facility (eg, textiles) should be laundered with an appropriate disinfectant. Porous materials that cannot be laundered (eg, wood, marble) should not be used. Avoid use of these materials in player areas, if possible.

✅ **Recommendation 7** Use electrostatic sprayers to perform nightly disinfection throughout the facility.

Rationale: Electrostatic sprayers apply a positive charge to the disinfectant, which results in greater adherence to negatively charged (eg, metallic) surfaces. Essentially, electrostatic sprayers allow you to effectively apply disinfectant to "hard-to-reach" surfaces without directly visualizing those surfaces, as the disinfectant will "wrap around" the surface completely. Given the number of surfaces in an athletic training facility, even the most diligent cleaning staffs are unlikely to be able to apply an appropriate amount of disinfectant to every surface every night. Electrostatic sprayers may provide an additional layer of protection for your facility. Please note that while electrostatic sprayers may be a useful adjunct to routine cleaning, use of these devices should NOT replace routine cleaning.

▶ **Best Practice** Apply disinfectant chemicals to surfaces for the appropriate amount of contact time.

✓ **Recommendation 1** Ensure disinfectant chemicals are left on surfaces for an adequate amount of time to achieve appropriate killing of microorganisms.

Rationale: "Contact time" refers to the amount of time that a surface needs to remain wet with the disinfectant in order for pathogens to be eradicated. Disinfectants are not effective if they are simply sprayed on surfaces and immediately wiped off. Contact time is printed on all EPA-registered disinfectants. EPA-registered contact times are generally very conservative (up to 10 minutes) and include the time required to kill hardy microbes like *Mycobacterium tuberculosis* and spores. In our experience, strict adherence to the EPA-registered contact time is rarely followed in healthcare settings for general disinfection purposes. In fact, hospital-grade disinfectant contact times of 1 minute are sufficient against the vast majority of healthcare-associated pathogens relevant to the athletic training environment (eg, vegetative bacteria like MRSA).[6,13,14] Thus, while we don't believe that adherence to such conservative contact times is necessary for routine use in a training facility, it is nevertheless important to ensure that disinfectant remains visibly wet for at least 1 minute. In the event that a player has an uncommon infection such as *C. difficile*, longer contact times may be needed (ie, 2-3 minutes, depending on the disinfectant).

Disinfectants are not effective if they are simply sprayed on surfaces and immediately wiped off.

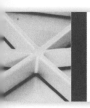

Standard cleaning protocols should contain the following information:
- Who is responsible for routine cleaning of the training facility?
- Which environmental cleaning products should be used for specific surfaces?
- When cleaning should take place (eg, time and frequency)?

▶ **Best Practice** Develop a standard cleaning and disinfection protocol that identifies who is responsible for routine cleaning, which products should be used on specific surfaces, and when cleaning should take place.

✓ **Recommendation 1** Develop a written protocol that addresses how often the facility is cleaned and by whom.

✓ **Recommendation 2** Use a professional cleaning company to perform routine cleaning of your facility, if possible.

✓ **Recommendation 3** Perform routine cleaning of all areas of the training facility a minimum of once daily.

✓ **Recommendation 4** Document that daily cleaning has been performed upon completion.

Rationale: The CDC describes cleaning and disinfecting environmental services as "fundamental in reducing the incidence of healthcare-associated infections."[7] Environmental cleaning agents kill bacteria and viruses that can make your players and staff sick. Environmental cleaning protocols standardize the approach for cleaning used at the healthcare facility.[7,15]

Environmental cleaning in healthcare settings is frequently inadequate. For example, studies using bioluminescent markers to document whether a specific surface was or was not physically cleaned demonstrate that as many as 50% of surfaces in hospitals are inadequately cleaned.[16] This study illustrates the limitations of environmental cleaning. Thus, we recommend that athletic facilities use a professional cleaning company to perform routine cleaning of the facility. Regardless of whether the housekeeper is employed by a professional cleaning company or not, housekeepers must receive specific education regarding appropriate chemical use and safety. The entire training facility should be thoroughly cleaned and disinfected at least once each day. Finally, we advocate for specific documentation of cleaning.

If a professional company is employed for cleaning and disinfection of the facility, we recommend consulting with the company to determine if and how daily cleaning will be documented. If housekeepers are directly employed by the facility, provide housekeepers with the protocol for cleaning and disinfection of the facility. One potential strategy is to use a daily cleaning checklist. If you are unable to hire a professional cleaning service, this checklist can nevertheless be completed by the person(s) responsible for cleaning the facility to encourage appropriate cleaning techniques. In acute care hospitals, checklists improve patient care,[17] ensure adherence to best practices, and remind staff which areas need to be cleaned. Daily cleaning checklists are recommended by the American Society for Health Care Engineering (ASHE) for all hospitals. Since our goal is to bring hospital-grade disinfection to athletic facilities, we believe that utilizing these checklists may be similarly helpful for athletic teams.[18]

Cleaning and Disinfection of Athletic Equipment

The main purpose of cleaning and disinfecting personal athletic equipment is to reduce the likelihood of reinoculating a player with a pathogen he/she may have picked up during the course of their athletic activity. For athletes who compete in contact sports, cleaning and disinfection of personal athletic equipment also reduce the likelihood of transmitting pathogens between athletes. Transmission of pathogens and germs via shared or individual-use equipment is a type of indirect transmission. In this section, we'll discuss best practices and recommendations for cleaning textiles and other athletic equipment to decrease the risk of indirect transmission of germs.

▶ **Best Practice** Disinfect laundry to prevent transmission of potentially infectious organisms.

✓ **Recommendation 1** Use disinfectants in all laundry cycles for all textiles and porous materials.

✓ **Recommendation 2** Use a professional laundry service to provide appropriate amounts of detergents and disinfectants in each cycle, if possible.

✓ **Recommendation 3** Develop and use preprogrammed laundry cycles for different types of laundry.

✓ **Recommendation 4** Use the checklist provided in *Appendix 2A* to ensure the laundry service meets appropriate standards for textile cleaning and disinfection.

Rationale: Overall, the risk of transmission of pathogens through clothing and textiles is extremely low. This very low risk can be essentially eliminated, however, with appropriate handling and disinfection of laundry.

Pathogens such as MRSA and *C. difficile* can persist on inanimate objects such as soiled clothing, but the risk of transmission of bacteria through laundry is small. Traditionally, laundry disinfection has been achieved through high-temperature wash cycles (>160°F). Hot temperatures, however, are infrequently achieved in industrial or home washers. Several carefully performed studies have demonstrated that levels of microbial killing similar to those achieved with high-temperature wash cycles can be achieved at lower water temperatures (22°C to 50°C or 72°F to 122°F) *when disinfectant solutions are added.*[19-21] The authors of these studies emphasized that the three critically important factors in achieving an appropriate reduction in the bacterial bioburden were:

1. Agitation and dilution
2. Addition of disinfectant
3. Passage through a drying cycle

Thus, low-temperature washing with appropriate disinfectants and drying is as effective as high-temperature washing for eliminating pathogens from laundry. As a result, laundry soiled with blood or body fluids can be effectively disinfected in standard laundry cycles that use disinfectants.

Many athletic facilities contract with professional laundry companies (eg, Proctor & Gamble, Ecolab, ISS, etc). These companies provide preset cycles for different types of laundry loads to ensure that appropriate amounts of chemicals and, most importantly, disinfectants are added. In our experience, however, many professional laundry companies do not routinely include disinfectants in ALL laundry cycles. If you use a professional laundry service, contact your service to ensure (1) they provide a disinfectant in their laundry cycles and (2) the disinfectant is included in *each* load. Some companies include a specific disinfectant while others rely on a color-safe bleach product with an appropriately high concentration of hydrogen peroxide; either approach is acceptable.

Although contracting with a professional service is not absolutely necessary, a well-defined and systematic approach to laundry disinfection is required to achieve adequate textile disinfection. If you're unable to contract with a professional laundry service, encourage your athletes to use a disinfectant with each load of athletic textiles. If they're laundering their jerseys or equipment at home, then adding a disinfectant is especially important, as home-based washing machines will not have an adequate temperature to disinfect laundry. Home-based washing machines rely on the home's hot water heater, which is typically set between 120°F and 140°F.

We recommend using the checklist in ***Appendix 2A*** to ensure that your laundry service is meeting the applicable standards set forth by the Healthcare Laundry Accreditation Council (HLAC).[21] If your laundry service is already HLAC accredited, this process does not need to be repeated.

✅ **Recommendation 5** Develop and use a policy to keep clean and dirty laundry separated at all times.

Rationale: Equipment managers (or other assigned staff) can use various methods to keep dirty laundry separated from clean laundry. These methods include using color-coded bins (eg, black bins are for dirty laundry, yellow bins are for clean laundry) or the use of separate, clearly designated or labeled areas where clean and dirty laundry are stored. Either method is equally effective. Regardless of which method is used, we recommend that equipment managers specifically write a policy to guide this process. This policy may simply include a summary of current practices if it allows for easy review and education of new employees.

⊘ Recommendation 6 Reusable athletic equipment that cannot be washed and dried in commercial washers and dryers should be appropriately disinfected after it is used, visibly soiled, or otherwise dirty.

Rationale: Some equipment includes a combination of porous and nonporous materials. Appropriate disinfection of this type of equipment is challenging. Fortunately, reusable athletic equipment (eg, helmets and pads) presents a minimal risk of transmission of infectious agents, especially when assigned to an individual. Routine drying, cleaning, and disinfection (wiping with a disinfectant) of such equipment are most likely safe and satisfactory. Importantly, there have been reports of skin burns among football players following the use of quaternary-ammonium disinfectants to clean shoulder pads. Therefore, equipment managers must be cautious when choosing which specific cleaning and disinfecting agent to use. While many agents can be used for this purpose, equipment managers or designated individuals should inspect the labels of the disinfectants under consideration to determine if skin contact is recommended. If not, equipment managers need to wipe the equipment with water after applying the disinfectant.

Cleaning with self-contained/closed units that utilize ozone as a disinfectant is a common practice in athletic facilities. We are unaware of any clinical data demonstrating that ozone disinfection of equipment leads to a decreased risk of transmission or infection (although it is a relatively effective disinfectant). Ozone disinfection requires high humidity, can be corrosive, and can be potentially toxic to humans (safe exposure level in the United States is <0.1 ppm), so effective containment of the gas and strict adherence to manufacturer's instructions must be achieved. Nevertheless, the use of ozone cleaning methods for equipment may have secondary benefits such as odor reduction/control and better acceptance by players.

Cleaning and Disinfection of Medical Equipment and Facilities

The main purpose of cleaning and disinfecting medical equipment and facilities is to reduce the likelihood of transmitting pathogens from one player to another via indirect transmission. Athletes spend a lot of time in athletic facilities, which puts them at greater risk of acquiring pathogens from the athletic facility environment. Moreover, there have been many documented outbreaks of infections related to athletic facilities. For example, outbreaks of *Pseudomonas aeruginosa* skin infections, norovirus, adenovirus, enterovirus, and hepatitis A have all been associated with therapy pools.[22,23] In this section, we discuss best practices and recommendations for cleaning and disinfecting medical equipment and facilities to decrease the risk of indirect transmission of germs in different locations throughout the facility.

Athletic Training Room Best Practices and Recommendations

▶ Best Practice Disinfect treatment and training equipment after each player use.

⊘ Recommendation 1 Clean and disinfect training and nonmedical treatment equipment after use by individual players.

Rationale: In addition to the regular nightly cleaning previously recommended and described, we recommend that training and nonmedical treatment equipment undergo cleaning and disinfection after use by an individual player. The vast majority of equipment described in this section are classified as "noncritical items," defined as surfaces or equipment that come into contact with intact skin but not mucous membranes.[6] Intact skin is an effective barrier against most bacteria and viruses. Thus, sterility of these items is *not* required. Instead, disinfection is sufficient to reduce the risk of pathogen transmission.

Cleaning and disinfection of surfaces and training (nonmedical) equipment in the training room performed by athletic trainers should follow the basic tenets and recommendations provided in the best practices described previously in this chapter.

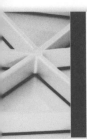

Don't Forget

Cleaning and disinfection should follow these principles:

- Use EPA-registered disinfection products.
- Use microfiber cloths to apply quaternary ammonium–containing disinfectant solutions.
- Ensure the disinfectant chemicals are applied with a sufficient "contact time" to provide appropriate activity against bacteria and viruses (eg, at least 1 minute).

Recommendation 2 Ensure that appropriate disinfectants are available in convenient and consistent locations in the training facility.

Recommendation 3 Assign responsibility for cleaning and disinfection of nonmedical equipment after use.

Rationale: Compliance with principles and policies of disinfection requires that disinfection products are stored in convenient and consistent locations so that they are quickly accessible when needed for routine cleaning and disinfection. Specifically, these cleaning products should be available in *each* area of the training facility where their use is indicated (eg, the taping, treatment, and rehabilitation areas of the training room; examination and procedure rooms; weight room; locker room; etc) rather than exclusively stored in a single or central location.

The responsibility of cleaning and disinfecting nonmedical equipment used in each area of the facility should be clearly and formally assigned to designated individuals. Athletic trainers and their designees should be primarily responsible for disinfecting equipment after use by individual players in the training room; other personnel may take responsibility for cleaning equipment in other areas of the facility (eg, food service areas, meeting rooms, lounges, and weight rooms). For example, strength and conditioning coaches may be responsible for disinfection of equipment in the weight room, and designated cleaning personnel may be given responsibility in the locker room.

Recommendation 4 Disinfect taping tables after each taping session (ie, not necessarily between each player within the same session).

Recommendation 5 Disinfect treatment tables after each use.

Rationale: We realize that it usually is not practical to disinfect taping beds and chairs between each player during high-volume taping sessions. Fortunately, routine taping sessions pose minimal risk to players; however, taping tables should be disinfected, at minimum, after each taping session. Additional disinfection should be performed after any player contacts surfaces with skin that is not intact. In contrast to taping sessions, treatment sessions generally involve player contact with treatment beds or tables for longer durations and are more likely to involve surface contact with skin. Therefore, these surfaces should be cleaned with an appropriate disinfectant after *each* player's treatment session.

✓ **Recommendation 6** Disinfect treatment equipment (eg, NormaTec, Game Ready, Graston devices, HawkGrips, ultrasound probes, and electrostimulation equipment) after each use.

✓ **Recommendation 7** Ensure each player uses individual electrostimulation pads.

✓ **Recommendation 8** Launder hydrocollator pads after each use.

Rationale: Nonmedical treatment equipment has close (and at times prolonged) contact with players' skin. Therefore, such items require cleaning and disinfection after each use. Quaternary ammonium–containing wipes may be easier to use than spray bottles of solution to clean some of these items. Electrostimulation pads cannot be routinely disinfected and consequently should be used by only one player. Hydrocollator pads should ideally be laundered after each use, particularly if they are applied directly to the skin without use of a clean towel barrier.

Special Recommendation for Athletic Trainers Who Work with Wrestlers

✓ **Recommendation** Disinfect wrestling mats between matches or practice sessions to reduce the risk of transmitting infections such as herpes simplex virus (HSV) and MRSA.

Rationale: Wrestling confers significant risk of athlete-to-athlete transmission of infectious diseases due to prolonged skin-to-skin contact and the high frequency with which athletes suffer abrasions. Many of the organisms that can be passed directly from athlete to athlete can also pass from athlete to wrestling mat to athlete. During practices or wrestling meets, subsequent athletes who use the wrestling mat may contract an infection. There are several studies that have demonstrated that wrestlers are commonly colonized with MRSA and that wrestling mats can become contaminated with MRSA or HSV during use.[1,24-26] In order to reduce the risk of transmission, we recommend that mats be disinfected with an EPA-approved disinfectant between practice sessions or matches. A study performed at Ohio Northern University between 2013 and 2014 demonstrated that (1) mats quickly became contaminated during use but (2) by using the "backward mopping" technique (applying disinfectant with a mop while walking backward so as not to step on the surface during the required contact time), the bioburden on the mat was reduced by over 75% throughout the course of the competition.[27]

Weight Room Best Practices and Recommendations

▶ **Best Practice** Perform routine disinfection in the weight room after each lifting session.

✓ **Recommendation 1** Disinfect all equipment after team workout sessions.

✓ **Recommendation 2** Provide clean towels to players as they enter the weight room. Instruct players to use these towels as barriers when using equipment.

✓ **Recommendation 3** Instruct players to wipe down equipment after each use.

✓ **Recommendation 4** If equipment becomes visibly soiled, use an appropriate EPA-registered disinfectant to clean and disinfect the equipment.

✓ **Recommendation 5** Inspect vinyl surfaces for cracks/defects and replace/repair if identified.

○ **Recommendation 6** Use electrostatic sprayers to perform nightly disinfection in the weight room.

Rationale: Players should use clean towels when using weight room equipment to decrease direct skin contact with surfaces. It may not be practical to clean surfaces with disinfectants after use by each player during high-volume workout sessions, but players should wipe equipment down with towels after each use. If equipment becomes visibly soiled, however, it should be cleaned with an appropriate disinfectant and wiped after the specified contact time. Strength coaches or other athletic staff should be responsible for appropriately disinfecting all weight room equipment at the conclusion of team workout sessions.

Bacteria can survive for extended time periods on vinyl surfaces.[28] This longevity may be prolonged further if vinyl surfaces are damaged. Vinyl surfaces need frequent inspection, and if defects are present, such equipment or flooring should be replaced or repaired.

Finally, the number of surfaces that players may potentially contact in the weight room is extraordinary. Given that many athletes are more likely to have MRSA colonization on their hands, weights and surfaces in the weight room may serve as a source of indirect transmission. Manual application of disinfectants on a large number of surfaces is difficult. As a result, the weight room is an ideal location for use of an electrostatic sprayer to apply disinfectant.

Hydrotherapy Room Best Practices and Recommendations
Please refer to Chapter 4 for additional recommendations related to hydrotherapy room best practices.

◉ **Best Practice** Contract with a commercial vendor or company to provide maintenance and regular cleaning of treadmill pools and other multiuse whirlpools in the hydrotherapy room.

○ **Recommendation 1** Use a commercial vendor or company to provide maintenance and regular cleaning of treadmill pools and other multiuse whirlpools in the hydrotherapy room.

Rationale: As described in *Chapter 4*, whirlpools have been implicated in prior outbreaks in athletic teams. Thus, cleaning and maintenance of whirlpools are keys to reducing the risk of transmission of potentially pathogenic bacteria. Although the daily monitoring of water temperatures, pH, and bromine or chlorine levels can be done by local staff, the responsibility of servicing filters, bromine or chlorine dispensers, and periodically draining and cleaning large whirlpools in hydrotherapy rooms is complex and is best done by commercial vendor technicians. These vendors should follow specific cleaning protocols and keep service logs.

○ **Recommendation 2** Require the commercial vendor to document compliance with CDC guidelines for environmental infection control of hydrotherapy tanks and pools.

Rationale: Medical treatment is provided in the hydrotherapy pools in training facilities. Thus, hydrotherapy tanks and pools must be maintained according to CDC guidelines.[29] The recommendations provided in this section outline some strategies to achieve this goal. However, we believe adherence to these guidelines should be regularly documented by commercial vendors as well. Documentation should be provided to and kept by the athletic training staff. In particular, the vendor should document the hydrotherapy equipment is in good working order. The vendor and athletic training staff must develop a plan to routinely check pH and chlorine residual levels and that pH and chlorine residual levels are maintained according to local and state health agencies. Most states use the following approach:

- For pH 7.2 to 7.8 (ideal is 7.5), ensure a minimum free chlorine concentration of 0.6 mg/L and a maximum concentration of 5 mg/L.
- For pH 7.8 to 8.2, ensure a minimum concentration of 1.5 mg/L free chlorine residual.

Maintenance and disinfection of hydrotherapy pools is mandated by state and local regulations in many areas. Refer to guidelines from your local and state health agencies to ensure you are following local regulations.

▶ **Best Practice** Appropriately disinfect individual-use/extremity whirlpools to reduce the risk of bacterial transmission between players.

✓ **Recommendation 1** Drain water from the extremity or individual whirlpools and disinfect with an EPA-registered disinfectant between uses.

✓ **Recommendation 2** Pour a hypochlorite-containing solution (eg, bleach) into drains of extremity and individual whirlpools as part of the cleaning process.

✓ **Recommendation 3** If drainage of extremity and individual whirlpools between uses is not possible or feasible during high-traffic periods, use disinfectants such as bromine tablets in the water.

Rationale: Many teams provide extremity or individual whirlpool treatments for players. According to CDC guidelines for infection control with hydrotherapy tanks and pools, individual-use pools should be drained and cleaned after each use, and equipment should be disinfected using an EPA-registered product.[29] Bacteria such as *Pseudomonas* predictably contaminate whirlpools and hydrotherapy equipment. Simple cleaning followed by complete drying of the equipment is effective in preventing this complication. However, *Pseudomonas* and other waterborne pathogens may persist in retained water in drains in these devices. Thus, we also recommend pouring additional disinfectant down the drain after disinfecting the surfaces. We agree with using EPA-registered, "hospital-grade" disinfectants to wipe down the surfaces after water is drained from these whirlpools (see above best practices for disinfection of nonporous surfaces). We recognize, however, that draining, cleaning, and refilling of extremity and individual whirlpools may not be feasible during high-traffic periods. If this process cannot be completed, we suggest using bromine or other powder-based disinfectants in these types of whirlpools to minimize the risk of bacterial transmission. Bromine tablets are available from vendors of pool supplies. These tablets also may be available from the vendor who maintains and chlorinates your large whirlpools.

▶ **Best Practice** Use appropriate disinfection strategies for footwear used in the hydrotherapy room.

✓ **Recommendation 1** Launder pool booties regularly.

✓ **Recommendation 2** Replace shoes used in treadmill pools regularly.

Rationale: The practice of sharing pool booties and shoes poses little risk to players if shared between players who have intact skin and no evidence of bacterial or fungal foot infections. Therefore, booties and shoes used in the hydrotherapy room are not required to be laundered or disinfected after each use. We recommend developing a schedule to routinely launder pool booties (eg, once each week). We also recommend developing a schedule to routinely replace pool shoes (eg, once each month).

Medical Examination/Procedure Room Best Practices and Recommendations

▶ **Best Practice** Disinfect treatment tables between player uses.

✓ **Recommendation 1** Apply disinfectant to treatment tables between player uses. If paper covers are used, also replace these between players.

Rationale: Treatment beds and tables used in examination or procedure rooms should be disinfected in the same manner as treatment tables in the training room. As explained in the best practices earlier in this chapter, adequate contact time is necessary before wiping off disinfectants, and microfiber cloths should be used to apply quaternary ammonium–containing disinfectants. Sheets or paper covers for treatment tables should be replaced between players. The use of sheets or paper covers should not replace the additional use of disinfectants.

▶ **Best Practice** Perform proper cleaning, disinfection, and sterilization (when necessary) of medical equipment to reduce the risk of transmission of infection.

✓ **Recommendation 1** Know the difference between "critical," "semicritical," and "noncritical" medical equipment.

Rationale: The CDC classifies medical equipment into three basic categories: critical items, semicritical items, and noncritical items.[6] Critical items, often used for medical procedures, require sterilization while less critical items require lower levels of disinfection. Less critical equipment can undergo higher level disinfection, but lower level disinfection cannot be used on critical or semicritical items.

Visible soiled surfaces (from body fluids, tissue, etc) must be cleaned before disinfection or sterilization for two reasons. First, organic residues reduce the effectiveness of disinfection and sterilization.[6] Second, organic materials from soiled surfaces inactivate or substantially reduce the efficacy of products used for disinfection and sterilization.[6]

Definition of Critical Items

According to the CDC, critical items "enter sterile tissue or the vascular system [and] must be sterile because any microbial contamination could transmit disease."[6] *Critical items at athletic training facilities include any equipment used in procedures where blood or body fluid exposures are expected (eg, needles for injections, surgical equipment, or suturing equipment).* The CDC states that critical items should be "purchased as sterile or sterilized between uses."[6] Hospitals and clinics typically sterilize reusable "critical items" in autoclaves after cleaning, though other sterilization methods are also available.

Definition of Semicritical Items

Semicritical items contact mucous membranes or nonintact skin. *Semicritical items at athletic training facilities include nail clippers and callus shavers.* According to the CDC, semicritical items should be "free from all microorganisms; however, small numbers of bacterial spores are permissible" because mucous membranes and nonintact skin are resistant to infection by most bacterial spores.[6] Athletic training facilities have several options as to how to safely use semicritical items. Semicritical items can be discarded after one use, sterilized between uses, or disinfected with an FDA-cleared high-level disinfectant between uses. Most hospitals and outpatient medical and surgical clinics disinfect reusable "semicritical items" with FDA-cleared high-level disinfectants.

Definition of Noncritical Items

The CDC defines noncritical items as items "that come into contact with intact skin but not mucous membranes." Noncritical items in the training environment include training equipment that comes into contact with bare skin and environmental surfaces such as floors, walls, computers, and examination beds. Equipment used on intact skin and scissors used to remove tape overlying intact skin are considered to be noncritical items.

✔ **Recommendation 2** Use single-use (disposable) "critical" and "semicritical" medical equipment whenever possible.

Rationale: Presterilized, single-use (disposable) "critical" and "semicritical" medical equipment is available from most medical equipment distributors. These items are increasingly used in hospitals and clinics because they are convenient, readily available, of high quality, and cost-effective in most environments.[30-32] In addition, athletic training staff can avoid the legal responsibility of adhering to burdensome federal guidelines needed for sterilization and high-level disinfection of non–single use medical equipment by disposing of critical and semicritical medical equipment after a single use.

Tips and Advice

- Provide nail clippers to players for individual use (and have a large supply handy).
- Dispose of callus shavers after each use. In theory, callus shavers can potentially lead to microscopic (or larger) cuts and scrapes on the skin that have a small amount of blood.

✔ **Recommendation 3** If single-use medical equipment is not available, send "critical" medical equipment to a commercial vendor for processing, cleaning, disinfection, sterilization, and subsequent packaging for reuse.

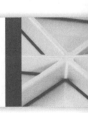

✓ **Recommendation 4** If non–single use medical equipment is not sent to a commercial vendor for processing, ensure that "critical" medical equipment is properly cleaned, disinfected, and sterilized between uses.

✓ **Recommendation 5** If an autoclave is used to perform sterilization of "critical" medical equipment on site, ensure that use of the autoclave is properly monitored and testing of its efficacy is documented.

Rationale: The sterilization of critical medical equipment is complicated and subject to stringent regulatory requirements. However, such sterilization is necessary as adequate processing of critical medical equipment is essential for player safety. Complex monitoring methods are employed in hospitals and clinics to ensure that critical equipment is processed and sterilized in autoclaves according to federal guidelines. Although adherence to these complex requirements is achievable at many athletic training facilities, we believe that the benefits of having an in-house autoclave are outweighed by burdensome regulatory requirements and the liability risks of noncompliance with these regulatory mandates. Furthermore, many collegiate and high-school athletic facilities may not have the means to purchase and maintain their own autoclave.

The juice is not worth the squeeze. In general, it's better to use disposable medical equipment or send out medical equipment for processing, disinfection, and sterilization instead of trying to perform high-level disinfection or sterilization within the athletic training facility.

Autoclaves must be monitored through a combination of mechanical, chemical, and biological techniques.[33] The mechanical measurements of the autoclave cycle (time, temperature, and pressure) must be monitored and documented with each cycle. Incorrect values for any of these parameters suggest inadequate sterilization. "Indicator tape" is typically used as a chemical indicator. These indicators are placed in and on the plastic packaging of all equipment placed into the autoclave and change color when the temperature reaches adequate sterilization levels. Biological indicators contain highly resistant bacteria that are only killed when an autoclave is functioning properly. The CDC recommends that biologic indicator monitoring be performed at least weekly.[6]

Autoclave users must also receive formal safety training on proper use of the equipment, adhere to manufacturer maintenance guidelines, maintain autoclave use logs, and record preventative maintenance or repairs. **An example autoclave use log is provided in Appendix 2D.**

We are unable to provide a single set of autoclave maintenance guidelines because these guidelines vary between autoclave devices and manufacturers. Thus, each team that uses an autoclave in the athletic training facility must closely follow the maintenance guidelines provided by the manufacturer of their individual autoclave.

Finally, *use of high-level disinfectants (eg, glutaraldehyde or Cidex) is not sufficient to achieve sterilization for "critical" medical equipment.*

✓ **Recommendation 6** If single-use medical equipment is not available, send "semicritical" medical equipment to a commercial vendor for processing, cleaning, and disinfection.

✓ **Recommendation 7** If non–single-use medical equipment is not sent to a commercial vendor for processing, ensure that "semicritical" medical equipment is properly cleaned and disinfected between uses.

Rationale: Proper use of FDA-cleared high-level disinfectants requires adherence to complex and burdensome requirements, including detailed monitoring, safety training, and record keeping. These steps and requirements vary depending on which disinfectant is used. Failure to follow these requirements can result in transmission of pathogens if medical instruments and equipment are reused. Although safe use of high-level disinfectants is achievable at professional athletic training facilities, we believe that the potential cost savings of disinfecting and reusing semicritical items are far less than the cost and inconvenience of:

1. Following these burdensome regulatory and safety requirements and
2. Exposure to safety risks if disinfection is not performed properly.

FDA-cleared high-level disinfectants include glutaraldehyde, hydrogen peroxide, ortho-phthaladehyde (OPA), and peracetic acid with hydrogen peroxide. The mechanisms of action and procedure of use of each of these chemicals are different. Each high-level disinfectant has advantages and disadvantages (**Table 6.1**).

Table 6.1 Comparison of the Characteristics of High-Level Disinfectants and Chemical Sterilants

	Hydrogen Peroxide (7.5%)	**Peracetic Acid (0.2%)**	**Glutaraldehyde (≥ 2.0%)**	**OPA (0.55%)**
High-level disinfection claim	30 min @ 20°C	NA	20-90 min @ 20°C-25°C	12 min @ 20°C
Sterilization claim	6 hr @ 20°C	12 min @ 50°C	10 hr @ 20°C-25°C	None
Activation required	No	No	Yes	No
Reuse life (days)	21	Single use	14-30	14
Shelf life stability	2 years	6 months	2 years	2 years
Disposal restrictions	None	None	Local	Local
Materials compatibility	Good	Good	Excellent	Excellent
Monitor MEC[a]	Yes (6%)	No	Yes (≥1.5%)	Yes (0.3%)
Safety	Serious eye damage	Serious eye and skin damage	Respiratory	Eye irritant, stains skin
Processing	Manual or automated	Automated	Manual or automated	Manual or automated
Resistant to organic material	Yes	Yes	Yes	Yes
OSHA exposure limit	1 ppm TWA[b]	None	None[c]	None

[a]MEC = minimum effective concentration (the lowest concentration of active ingredients at which the product is still effective).
[b]TWA = time-weighted average for an 8-hr workday.
[c]The ceiling limit recommended by the American Conference of Governmental Industrial Hygienists is 0.05 ppm. A list of FDA-cleared high-level disinfectants can be found at the following FDA website: https://www.fda.gov/MedicalDevices/DeviceRegulationandGuidance/ReprocessingofReusableMedicalDevices/ucm437347.htm.
Modified from U.S. Food & Drug Administration. https://www.fda.gov/MedicalDevices/DeviceRegulationandGuidance/ReprocessingofReusableMedicalDevices/ucm437347.htm.

✓ **Recommendation 8** If "semicritical" medical equipment is processed for repeat use in the athletic training facility, use an EPA-cleared "high-level" disinfectant such as glutaraldehyde (eg, Cidex, Wavicide, etc).

✓ **Recommendation 9** If a high-level disinfectant (ie, glutaraldehyde) is used to perform disinfection of "semicritical" medical equipment on site, staff must be trained in their proper use. Such training must be documented, and logs must be kept when disinfection is performed.

Rationale: The most frequently used high-level disinfectant for basic semicritical medical equipment is glutaraldehyde (eg, Cidex, Wavicide, etc). This compound is highly effective, is noncorrosive to metal, and does not damage lensed instruments, rubber, or plastics. Staff members involved in reprocessing semicritical medical equipment must receive specific training on the use of glutaraldehyde in order to understand important use, safety, and disposal requirements. *Complete information regarding the use of glutaraldehyde in medical facilities can be found at https://www.osha.gov/Publications/glutaraldehyde.pdf.*

Aqueous solutions of glutaraldehyde are acidic. Solutions of glutaraldehyde must be "activated" (made alkaline) in order to become sporicidal and thus qualify as a "high-level disinfectant." Once activated, these solutions have a shelf life of 14 to 30 days (depending on the specific product) because of the polymerization of the glutaraldehyde molecules at alkaline pH levels. This polymerization blocks the active sites (aldehyde groups) of the glutaraldehyde molecules that are responsible for its biocidal activity. Antimicrobial activity, however, depends not only on age but also on dilution and organic stress.

Two percent alkaline glutaraldehyde (the formulation available from most manufacturers) is highly effective in killing vegetative bacteria in less than 2 minutes; *M. tuberculosis*, fungi, and viruses in 10 to 30 minutes; and spores of *Bacillus* and *Clostridium* species in 3 hours.[6] Dilution and degradation of glutaraldehyde occur over time; 1.0% to 1.5% glutaraldehyde is the minimum effective concentration (MEC) for >2% glutaraldehyde solutions. Thus, chemical test strips or liquid chemical monitors must be used to determine whether an effective concentration of glutaraldehyde is present.[34,35] Frequency of testing should be based on how frequently the solutions are used. In general, glutaraldehyde solutions should be tested prior to first use of the chemical each day. Chemical test strips deteriorate over time. Thus, test strips must be replaced at designated times depending on the manufacturer's instructions. Finally, the results of test strip monitoring must be documented in a logbook (see **Appendix 2D**).

Inappropriate, potentially harmful exposure to glutaraldehyde occurs when equipment is processed in poorly ventilated rooms, when spills occur, or when open immersion baths are used. The Occupational Safety and Health Act (OSHA) has not defined a specific "permissible exposure limit" (ie, a maximum allowable amount of exposure) for glutaraldehyde. Adverse health effects can occur following exposure to glutaraldehyde, including irritation of eyes, nose, throat, and respiratory tract, skin burns, nausea, headache, and dizziness. *A safety fact sheet from OSHA regarding glutaraldehyde can be found at https://www.osha.gov/SLTC/etools/hospital/hazards/glutaraldehyde/glut.html.*

If glutaraldehyde is used in immersion trays, tight-fitting lids must be used in order to minimize exposure to glutaraldehyde fumes.[36] In addition, manufacturers typically recommend that the disinfectant be used in "well-ventilated areas," defined as a room with 10 or more air exchanges per hour.

Because glutaraldehyde is considered to be a hazardous chemical, OSHA's Hazard Communication Standard (HazCom) requires that information concerning any associated health or physical hazards be provided to employees. Any employee who may be "exposed" to glutaraldehyde must be provided information and be trained prior to working with the hazardous chemical. The training must include:

- **Written program**—A written program that informs the employee of the hazard and ways to avoid harm. This document must include verification that each athletic trainer or staff member who uses glutaraldehyde has received appropriate training and has reviewed the written program.
- **Labels**—Containers of glutaraldehyde must be labeled, tagged, or marked with the identity of the material and appropriate hazard warnings.
- **Material Safety Data Sheets (MSDSs)**—Employers must have an MSDS for each hazardous chemical they use. Each MSDS must be readily accessible to employees.

Glutaraldehyde remains toxic after use for high-level disinfection. Thus, personnel can be harmed if spills or splash exposures occur during disposal of used chemicals. In addition, glutaraldehyde can contaminate water supplies if it is poured into sink drains after use. Some states have specific regulations requiring the disposal of high-level disinfectants such as glutaraldehyde. For example, California now requires that glutaraldehyde be neutralized prior to disposal into sink drains. These neutralizers (which typically consist of glycine) are available from many chemical manufacturers.

▶ **Best Practice** Separate "clean" and "dirty" areas and materials at all times.

✓ **Recommendation 1** Use physically separated areas to store "clean" unused medical equipment and used medical equipment (that has not yet been cleaned and/or disinfected).

✓ **Recommendation 2** Do not store materials used for medical care (clean) in the same areas used to store cleaning materials (dirty).

✓ **Recommendation 3** Do not store medical equipment under sinks.

Rationale: "Clean" areas are defined as areas where medical procedures or medical care are provided. For example, a "procedure table" that includes an area where skin disinfectants, sterile needles, syringes, and medications or injections are used or administered is considered a clean area. Similarly, areas where the above materials and equipment are stored are considered to be clean areas as well. Contaminated medical equipment should never be left or stored in these areas after use.

Similarly, equipment used for medical care should not be stored in the areas or locations where materials used for cleaning and disinfection are stored or located. These recommendations are strictly enforced in healthcare facilities by accreditation groups such as the Joint Commission. Given that space is at a premium in most athletic training facilities, advanced planning and deliberation must be used to avoid this common error.

Tips and Advice

- Do not store medical equipment under sinks.
- Boxes used for shipping are considered "dirty." After medical supplies are removed from "dirty" shipping boxes, they are considered "clean."
- Add a sign stating "no medical equipment" in "dirty" areas where cleaning materials and disinfectants are stored.

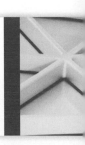

Tips and Advice: Storage of Medications

Many facilities include a small pharmacy or stockpile of routinely used prescription medications. While risks of infection related to the use of these medications are minimal, follow these best practices and recommendations to reduce risks related to the dispensing of medications.

⊙ **Best Practice** Develop and follow written policies concerning storage and dispensing of prescription medication in the team facility by medical staff.

✓ **Recommendation 1** Maintain dispensing logs for all prescription medications provided at the facility.

✓ **Recommendation 2** Store medications requiring refrigeration in secure refrigerators that contain signage prohibiting their use for concurrent storage of food or specimens.

✓ **Recommendation 3** Regularly monitor the temperature of these refrigerators to ensure maintenance of appropriate temperature control.

Rationale: The use of drug-dispensing logs should be a standard of care for all teams. Cross-contamination of medications may occur if food or clinical specimens are concurrently stored in the same refrigerators. Prominently placed signage prohibiting the storage of food or specimens in refrigerators used to store medications is the standard of care in all healthcare facilities. As temperature control is important for the safe storage of some medications such as tetanus vaccines, we recommend using continuous temperature monitors with alarms when such medications are stored on-site in a training facility.

✓ **Recommendation 4** Monitor for and discard outdated prescription medication.

Rationale: Some antibiotics and vaccines may lose potency if used beyond their expiration date. Others, such as tetracyclines, can become toxic beyond their expiration date. In order to prevent accidental administration of an outdated medication, we recommend performing periodic (eg, quarterly or semiannual) checks to evaluate expiration dates of medications stored in locked cabinets.

Blood/Body Fluid Spills

⊙ **Best Practice** Perform appropriate disinfection of surfaces that are known or suspected to be contaminated with blood or infectious body fluids.

✓ **Recommendation 1** Use a bleach-containing cleaning product (or other effective disinfectant) to clean or remove blood or body fluid spills.

Rationale: Solutions containing a 1:10 dilution of household bleach (5.25%-6.15% aqueous sodium hypochlorite) are highly effective in eradicating bloodborne viruses such as hepatitis B, hepatitis C, and HIV. Because solutions of bleach diluted with tap water lose potency after storage in opaque bottles for greater than 1 month, we recommend that teams purchase commercially available bottles of appropriately diluted bleach to be used when blood spills occur. Alternatively, most commercially available "kits" contain chemicals required for appropriate disinfection following a blood or body fluid spill.

A "spill" is defined as ANY amount of blood or body fluid on a surface.

✅ **Recommendation 2** Ensure blood or body fluid spill kits are available in the facility and that training staff know where they are and how to use them.

✅ **Recommendation 3** Dispose of contaminated supplies, materials, and linens in red bags or containers labeled "Infectious Waste" or marked with a biohazard label.

Rationale: Spill "kits" are not technically required by OSHA standards, but we believe they simplify the process of handling a blood or body fluid spill. In other words, use of spill kits can help ensure that the correct chemicals are conveniently and immediately available for use if a blood or body fluid spill occurs.

Use of spill kits can help ensure that the correct chemicals are conveniently and immediately available for use if a blood or body fluid spill occurs.

Kits typically include standard red bags with labels for disposal of contaminated items. All contaminated items should be placed in these bags to ensure that everyone in the facility realizes the materials in the bag may be contaminated with bloodborne pathogens. We suggest traveling with a blood or body fluid spill kit to ensure access to these materials at away games.

Approach to Outbreaks and Exposures

Outbreaks of infections can and frequently do occur among athletes. *Chapter 5 outlines multiple strategies for responding to outbreaks or "epidemics" of infection, depending on the pathogen causing the outbreak.* Transmission of germs during an outbreak scenario can occur through several routes, including person to person, aerosols, and environmental surfaces. This section provides additional steps to be taken with environmental disinfection when an outbreak has been identified among athletes.

▶ **Best Practice** Perform "enhanced" cleaning and disinfection of all treatment and training areas in the facility when a cluster of infections has been identified.

✅ **Recommendation 1** Increase the frequency of environmental cleaning and disinfection when an outbreak of infection has been identified.

✅ **Recommendation 2** Ensure that cleaning and disinfection in the athletic facility is documented.

Rationale: Multiple steps may be required to stop outbreaks of infection. During any outbreak, the routine steps used for cleaning and disinfection of the facility must first be reviewed for adequacy:

- Who is responsible for cleaning and disinfection?
- What products are being used?
- How often are surfaces cleaned?

Guidance for the best approach to these questions is provided above.

In most cases, it is prudent to increase the frequency of routine cleaning from the baseline during an outbreak. At baseline, we recommend that frequently used surfaces (eg, weight equipment) undergo cleaning disinfection at least once each day. During an outbreak of infections, cleaning and disinfection of equipment should be performed more frequently (eg, multiple times each day and/or after each weight training session).

Simply saying that changes to cleaning and disinfection are needed is insufficient. During an outbreak, the steps used to clean and disinfect the facility should be documented to ensure they have been successfully completed as prescribed. This approach helps ensure that responsible parties are sufficiently educated to complete the tasks required during the high-risk outbreak scenario.

✓ **Recommendation 3** Temporarily use a bleach-containing or hydrogen peroxide–containing disinfection agent to perform all cleaning and disinfection in the training facility whenever two or more players or staff develop diarrheal illness.

✓ **Recommendation 4** Continue to use "enhanced cleaning and disinfection" for at least 1 week after the last case of diarrheal illness has resolved.

Rationale: As outlined in **Chapters 1 and 4**, norovirus is the most common cause of diarrheal illness and is highly contagious. However, quaternary ammonium–containing disinfectant solutions do not kill norovirus. As a result, outbreaks of diarrheal illness require careful evaluation of the disinfection products used in the facility.

Outbreaks of norovirus infections are common, occurring periodically in athletic teams, cruise ships, day cares, hospitals, and college campuses. Norovirus transmission in such outbreaks occurs by multiple routes, including aerosols produced during vomiting or flushing toilets, direct contact, food ingestion, and via contact with contaminated environmental surfaces. Thus, when two or more players have a diarrheal illness, facilities that use a quaternary ammonium–containing disinfectant for routine cleaning must change to a disinfectant with activity against norovirus (eg, bleach-based or hydrogen peroxide–based). If possible, the disinfectant should be used for all cleanings in all settings.

It is usually not possible to determine if an individual player or group of players with a diarrheal illness is infected with norovirus or one of a multitude of other viral pathogens that cause gastroenteritis. However, diarrheal illness in such instances should be presumed to be due to norovirus, particularly if affected individuals have both vomiting and diarrhea. Indeed, the measures outlined above can be assumed to be effective in limiting the spread of **all** common viral causes of gastroenteritis. Disinfection with bleach- or hydrogen peroxide–based disinfectants should continue for at least 1 week after all players have returned to full health and are symptom free with no diarrhea.

Remember, disinfectants come in two types: sporicidal and nonsporicidal. Diarrheal illnesses require disinfection with a sporicidal disinfectant like bleach or hydrogen peroxide.

REFERENCES

1. Oller AR, Province L, Curless B. *Staphylococcus aureus* recovery from environmental and human locations in 2 collegiate athletic teams. *J Athl Train.* 2010;45(3):222-229.
2. Freedberg DE, Salmasian H, Cohen B, Abrams JA, Larson EL. Receipt of antibiotics in hospitalized patients and risk for *Clostridium difficile* infection in subsequent patients who occupy the same bed. *JAMA Intern Med.* 2016;176(12):1801-1808.
3. Shaughnessy MK, Micielli RL, DePestel DD, et al. Evaluation of hospital room assignment and acquisition of *Clostridium difficile* infection. *Infect Control Hosp Epidemiol.* 2011;32(3):201-206.
4. Edmiston CE Jr, Seabrook GR, Johnson CP, Paulson DS, Beausoleil CM. Comparative of a new and innovative 2% chlorhexidine gluconate-impregnated cloth with 4% chlorhexidine gluconate as topical

antiseptic for preparation of the skin prior to surgery. *Am J Infect Control.* 2007;35(2):89-96.

5. Rutala WA, Cole EC. Antiseptics and disinfectants–safe and effective? *Infect Control.* 1984;5(5):215-218.

6. Rutala W, Weber DJ; the Healthcare Infection Control Practices Advisory Committee (HICPAC). Guideline for Disinfection and Sterilization in Healthcare Facilities; 2008. Available at https://www.cdc.gov/infectioncontrol/pdf/guidelines/disinfection-guidelines-H.pdf. Accessed August 30, 2019.

7. *Guidelines for Environmental Infection Control in Healthcare Facilities: Centers for Disease Control and Prevention and the Healthcare Infection Control Practices Advisory Committee (HICPAC)*; 2003. Available at https://www.cdc.gov/infectioncontrol/pdf/guidelines/environmental-guidelines-P.pdf. Accessed August 30, 2019.

8. Smith DL, Gillanders S, Holah JT, Gush C. Assessing the efficacy of different microfibre cloths at removing surface micro-organisms associated with healthcare-associated infections. *J Hosp Infect.* 2011;78(3):182-186.

9. *Using Microfiber Mops in Hospitals: Environmental Protection Agency. Environmental Best Practices for Health Care Facilities*; 2002. Available at https://archive.epa.gov/region9/waste/archive/web/pdf/mops.pdf. Accessed August 30, 2019.

10. Grieme L, Thompson K, Carbone H. Evaluation of quat absorption and efficacy of cleaning cloths. *Am J Infect Control.* 2009;37(5):E23-E24.

11. MacDougall KD, Morris C. Optimizing disinfectant application in healthcare facilities. *Infect Control Today.* 2006:62-67.

12. Disinfection, sterilization and antisepsis: principles, practices, current issues, and new research. Paper presented at: Association for Professionals in Infection Control and Epidemiology 2007; Tampa, FL.

13. Rutala WA, Barbee SL, Aguiar NC, Sobsey MD, Weber DJ. Antimicrobial activity of home disinfectants and natural products against potential human pathogens. *Infect Control Hosp Epidemiol.* 2000;21(1):33-38.

14. Silverman J, Vazquez JA, Sobel JD, Zervos MJ. Comparative in vitro activity of antiseptics and disinfectants versus clinical isolates of Candida species. *Infect Control Hosp Epidemiol.* 1999;20(10):676-684.

15. Guh A, Carling P. *Options for Evaluating Environmental Cleaning*; 2010. Available at https://www.cdc.gov/HAI/pdfs/toolkits/Environ-Cleaning-Eval-Toolkit12-2-2010.pdf. Accessed August 30, 2019.

16. Cooper RA, Griffith CJ, Malik RE, Obee P, Looker N. Monitoring the effectiveness of cleaning in four British hospitals. *Am J Infect Control.* 2007;35(5):338-341.

17. Gillespie BM, Chaboyer W, Thalib L, John M, Fairweather N, Slater K. Effect of using a safety checklist on patient complications after surgery: a systematic review and meta-analysis. *Anesthesiology.* 2014;120(6):1380-1389.

18. *Using the Health Care Physical Environment to Prevent and Control Infection: A Best Practice Guide to Help Health Care Organizations Create Safe, Healing Environments*; 2018. Available at http://www.ashe.org/resources/UseHealthCarePhysEnvironPreventandControlInfection.shtml. Accessed August 30, 2019.

19. Blaser MJ, Smith PF, Cody HJ, Wang WL, LaForce FM. Killing of fabric-associated bacteria in hospital laundry by low-temperature washing. *J Infect Dis.* 1984;149(1):48-57.

20. Christian RR, Manchester JT, Mellor MT. Bacteriological quality of fabrics washed at lower-than-standard temperatures in a hospital laundry facility. *Appl Environ Microbiol.* 1983;45(2):591-597.

21. *Accreditation Standards for Processing of Reusable Textiles for Use in Healthcare Facilities*; 2016. Available at https://www.hlacnet.org/. Accessed August 31, 2019.

22. Bonadonna L, La Rosa G. A review and update on waterborne viral diseases associated with swimming pools. *Int J Environ Res Public Health.* 2019;16(2):E166.

23. Zacherle BJ, Silver DS. Hot tub folliculitis. A sheep in wolf's clothing. *Arch Intern Med.* 1982;142(9):1620.

24. Herzog MM, Fraser MA, Register-Mihalik JK, Kerr ZY. Epidemiology of skin infections in men's wrestling: analysis of 2009-2010 through 2013-2014 National Collegiate Athletic Association Surveillance Data. *J Athl Train.* 2017;52(5):457-463.

25. Fritz SA, Long M, Gaebelein CJ, Martin MS, Hogan PG, Yetter J. Practices and procedures to prevent the transmission of skin and soft tissue infections in high school athletes. *J Sch Nurs.* 2012;28(5):389-396.

26. Champion AE, Goodwin TA, Brolinson PG, Werre SR, Prater MR, Inzana TJ. Prevalence and characterization of methicillin-resistant *Staphylococcus aureus* isolates from healthy university student athletes. *Ann Clin Microbiol Antimicrob.* 2014;13:33.

27. Young LM, Motz VA, Markey ER, Young SC, Beaschler RE. Recommendations for best disinfectant practices to reduce the spread of infection via wrestling mats. *J Athl Train.* 2017;52(2):82-88.

28. Coughenour C, Stevens V, Stetzenbach LD. An evaluation of methicillin-resistant *Staphylococcus aureus* survival on five environmental surfaces. *Microb Drug Resist.* 2011;17(3):457-461.

29. *Guidelines for Environmental Infection Control in Health Care Facilities - Hydrotherapy Tanks and Pools*; 2016. Available at https://www.cdc.gov/healthywater/swimming/aquatics-professionals/hydrotherapy-tank-pool-operation.html. Accessed September 4, 2019.

30. Chapman RA, Somani BK, Robertson A, Healy S, Kata SG. Decreasing cost of flexible ureterorenoscopy: single-use laser fiber cost analysis. *Urology.* 2014;83(5):1003-1005.

31. O'Flynn P, Silva S, Kothari P, Persaud R. A multicentre audit of single-use surgical instruments (SUSI) for tonsillectomy and adenoidectomy. *Ann R Coll Surg Engl.* 2007;89(6):616-623.

32. Zimlichman E, Henderson D, Tamir O, et al. Health care-associated infections: a meta-analysis of costs and financial impact on the US health care system. *JAMA Intern Med.* 2013;173(22):2039-2046.

33. *Summary of Infection Prevention Practices in Dental Settings*; 2016. Available at https://www.cdc.gov/oralhealth/infectioncontrol/summary-infection-prevention-practices/index.html. Accessed September 1, 2019.

34. Kleier DJ, Averbach RE. Glutaraldehyde nonbiologic monitors. *Infect Control Hosp Epidemiol.* 1990;11(8):439-441.

35. Kleier DJ, Tucker JE, Averbach RE. Clinical evaluation of glutaraldehyde nonbiologic monitors. *Quintessence Int.* 1989;20(4):271-277.

36. Weber DJ, Rutala WA. Lessons from outbreaks associated with bronchoscopy. *Infect Control Hosp Epidemiol.* 2001;22(7):403-408.

Appendix 1 – Policies

Appendix 1A Methicillin-Resistant *Staphylococcus aureus* Fact Sheet for Athletes

What Is MRSA?

MRSA stands for methicillin-resistant *Staphylococcus aureus*. This germ (bacteria) is resistant to many common antibiotics. In the past, MRSA usually infected patients in hospitals or nursing homes. Now MRSA can cause infections in otherwise healthy people, including professional and amateur athletes. In general, MRSA is present on the skin of a small percentage of people in the community; MRSA "colonizes" or lives on the skin, groin, nose, hands, and/or arm pits in approximately 1 in 50 people (2%). MRSA lives on the skin of 5% to 10% of athletes who are otherwise completely well.

What Types of Infections Does MRSA Cause?

MRSA usually causes skin infections, but these germs can rarely also cause severe pneumonia and other types of infections. MRSA skin infections can appear as simple pimples, boils, abscesses, or infected cuts. These infections may occur without an obvious cause and are sometimes mistakenly assumed to be a "spider bite."

Who Gets MRSA?

Infections caused by MRSA occur in people from all walks of life including children. MRSA can easily spread between family members or other close contacts (even if the other person is not sick). In fact, outbreaks are well known to occur in families, members of sports teams, prison inmates, and military recruits. MRSA infections can also happen after a surgery or other medical procedures.

How Does MRSA Spread?

MRSA germs typically spread by direct skin-to-skin contact. They can also spread by contact with contaminated items such as medical equipment, lotions, or surfaces. The germs frequently live on the skin or mucous membranes without causing infection and then later cause infection when the skin has been injured in some way. Sharing personal items like towels, sheets, razors, clothes, or improperly cleaned sports equipment with others can increase the chance of acquiring MRSA or spreading it to others. Cuts in the skin from body shaving, turf burns, or other cuts and scrapes increase the chance for MRSA to spread and cause infection. MRSA is not spread through coughing or sneezing, and simple hygienic measures such as showering and frequent handwashing reduce the risk of transmission.

How Is MRSA Diagnosed?

MRSA infection is diagnosed by culturing the germ from pus or swabs taken of infected tissue.

How Is MRSA Treated?

Many antibiotics normally used to treat sensitive staph germs (sometimes called methicillin-susceptible *Staphylococcus aureus* or MSSA) do not work against MRSA. However, MRSA skin infections can be treated with oral antibiotics such as trimethoprim-sulfamethoxazole, linezolid, tedizolid, clindamycin, or doxycycline. Severe infections can be successfully treated with IV antibiotics. If you are given antibiotics for an infection, it is important that you finish all of them, even if your infection seems to be getting better. You should not share antibiotics with other people or save them for later. If pus is present, it may need to be drained. Never try to drain an abscess without a medical professional. You can make things worse. A doctor can determine the best treatment. Medicated soaps with chlorhexidine gluconate can be used to reduce the amount of MRSA on your skin.

What Can You Do to Prevent the Spread of MRSA?

- Frequent handwashing with alcohol-based hand sanitizers or liquid soap is the most important way to prevent MRSA (at home and on the field).
- Shower with soap after all practices. Practices lead to the most skin-to-skin contact with other players. Showering after practices can reduce the chances you acquire MRSA from this contact.
- Always shower before using the hydrotherapy room.
- Do not use hydrotherapy pools if you have open wounds.
- Cuts and wounds should be kept clean, dry, and covered.

Prompt Care and Treatment Are Important

Early diagnosis and treatment can reduce the chances of developing a severe infection. Treatment of minor infections with antibiotic ointments or pills alone often works. Report to your athletic trainer ASAP if you have:

1. Anything that looks like a pimple or boil
2. Red and/or painful areas of skin
3. Fever, chills, or cough
4. A cut or scrape that gets worse instead of better or an injury that drains pus or fluid

Preventing Spread of MRSA to or From Family Members

All of the preceding recommendations help prevent the spread of MRSA to and from family members. Athletes with family members who develop boils or pimples or infected cuts or skin injuries that appear to be infected should be sure that their family members seek medical care in order to get a correct diagnosis and prompt treatment. Players with young children should be especially vigilant for any skin infections "brought home" by their children.

Appendix 1B Methicillin-Resistant *Staphylococcus aureus* Fact Sheet for Athletes (Shortened Version)

What Is MRSA?

MRSA stands for methicillin-resistant *Staphylococcus aureus*. MRSA is a germ (bacteria) that is resistant to common antibiotics. MRSA lives on the skin or mucous membranes of 1 in 50 otherwise-healthy people in the community. MRSA lives on the skin of 5% to 10% of athletes.

Why Do Athletes Get MRSA?

Athletes have frequent skin-to-skin contact and frequent skin abrasions. These two factors combine to put athletes at increased risk for MRSA infections. In addition, MRSA infections can also occur after surgery or medical procedure.

How Is MRSA Treated?

Most MRSA infections require specific antibiotics. If pus is present, it may need to be drained. Report to your athletic trainer ASAP if you have:

1. Anything that looks like a pimple or boil
2. Red or painful areas of skin
3. Fever, chills, or cough
4. A cut or scrape that gets worse instead of better or an injury that drains pus or fluid

What Can You Do to Prevent the Spread of MRSA?

1. Improve your hygiene.
   a. Frequent handwashing with alcohol-based hand sanitizers or liquid soap is the most important way to prevent MRSA (at home and on the field).
   b. Shower with soap after all practices.
2. Always shower before using the hydrotherapy room.
3. Do not enter hydrotherapy pools if you have open wounds.
4. Cuts and wounds should be kept clean, dry, and covered.

Appendix 1C Policy for Care of Cuts, Abrasions, and Other Skin Trauma

Components of Policy

Policy statement: Prompt and appropriate care of skin trauma decreases the risk of subsequent infection and promotes prompt wound healing.

STEPS FOR SYSTEMATIC IMPLEMENTATION

1. Cleanse all fresh wounds with 4% chlorhexidine gluconate (CHG) and water
2. Apply mupirocin or a silver-containing ointment to the wound
3. Cover the wound with a hydrocolloid dressing
4. Check the wound, cleanse the wound, and change the dressing daily

Rationale

WOUND CLEANING

The mainstay of treatment of superficial cutaneous injuries such as cuts and scrapes currently is (and will almost certainly remain) careful cleaning using one of the following:

- Regular soap and water
- A solution containing a quaternary ammonium compound such as benzethonium chloride (eg, dermal skin cleanser) or benzalkonium chloride *and/or*
- Other antibacterial topical antiseptic agents such as chlorhexidine- or iodophor-containing soaps or solutions

Many antiseptic solutions contain alcohol in varying concentrations. Such alcohol-containing compounds provide rapid antibacterial effects; however, they also produce local burning. Soap and water, 4% CHG, 10% betadine solution, and surgical scrub reagents are safe and effective agents for cleaning abrasions and cuts. We discourage the use of hydrogen peroxide for standard cut care because it may impair wound healing and because it is not more effective than the agents listed above.

Although soap and water are adequate cleaning agents, we recommend the general use of an antiseptic agent for standard wound care.

Specifically, we advise using 4% CHG (Hibiclens or Betasept wash) instead of betadine/iodophors for the following reasons:

- It has in vitro bactericidal activity against methicillin-resistant and methicillin-susceptible staphylococci, streptococci, and most bacteria that colonize normal skin[1]
- It is well tolerated and safe
- Unlike betadine/iodophors, its activity is not diminished by the presence of organic debris or material such as blood
- It produces a prolonged antibacterial effect after application
  - CHG "sticks" are now available for use and should replace Betadine sticks in all settings
- While bacterial resistance to chlorhexidine has been demonstrated,[2] this occurs only rarely and its clinical significance in everyday practice is currently insignificant

Commercially available 4% CHG-containing cloths provide a clinically proven dose of chlorhexidine to skin.[3] Even though these products have not been FDA-approved for use for wound care, they are widely used in hospitals and surgical centers, and their safety is proven. A recent evaluation of seven animal studies and three human studies of chlorhexidine-containing products demonstrated that they are associated with few adverse effects on healing.[4] We believe there is a practical and scientific basis to support the use of these cloths for wound care.

ANTIBACTERIAL OINTMENT

Many athletic trainers and medical professionals routinely apply antibacterial ointments prior to the placement of a clean dry dressing. These agents are safe and probably effective. Although topical antibacterial ointments are probably not required for every cut or abrasion, we recommend their use especially if the skin injury is extensive, deep, or otherwise a concern. Choices for topical therapy include the following:

- Mupirocin
- Silver sulfadiazine creams and silver nanoparticle creams
- Bacitracin
- Bacitracin/polymyxin B or bacitracin, neomycin, and polymyxin B

Of the four therapeutic options listed above, we prefer mupirocin for the following reasons:

- It has established activity against MRSA, other strains of *S. aureus,* and common skin pathogens such as streptococci
- It is safe and has few, if any, significant side effects
- MRSA is the predominant pathogen causing skin and soft-tissue infections in the United States; thus, using an agent with proven activity against MRSA for primary prevention is logical
- Although emergence of antimicrobial resistance is a concern when mupirocin is used, the likelihood that regular use of mupirocin as topical therapy will result in the emergence of resistance in a small closed population such as a team is unlikely

Silver-containing creams and ointments can be used in place of mupirocin but are typically more costly. While older silver sulfadiazine creams frequently became dry, crusty, and difficult to use, these issues have been obviated by the new nanoparticle formulations of silver ointment.

Bacitracin, bacitracin/polymyxin B, Neomyocin, double-, and triple-antibiotic creams are often used for topical therapy. However, we prefer mupirocin over these other agents for the following reasons:

- Bacitracin topical activity is inferior to mupirocin against MRSA and other common bacterial pathogens.
- Bacitracin, neomycin, and polymyxin B and bacitracin/polymyxin B ointments are not effective against MRSA and can lead to allergic reactions that may be confused with an infection.

WOUND DRESSING

The choice and type of dressing to apply to skin injuries are primarily a matter of clinical judgment and preference. Although Band-Aid and other "breathable" bandages are fine for small and minor skin injuries, hydrocolloid dressings such as DuoDERM are preferable to gauze for deeper and more extensive skin injuries. DuoDERM protects the injured skin from drying; it can be left in place for long periods; and it is easy and painless to remove. Hydrocolloidal dressings containing CHG are available, but little data are available to evaluate their superiority/inferiority compared to standard DuoDERM dressings.

REFERENCES

1. McDonnell G, Russell AD. Antiseptics and disinfectants: activity, action, and resistance. *Clin Microbiol Rev*. 1999;12(1):147-79.
2. Cookson BD, Bolton MC, Platt JH. Chlorhexidine resistance in methicillin resistant *Staphylococcus aureus* or just an elevated MIC? An in vitro and in vivo assessment. *Antimicrob Agents Chemother*. 1991;35(10):1997-2002.
3. Vernon MO, Hayden MK, Trick WE, Hayes RA, Blom DW, Weinstein RA for the Chicago Antimicrobial Resistance Project (CARP). Chlorhexidine gluconate to cleanse patients in a medical intensive care unit: the effectiveness of source control to reduce the bioburden of vancomycin-resistant enterococci. *Arch Intern Med*. 2006;166:306-312.
4. Drosou A, Falabella A, Kirsner RS. Antiseptics on wounds: an area of controversy. *Wounds*. 2003;15(5):149-166.

Appendix 1D Sample Policy for Vaccinations Among Players and Team Personnel

Components of Policy

Policy statement: Vaccines are highly effective and safe. As such, vaccination is a cornerstone of infection prevention efforts. Five highly transmissible and potentially serious infections can be easily prevented among athletes using safe vaccines: influenza, *Bordetella pertussis* (pertussis or "whooping cough"), meningococcal meningitis, mumps, and hepatitis A.

STEPS FOR SYSTEMATIC IMPLEMENTATION

1. Influenza
   a. Require that all players receive annual influenza vaccination.
   b. Require that all athletic trainers and team physicians receive annual influenza vaccination.
   c. Document annual receipt of the vaccination.
2. Pertussis
   a. When a player requires a tetanus booster, replace the tetanus booster with Tdap to also vaccinate against pertussis.
   b. Alternatively, provide Tdap vaccination to all players who are uncertain if they have received it.
3. Meningococcus
   a. Provide meningococcal vaccine to players who have not previously been immunized.
   b. Immunize players if they are uncertain if they have received the vaccine or not.
4. Mumps
   a. Provide measles, mumps, and rubella (MMR) vaccine to players who have not previously been immunized.
   b. Immunize players who did not attend college in the United States.
5. Hepatitis A
   a. Provide hepatitis A vaccine to players who have not previously been immunized.

Rationale

INFLUENZA

Influenza is a common and partially preventable respiratory infection that is readily transmitted from person to person. Influenza infection significantly reduces respiratory capacity and athletic performance even in players with relatively mild infections. A small but important percentage of young and otherwise healthy individuals who acquire influenza may develop severe infections that require hospitalization and, occasionally, intensive care. Influenza vaccines have proven benefits that are important for teams. *Most importantly, players who receive influenza vaccines are less likely to have fever or influenza-like illness, are less likely to miss work, and are less likely to spread influenza to teammates.*

We believe the best and most effective approach is to require that all players receive influenza vaccination. This approach is now widely used in most hospitals in the United States. We acknowledge, however, that this approach may not be feasible in your team without union and player approval. Thus, we recommend developing and implementing a highly visible and active campaign designed to increase compliance with influenza vaccination among players. Potential components of such a campaign include the following measures:

- Influenza vaccination "blitzes," in which vaccination is provided by practitioners at the team facilities on specific days and times, so that influenza vaccination can be immediately provided on-site to whomever consents. However, don't limit access to these blitzes. Make sure it is clear the vaccination is available any time.
- Influenza vaccination "stations" placed in strategic, high-traffic locations (eg, cafeteria, training room, outside locker room) so that individuals can be immunized during the course of their normal activities without an appointment or clinic visit.
- Providing educational materials to players at the beginning of influenza season describing the benefits of the vaccination and debunking the myths about the vaccine.
- Recruitment of player champions to promote the use of the vaccination. Promotion can include the following simple message: "*Don't hurt the team*—Get the vaccine so you don't miss practice or game time. Get the vaccine so you don't get the rest of us sick".
- Demonstration of receipt of the vaccination by team leaders and coaches (ie, lead by example).
- Identify players with young children and/or pregnant partners and target for vaccination in order to keep their families safer.

Vaccination can be given intranasally or via intramuscular (IM) injection. These methods are equally effective. Injections can be given using either trivalent (covers three types of flu) or quadrivalent (covers four types of flu) vaccine. We suspect the quadrivalent vaccine is more effective, but supplies may be limited.

PERTUSSIS

Pertussis is highly contagious. It can spread rapidly, and it frequently causes outbreaks or clusters of infection in populations in close quarters such as sports teams. For example, some high schools have postponed or canceled games due to outbreaks of pertussis among players. While an infection of a single player may be easy to deal with, having a teamwide outbreak can be devastating.

Acellular pertussis vaccine can be administered to both adults and children. "Acellular" refers to the fact that the immune response is triggered by immunogenic proteins, toxins, and other cellular components and not due to an intact bacterium. *As such, pertussis vaccine cannot and does not cause pertussis.* Also this vaccine is safe and effective. Pertussis immunization is available as part of Tdap vaccine, which contains tetanus toxoid, diphtheria, and acellular pertussis antigens. The Centers for Disease Control and Prevention's (CDC) Advisory Committee on Immunization Practices (ACIP) recommends that *all* persons over 11 years of age receive Tdap *once*. Given the high amount of trauma incurred by players on a regular basis, we assume that most players have received tetanus vaccine at least every 10 years. If an individual player is now due for his next Td booster or if a Td booster is needed as a component of wound management, simply replace the Td booster with Tdap.

MENINGOCOCCUS

Meningococcal vaccine is required for attendance at most American universities. The meningococcal vaccine is effective and safe. In addition, it is safe to reimmunize players who are not certain if they have or have not previously received this vaccine. This policy and the high effectiveness of meningococcal vaccines have led to a 21% decrease in the incidence of meningitis in developed countries from 1993 to 2011. We recommended that teams assess the prior receipt of meningococcal vaccine in new players because some universities and colleges may not have monitored compliance with meningococcal vaccination mandates. Similarly, players from other countries (eg, Australia) may not have received meningococcal vaccine. Vaccine should be offered to team members who have not received this vaccine.

MUMPS

Measles-mumps-rubella vaccine is also required for attendance at American universities. Mumps vaccines are safe and effective. In 1989, the CDC's ACIP recommended that all school-age children in the United States receive two doses of combined MMR vaccine. Following widespread adoption of these recommendations, the reported incidence of mumps in the United States decreased by 99% (from 185,691 cases in 1988 to 231 cases in 2003). However, the number of cases of mumps increased significantly in recent years as a direct consequence of declining vaccination rates.

However, several mumps outbreaks occurred in multiple locations including college campuses in the United States in 2006. These findings prompted the ACIP to revise their earlier recommendations. As a result, ACIP now recommends an additional dose of MMR for (1) students at the time of entry into college who lack documentation of prior receipt of two doses of MMR; (2) healthcare and day care workers who are at increased risk of exposure who similarly lack documentation; or (3) any individual exposed during an outbreak. In the event that a player did not attend a US college, we recommend immunizing the player with a booster of MMR vaccine.

HEPATITIS A

Outbreaks of hepatitis A continue to occur in the United States even though the overall incidence of hepatitis A has declined following the introduction of vaccine in approximately 2000. Due to these outbreaks, the CDC now supports the use of hepatitis A vaccine after known or possible exposure to a single case of hepatitis A. Some experts have recommended vaccination in athletes involved in close-contact sports. We agree with this recommendation.

Appendix 1E Five Common Myths About the Flu Vaccine[1]

I Don't Need the Flu Vaccine Because...

1. **"I am healthy and influenza is not serious." WRONG.** Even if you do not develop severe or classic flu symptoms (eg, fever, cough, muscle or body aches, sore throat, fatigue, runny or stuffy nose, or headache), you can transmit flu to others. Even healthy people can have severe cases of flu and complications such as pneumonia and brain inflammation. More than 650,000 people die from the flu each year.

2. **"The vaccine causes the flu." WRONG.** This widespread myth is as wrong as it gets. In other words, no one has EVER contracted the flu after getting the flu shot. It is biologically impossible. When people claim they got the flu from the vaccine, they have simply been infected by a virus (flu or otherwise) prior to receiving the flu shot.

3. **"The vaccine causes side effects." WRONG.** The flu vaccine is proven to be safe. Severe side effects are extraordinarily rare. Alternative, egg-free flu shots are available for people with severe anaphylactic reactions to eggs.

4. **"The vaccine doesn't work." WRONG.** While it is not as effective as many other popular vaccines, "not as effective" is not the same thing as "not effective." In fact, the flu vaccine is approximately 50% effective in preventing flu. In addition, if you do become sick with the flu after vaccination, your symptoms will be greatly reduced.

5. **"I'm pregnant or live with someone whose immune system is compromised." WRONG.** Pregnant women have weakened immune systems during pregnancy and have higher rates of complications from flu. As a result, pregnant women should *always* get the flu vaccine. If you live with a pregnant woman or someone else with a weakened immune system, you can help preserve the health of the person you are living with by obtaining the flu shot. Since you cannot get flu from the flu shot, you also can't spread flu because you received the flu shot.

REFERENCE

1. World Health Organization. *5 Myths About the Flu Vaccine*. Available at https://www.who.int/influenza/spotlight/5-myths-about-the-flu-vaccine. Accessed January 9, 2020.

Appendix 1F Tiered Response Protocol When MRSA Cases Occur in the Facility

Tier 1. Standard Care

Follow general recommendations provided throughout the book.

Tier 2. One Case of MRSA in the Facility

In addition to all recommendations made in tier 1, we recommend the following:

- Educate and alert players that the first case has occurred and that, by definition, they are now also at higher risk for infection.
    - This information:
        - Provides full disclosure to players who are logically concerned about their health.
        - Provides stimulus for improved hygienic practices.
        - Overcomes the perception of secrecy regarding MRSA.
- Specifically recommend that all players present to training staff with any skin abrasion, cuts, or infection.
- Enforce no exception policy for handwashing.
    - All players and staff must wash hands upon first entering facility and upon leaving.
- Enforce no exception policy for postpractice showering.
    - All players must shower following practices and prior to further use of the training facility.
- Perform decolonization strategy on the player with infection, including the following regimen:
    - Mupirocin ointment to the bilateral nares two times each day.
        - Helpful tip: use a cotton-tip applicator to apply the ointment to one nostril, turn the applicator over and use the other end to apply to the other nostril. This avoids contamination of the mupirocin bottle.
    - Chlorhexidine bath each day.
    - NOTE: Begin regimen as the player completes antibiotic treatment for the infection. Be sure to continue these two agents for 5 more days after completing the oral antibiotic.
- Monitor frequency of cleaning of training equipment (eg, weight room). Ensure that equipment is thoroughly cleaned a minimum of once daily.
    - Provide numerous bottles of cleaning sprays throughout training facility and encourage all players and/or staff to wipe down equipment after use; OR
    - Provide disposable pop-up wipes of disinfectant (eg, bleach, chlorox, or ammonia) to wipe down equipment after each use.
- Ban players with skin infections from whirlpool therapy.
- Ban sharing of ANY equipment, including towels, water bottles, soap, etc.
- Ensure no bar soap is available in showers.
- Enforce strict policy for towel usage—only use one towel per player. No towels should be used for more than one day.
- Discard tubs of communal balms and lotions and restrict use to single-use products or products that can be dispensed via pumps.
- Remove player with infection from team activities.

OPTIONAL: Perform intensive "source control" daily on all players. That is, use chlorhexidine-containing cloths to wipe skin following the posttraining shower of each player.

Tier 3. Two or More Cases of MRSA in the Facility

In addition to all recommendations made in tiers 1 and 2, we recommend the following:

- If not begun in tier 2, begin intensive "source control" daily on all players. Players should disinfect their skin using CHG-containing cloths for 14 days. Provide 4 to 10 CHG-containing cloths to each player each day and instruct them to wipe their skin following their postpractice shower. **See Appendix 1J** for additional information about how to use CHG-containing cloths.
- Replace soap in showers with chlorhexidine-containing soap.
    - Note: chlorhexidine-containing soap can be drying to skin; thus, encourage players to use moisturizing lotion, but ensure that EACH player has own supply and that lotion is not shared among players.
- Provide players with take home supply of chlorhexidine-containing solution (either liquid or on cloths) for home application. For maximal efficacy, chlorhexidine should be allowed to dry (and not washed off) skin.
- Ban all shaving (below the neck) for nonmedical purposes.
- Identify monitors to observe practices during busy treatment periods to ensure athletic trainers wash hands between player contacts and that all treatment tables undergo appropriate disinfection between uses.
- Furthermore, increase frequency of cleaning of training equipment (eg, weight room).
    - Enforce policy that players must wipe down equipment with disposable wipes (not towels) after each usage.

ADDITIONAL RECOMMENDATIONS FOR ALL TIERS—RECOMMENDED MEASURES WHEN ONE OR MORE CASES OF MRSA INFECTION OCCUR IN THE HOUSEHOLD OF A PLAYER

Athletes who have family members with boils, pimples, infected cuts, or minor skin injuries should insist that their family members seek medical care in order to get a correct diagnosis and prompt treatment. Other measures include:

- All family members should wash hands with soap and water or practice hand hygiene with an alcohol-containing hand rub before and after dressings are changed.
- Infected wounds should be covered at all times.
- Family members should avoid handling soiled bandages.
- Family members should not share hand or bath towels, clothes, or any other common personal hygiene objects such as razors, toothbrushes, or eating utensils.
- Special cultures (eg, nasal swabs) are NOT recommended when a single or multiple family members have an infection due to MRSA. However, when more than one family member is infected, we advise the use of topical nasal mupirocin and chlorhexidine showers for a total of 5 days by each family member. If MRSA infections continue to recur, consultation with a local infectious diseases specialist is recommended.
- Any skin lesion that drains pus (even a minor cut or pimple) should be cultured and treated if one of more family members has or has recently had an infection due to MRSA.
- All family members should shower with CHG surgical wash daily until all family members are well and free of infection for 2 weeks.

Appendix 1G Tiered Response Protocol When Cases of Diarrheal Illness Occur in the Facility

Tier 1. Standard Care

Follow general recommendations provided throughout the book.

Tier 2. One Case of Diarrhea in the Facility

In addition to all recommendations made in tier 1, we recommend the following:

- *Immediately send any player with diarrheal illness home. This is the most important measure to prevent a team outbreak.* The duration of most diarrheal illnesses is short, and the player can return to practice when symptoms have resolved.
- Educate and alert players that the first case has occurred and that, by definition, they are now also at higher risk for infection.
- Specifically recommend that all players with symptoms of diarrhea or vomiting present to the training staff.
- *Enforce no tolerance policy for handwashing.*
    - All players and staff must wash hands upon first entering facility and upon leaving.
    - *The affected player and contacts (e.g., athletic trainers providing care) should use soap and water for hand hygiene instead of alcohol-based products, as alcohol is not effective against some diarrheal pathogens.* Soap and water should be used for handwashing by the player and contacts until the player has been asymptomatic for at least 72 hours.
- Wear gloves for all interactions with player with diarrhea.
    - Use soap and water to wash hands after removing gloves.
- Disinfect all toilets with a hypochlorite-, phenol-, or hydrogen peroxide–containing solution. Also use one of these disinfectants to clean other areas any player has contacted while symptomatic.
- Athletic trainers and other staff should wear gloves when treating any player with a diarrheal illness.
- Enforce a ban on all food and food containers from the bathroom and treatment areas.

Tier 3. Two or More Cases of Diarrhea in the Facility

In addition to all recommendations made in tiers 1 and 2, we recommend the following:

- *Hand hygiene should be performed throughout the facility with soap and water, instead of alcohol-based products, as alcohol is not effective against some diarrheal pathogens.* Soap and water should be preferentially used for handwashing until no player has had symptoms of acute illness for 72 hours.
- Disinfect all areas of the facility with a hypochlorite-, phenol-, or hydrogen peroxide–containing solution. Use this solution for all cleaning at the facility until no further personnel have had diarrhea or vomiting for 72 hours.
- Strictly enforce a policy of no food in locker room, bathroom, and treatment areas.

ADDITIONAL RECOMMENDATIONS FOR ALL TIERS WHEN ONE OR MORE CASES OF DIARRHEA OCCUR IN THE HOUSEHOLD OF A PLAYER

- All household members should wash hands frequently with soap and water.
- Family members should not share hand or bath towels, clothes, or any other common personal hygiene objects, such as toothbrushes and eating utensils.
- Toilets, bathroom surfaces, and other common areas the affected family member has contacted while symptomatic should be cleaned with a hypochlorite (ie, bleach) solution.
- The player with an affected family member MUST wash hands upon entry to the training facility.

Appendix 1H   Tiered Response Protocol When Cases of Influenza-like Illness Occur in the Facility

Tier 1. Standard Care

Follow general recommendations provided throughout the book.

Tier 2. One Case of Influenza-like Illness in the Facility

In addition to all recommendations made in tier 1, we recommend the following:

- Educate players about using "cough etiquette"
  - Cover the mouth with a tissue or a body part when coughing.
  - Promptly clean hands when contaminated with respiratory secretions.

Tier 3. Two or More Cases of Influenza-like Illness in the Facility

Higher level (tier 3) recommendations for managing clusters of respiratory illness in players and/or staff must be individualized based on the likely or known diagnosis, the time of year, the presence or absence of a known outbreak of respiratory infection in the community, and the severity of observed illness. In general, we advise teams to seek advice about management of such clusters from local or regional experts in infectious diseases and epidemiology. However, the following general guidelines can be utilized in assessing and managing such outbreaks:

- Make an etiologic or probable diagnosis whenever possible. Such efforts may include cultures for influenza or pertussis when appropriate.
  - Use PCR-based tests to diagnose influenza.
  - Send both culture and PCR for suspected pertussis if player has less than 4 weeks of cough. If the player has cough for more than 4 weeks, test for pertussis using serologic tests.
- Encourage symptomatic and ill individuals to avoid direct contact with healthy individuals whenever possible.
- In general, it is best to remove symptomatic/ill individuals from the training facility until the acute phase of their illness is over.
- Do not provide antimicrobial therapy when the likely pathogen is viral.
- Make return to team activities on a case-by-case basis.
  - In general, players with viral respiratory illness can return to training when they have been afebrile for >24 hours.
- Decisions about the utility and type of prophylaxis (eg, for influenza or pertussis) or the implementation of a teamwide vaccine program should be made by team physicians with input from infectious disease experts/epidemiologists or the local health department. Prophylaxis or vaccine use may need to be extended to household contacts of players or staff in selected cases.

Appendix 1I Tiered Response Protocol When Cases of Hand, Foot, and Mouth Disease Occur in the Facility

Tier 1. Standard Care

Follow general recommendation provided throughout the book.

Tier 2. One or More Cases of HFMD in the Facility

In addition to all recommendations made in tier 1, we recommend the following:

- Educate players about HFMD, including information regarding transmission, the importance of hand hygiene, and children as likely source of initial case.
- Perform a thorough cleaning of the facility with particular emphasis on areas that hands encounter (eg, weights, footballs, meeting room chairs, and armrests). Look for and disinfect other items that may be passed hand to hand, including phones and tablets.
- Avoid sharing towels, even on the practice field.
- Implement "no exception" policy for hand hygiene.
- Discard and replace gloves used by players.

The benefit of isolation is controversial. Isolate infected players if possible. However, if the player cannot be removed from team activities, he or she may continue to participate as long as afebrile and any vesiculopapular lesions can be covered.

Appendix 1J Sample Protocol for Source Control Using 2% Chlorhexidine Gluconate

The antiseptic CHG is routinely used for surgical skin preparation because of its broad spectrum of activity against both bacteria and viruses. Topical CHG is also used to prevent recurrent infections due to MRSA in a process called decolonization. For example, daily baths using CHG-impregnated cloths are widely used in patients in intensive care units to prevent infections caused by MRSA and other multidrug-resistant organisms. Daily bathing with CHG-impregnated cloths reduces the MRSA "disease burden" by 37% among ICU patients compared to patients receiving routine care.

This protocol outlines an additional use of CHG, named "source control," to decrease the overall burden of potentially pathogenic bacteria on skin in a larger group or population. We recommend that all players undergo routine source control throughout the season by bathing with CHG-containing soap three times each week.

Showering With Antiseptics Containing CHG

Liquid, detergent-based preparations containing 2% to 4% CHG have been widely used for prevention of postoperative infections. CHG liquid soaps are supplied in unit doses ranging from 25 to 250 mL; the most commonly used commercially available unit dose is 4 ounces (approximately 120 mL). Liquid CHG preparations are typically used in the following manner: after an initial rinse in the shower, undiluted topical CHG liquid is applied to the skin, lathered, rinsed, reapplied, and then rinsed a final time. Although showering with CHG is widely recommended for preoperative patients, its effectiveness remains unproven. CHG is most effective when allowed to dry on the skin. However, when a case or cluster of MRSA infections occurs among players, we recommend "advanced" source control, as described below.

Advanced Source Control Using CHG-Impregnated Cloths

Two percent CHG-impregnated cloths are more effective and have a lower risk of side effects than liquid CHG preparations. These cloths are commercially available in alcohol-free prepackaged unit doses sufficient for bathing a single person. Four to ten 7.5 × 7.5 inch cloths are needed to bath a single, standard-sized (70 kg) adult. More cloths will likely be needed for larger players.

No rinsing is needed after application (Figure A1J.1). CHG dries on the skin. If used after showering, they should be applied only after the skin is dry and cool. Warmers can be used to heat the cloths prior to application. Importantly, these effective, disposable, safe cloths are available as a prepackaged product that provides a consistent and effective concentration of CHG.

When and How Should CHG Be Administered for Advanced Source Control?

We recommend teamwide use of advanced source control using CHG-containing wipes when two or more players have been diagnosed with MRSA infections in a team training facility. Unfortunately, there is no reliable data regarding ideal time of day for CHG administration for nonhospitalized individuals. We recommend applying prepackaged body wipes to athletes after the postpractice shower. CHG should not be applied to the face; we recommend instructing athletes to apply wipes to all skin surfaces below the chin.

Ideal Frequency and Duration to Administer CHG

Two studies in military recruits using three times weekly CHG cloths demonstrated a statistically significant reduction in acquisition of MRSA (3.3% vs 6.5%) colonization.[1,2] One study focused on duration of CHG activity on patients' skin using 2% chlorhexidine-impregnated cloths. In that study, CHG retained antibacterial activity in 90% of hospitalized patients 24 hours after administration.[3] To our knowledge, there are no studies that examine the ideal frequency to administer CHG in team settings. Based on available data, however, we believe that daily application is appropriate. Similarly, there are no data on the duration of topical treatments in nonhospitalized patients. *We recommend daily applications **for all players** for a minimum of 2 weeks. Then resume routine source control for the remainder of the season* (Figure A1J.2).

Side Effects of CHG

Descriptions of adverse reactions to topical application of CHG range in severity from local skin rash (dermatitis) to anaphylaxis. However, severe reactions are extraordinarily rare. CHG rarely has also been associated with asthma. Patients with severe reactions usually develop a

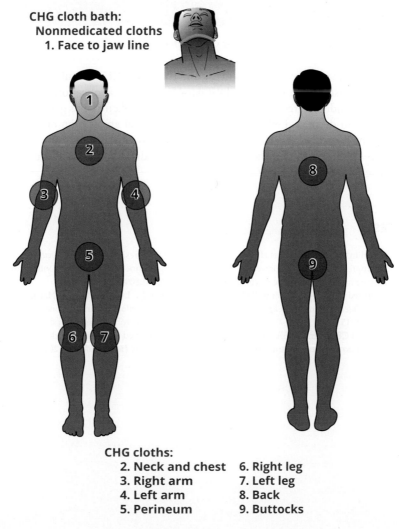

CHG cloth bath:
Nonmedicated cloths
1. Face to jaw line

CHG cloths:

2. Neck and chest	6. Right leg
3. Right arm	7. Left leg
4. Left arm	8. Back
5. Perineum	9. Buttocks

Figure A1J.1 Anatomic location for use of chlorhexidine gluconate (CHG)-containing cloths.

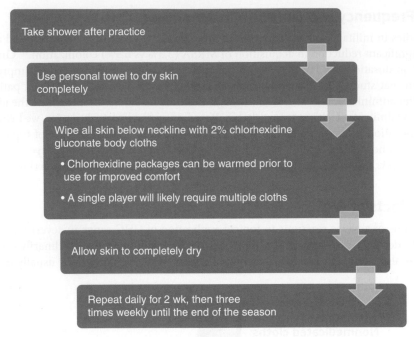

Figure A1J.2 Chlorhexidine gluconate (CHG) body cloth protocol.

simple rash before more severe reactions manifest. Therefore, CHG should be avoided in any patient who has a history of rash after administration. Direct application to mucous membranes should be avoided. Direct application of CHG over broken skin is generally considered safe but may lead to decreased efficacy. Occasionally, topical application of CHG can result in a "sticky feeling" on skin. This sticky feeling is related to a moisturizer on CHG cloths and typically resolves completely after the skin is completely dry. Overall, side effects from CHG remain low when used appropriately.

REFERENCES

1. Whitman TJ, Herlihy RK, Schlett CD, et al. Chlorhexidine-impregnated cloths to prevent skin and soft-tissue infection in marine recruits: a cluster-randomized, double-blind, controlled effectiveness trial. *Infect Control Hosp Epidemiol.* 2010;31(12):1207-1215.
2. Whitman TJ, Schlett CD, Grandits GA, Millar EV, et al. Chlorhexidine gluconate reduces transmissoin of methicillin-resistant *Staphylococcus aureus* USA300 among Marine recruits. *Infect Control Hosp Epidemiol.* 2012;33(8):809-816.
3. Popovich JK, Lyles R, Hayes R, Hayden MK et al. Relation of chlorhexidine gluconate skin concentration to microbial density on skin of critically ill patients bathed daily with chlorhexidine gluconate. *Infect Control Hosp Epidemiol.* 2012;33(9):889-896.

Appendix 1K   Policy for the Appropriate Use of the Hydrotherapy Room

Policy statement: Hydrotherapy pools can act as vectors to transmit serious bacterial pathogens. Appropriate player use of the hydrotherapy room can greatly reduce the risk of bacteria among players.

Policy Components

1. Players with open wounds are not allowed in the pools unless the wounds are covered with impermeable dressings.
2. Players must shower prior to using the hydrotherapy pools.
3. Players with known MRSA infections are not allowed in the pools until the infection is completely resolved.
4. Clean, laundered towels will be available for player use at all times.

STEPS FOR SYSTEMATIC IMPLEMENTATION

1. Player will receive education about the hydrotherapy room policies each year
2. The pool will be drained if a player with an open, uncovered wound enters
3. The pool will be drained if a player with a known skin infection enters

A sign will be posted in the hydrotherapy room to remind players of the policy.

Rationale

PLAYER ACCESS

Whirlpools have been implicated in previous outbreaks of MRSA among athletes. For example, one MRSA outbreak of 10 college football players (2 of whom required hospitalization) was linked to a whirlpool. Players who used the whirlpools during or after players with MRSA infections entered the water had a 12-fold higher risk of MRSA infection. Pool environments can also spread other pathogens like *Pseudomonas*, *Cryptosporidium*, and *Legionella*.

Open sores or breaks in the skin can become infected by bathing in contaminated pool water. The CDC recommends that individuals with an open wound avoid going into swimming pools. However, we understand that hydrotherapy can be essential for athlete rehabilitation.

Therefore, athletes with open wounds who require hydrotherapy should always cover open wounds with impermeable dressings. If a player with an uncovered open wound or known skin infection uses a hydrotherapy pool, we recommend draining, drying, and disinfecting the pool. Subsequent players may be at risk for infection.

Other body fluids can also contaminate pools. The CDC recommends adjusting free chlorine levels following known stool or vomit contamination. Pool volumes, however, may be significantly different in public pools than in a small hydrotherapy pool. We recommend draining, drying, and disinfecting the pool in the unlikely and rare event of contamination from body fluids such as vomit or stool.

Over half of swimming pools contain fecal bacteria. Such contamination not only spreads bacteria but also can interfere with disinfection chemicals. Showers remove perianal fecal material, sweat, excess skin cells, and dirt before bathers enter the pool. Thus, showering before entering a hydrotherapy pool reduces the risk of contamination and helps maintain the cleanliness of the pools. In fact, showers prior to pool entry are required by some state and local regulations.

TOWELS

Sharing towels places athletes at higher risk of developing MRSA and other infections. In one study, football players who shared towels were over eight times more likely to develop MRSA than those who did not. Thus, clean laundered towels must be readily available for use by players exiting the hydrotherapy pools.

Appendix 1L Bloodborne Pathogen Exposure Control Plan

Team: _____

Date Effective: _____

Policy Version: _____

Overview

Employees in this facility are at risk of exposure to a bloodborne pathogen through accidental exposure to body fluids as part of routine care, handling of equipment, and/or routine cleaning and disinfection activities. This Exposure Control Plan has been developed to eliminate or minimize employee exposure to BBPs.

Bloodborne Pathogens

Bloodborne pathogens (BBPs) are organisms that may be present in blood and other body fluids that can be transmitted from one person to another. The three primary BBPs of interest are hepatitis B, hepatitis C, and human immunodeficiency virus (HIV).

The following activities may lead to an exposure to a BBP:

1. Wound care
2. Medical procedures, particularly procedures involving needles, scalpels, or any equipment that can easily penetrate skin
3. Transport and disposal of biohazard waste
4. Handling of equipment
5. Cleaning and disinfection of equipment

Exposure Risk Determination

The following positions or employees are at risk for exposure:

1. Athletic trainers
2. Team physicians
3. Physical therapists
4. Equipment managers
5. Strength and conditioning coaches
6. Environmental services/facility managers

Methods of Compliance

Several strategies can be used to eliminate or reduce the risk of exposure to BBPs.

UNIVERSAL PRECAUTIONS

1. Treat all blood, cultures, soiled bandages, and other potentially infectious materials as if they are infectious
2. Work in the safest way available to minimize splash, spray, splatter, or droplets of blood
3. Use appropriate personal protective equipment (PPE)

PERSONAL PROTECTIVE EQUIPMENT

When used appropriately, PPE prevents exposure to BBP. PPE includes gloves, gowns, face-masks, and eye shields.

1. Always use gloves when:
    a. Performing care that may lead to contact with blood, body fluids, broken skin, or mucosal membranes (eg, eyes, nose, and mouth).
    b. Touching potentially contaminated or infected areas of the body.
    c. Disposing of waste materials.
    d. Handling or disposing of biohazardous waste (eg, used bandages).
    e. Handling soiled laundry.
2. Always use protective gowns when performing care or procedures that may lead to spray, splatter, or splashing of blood or body fluids.
3. Always use protective eyewear performing care or procedures that may lead to spray, splatter, or splashing of blood or body fluids.

Always perform hand hygiene after removal of PPE. If PPE is penetrated or compromised in any way, remove and replace as soon as safe to do so.

HAND HYGIENE

HH is heavily emphasized at this facility as a key strategy to prevent transmission of infections, including infections caused by BBP. All employees are instructed to perform hand hygiene frequently, including:

1. When removing gloves and PPE.
2. Following inadvertent contact with blood and/or body fluids.
3. When entering the examination room, training room, and cafeteria.
4. When exiting the bathroom.
5. Before eating, preparing food, or preparing drinks.
6. After contact with any player or player equipment.
7. After collecting specimens (eg, urine).
8. After cleaning or disinfecting equipment.

WORK PRACTICE CONTROLS

Never bring food into or eat in locations where infectious materials may be present, including training rooms, examination rooms, and procedure rooms.

All employees with potential exposure to BBP should receive the hepatitis B vaccine. At this time, no vaccines exist for hepatitis C or HIV.

EDUCATION

Per OSHA standards, employees must receive annual education on strategies to prevent exposures to BBP. Employees in our facility will receive this education via _____.

Plan for Blood or Body Fluid Exposures

In the event of exposure during a job-related duty, the following procedure should be followed:

1. Treat the site of exposure as soon as possible
    a. For exposures to the skin, wash the site of exposure with soap and water
    b. Flush exposed mucous membranes with water
    c. Flush eye mucosa with saline
2. Do not apply caustic agents or disinfectants
3. Report the incident

All exposures to blood and body fluid involving mucous membranes or nonintact skin that occur at this facility must be evaluated by medical professionals to determine if postexposure prophylaxis and/or other therapy is required. Mucous membranes include the membranes of the eyes, nose, and mouth.

Injury Type	Pathogen		
	Hepatitis B	Hepatitis C	HIV
Intact skin	No action	No action	No action
Mucous membrane	Evaluation required	No action	No action
Penetrating injury	Evaluation required	Evaluation required	Evaluation required

For events with "evaluation required," the treatment plan is dependent on a number of factors: if exposure source is known to have an infection, if the exposed individual has been vaccinated for hepatitis B, and the severity of exposure.

During this process, blood testing may be required for the source patient.

Members of our team and staff will receive postexposure evaluation by calling the "needlestick hotline" as outlined below:

Affiliated Medical Center: _____

Affiliated Medical Center "Needlestick Hotline": _____

In the event that we cannot contact the hotline outlined above, we will call the CDC exposure prophylaxis hotline at *1-888-448-4911* (available 24 hours a day).

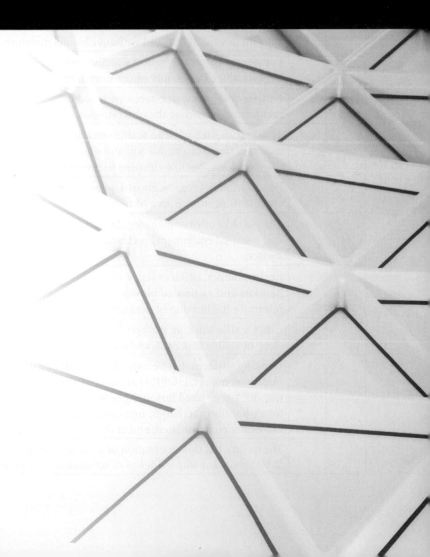

Appendix 2 – Checklists

Appendix 2A Checklist: Recommendations for Laundry Best Practices—Facilities Standards

This checklist of best practices should be completed by your laundry service or whomever in your team staff is laundering athletic textiles.

YES	NO	STANDARD
		The laundry facility's physical layout ensures an efficient workflow for processing of soiled textiles to clean textiles.
		The laundry facility's maintenance procedures minimize environmental contamination and protect the material and hygienic integrity of the processed textiles.
		Handwashing facilities are located in all work areas and in personnel support areas (laundry room, offices, dirty laundry area, clean laundry storage area, etc).
		Emergency eyewash equipment is available with unobstructed access (ie, requiring no more than 10 sec to reach) in all areas where soiled textiles are processed.
		The textile staging and storage areas for cleaned, processed textiles are free of vermin; devoid of lint; and without obvious moisture contamination.
		Policies and protocols reflect a facility-specific strategy for ensuring the hygienically clean quality of the stored, processed textiles.
		Policies and protocols establish a schedule of visual inspection of the stored textiles and recording the observations.
		The bottom shelf of clean textile storage is made of solid, nonporous material, free from visible soil and dirt, and at a minimum of 8 inches from the floor for accessible cleaning to prevent contamination.
		Porous material (eg, cardboard, paper, etc) is not used as a shelf liner in the clean textiles storage area or to store clean textiles.
		The physical environment (eg, floors, walls, ceilings, vents, working surfaces, and installed equipment) is cleaned on a regular schedule appropriate for the surface.
		Environmental surfaces (eg, walls, ceilings, vents, and equipment) undergo periodic and as-needed blowdown processes from ceiling downward to minimize the buildup of dust and lint.
		Clean textile working surfaces (eg, counters, benches, tables, etc) are kept clean of visible soil, dust, and lint.
		Working surfaces that become contaminated with blood or other potentially infectious material (OPIM) are decontaminated, cleaned, and disinfected with EPA-registered hospital-grade disinfectants after completion of soiled textile handling activities; immediately or as soon as feasible when surfaces are visibly contaminated; and at the end of the work shift.
		The facility has documentation of a current integrated pest management (IPM) program with evidence of scheduled treatments.

		Facility documents include evidence of compliance with local regulations or the authority having jurisdiction (AHJ) as they pertain to air, water, and chemicals management, if applicable.
		Wastewater and/or air quality permit compliance is documented, if applicable.
		Compliance with hazardous chemical (eg, hydrogen peroxide) regulations (ie, Department of Homeland Security Chemical Security Assessment Tool [CSAT], local hazardous materials license or permit) is documented and available for review, if applicable.

Appendix 2B Checklist: Recommendations for Laundry Best Practices—Equipment Standards

This checklist of best practices should be completed by whomever services the laundry equipment at your facility.

YES	NO	STANDARD
		Equipment safety documentation includes safety instructions that describe the potential hazards associated with the equipment use; appropriate safeguards; and complies with American National Standards Institute (ANSI) Z8.1. (Commercial Laundry and Dry Cleaning Equipment and Operations—Safety Requirements) regarding safe operation and maintenance of equipment.
		Maintenance personnel have access to equipment manuals to inform them on installation, operation, preventive maintenance, repairs, replacements, and illustrations of the equipment components.
		The laundry service provides evidence and documentation of an ongoing maintenance program, including work orders and a current inspection tag if one has been issued from inspection.
		Equipment preventive maintenance is documented and kept on file.
		Equipment installation involves trained or qualified installers, appropriate utilities and support services, compliance with the equipment manufacturer's instructions, and properly functioning safety equipment specified by the manufacturer.
		The performance of each piece of equipment meets the manufacturer's specifications prior to use following installation or servicing.
		Machinery connected to utilities appears to be properly installed and operating correctly.
		The laundry service or facility can ensure that all equipment is safely and correctly connected to utilities (ie, water, electrical power, gas, and/or steam) as appropriate and that the connection includes the proper controls for the incoming utilities.
		The laundry service or facility has assessed whether pretreatment of the water to be used for processing is needed and, if necessary, the appropriate type of pretreatment is performed.
		If pretreatment is performed, compatibility between the pretreatment and chemicals to be used in processing is documented.
		If the water hardness is 2 grains/gallon (34.2 parts per million [ppm]) or higher, the water is softened.
		Mechanical systems function according to manufacturer's specifications, including, but not limited to, valve openings and closures, water level in inches for each level setting, tilting for loading and unloading, temperature sensor design, correct operational safety features, and speed and direction of drum rotation.
		Automated controls are verified, calibrated, and checked at least annually.
		The performance of the chemical delivery system is checked at least monthly by verifying chemical delivery rates (eg, correct chemical delivered in correct amount during the correct cycle) and/or by conducting chemical titrations (eg, activity, concentration, and loading).

Appendix 2C Checklist: Recommendations for Laundry Best Practices—Personnel Standards

This checklist of best practices should be completed by whomever oversees personnel who handle athletic textiles.

YES	NO	STANDARD
		Personnel involved in processing of laundry receive standard safety training in all aspects of laundry operations applicable to their respective position(s), including, but not limited to, safe operations of equipment per manufacturer's instructions and notification procedures when malfunctions occur.
		The laundry service or facility sorts and processes textiles used for environmental cleaning and disinfection (eg, cleaning cloths, microfiber cloths, mop heads, etc) in separate wash loads from textiles intended for player or staff use.
		The laundry service or facility has policies and procedures to prevent athletic textiles from being handled by or exposure to personnel with potential health issues (ie, illness, open wounds or sores, and skin injuries).
		Personnel adhere to good work practices to minimize or eliminate exposures to blood, other potentially infectious material (OPIM), chemical, and mechanical hazards. This includes, but is not limited to, use of personal protective equipment (PPE) when handling contaminated and soiled textiles and understanding safe operation of equipment.
		Eating, drinking, smoking, applying cosmetics or lip balm, and handling contact lenses are prohibited in work areas where there is a reasonable likelihood of occupational exposure to bloodborne pathogens (BBPs).
		Personnel handle chemicals safely in accordance with Safety Data Sheets (SDSs) in the laundry facility.
		SDS information is readily accessible to personnel in a location for immediate access where chemicals are handled.
		Personnel who are exposed to hazards (eg, biological, chemical, mechanical, etc) report such occurrences to their supervisor according to the provider's policies and procedures.
		Personnel wash their hands after restroom use; before eating; when hands become inadvertently contaminated with blood, OPIM, or other body substances; before donning gloves; and after removal of gloves.

Appendix 2D Sample Autoclave Sheet

DATE	ITEMS STERILIZED	STERILIZATION TIME	TIME		ELAPSED TIME	MAX TEMP	MAX PRESSURE	QC CHECKS				TECH
			IN	OUT				TAPE	CLOCK	SPORE +/−	SPORE REF #	

Index

Appendix 3 – Cards

CELLULITIS

Bacterial infection of the upper skin layers

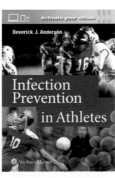

© Wolters Kluwer. All Rights Reserved.

Wolters Kluwer

CELLULITIS

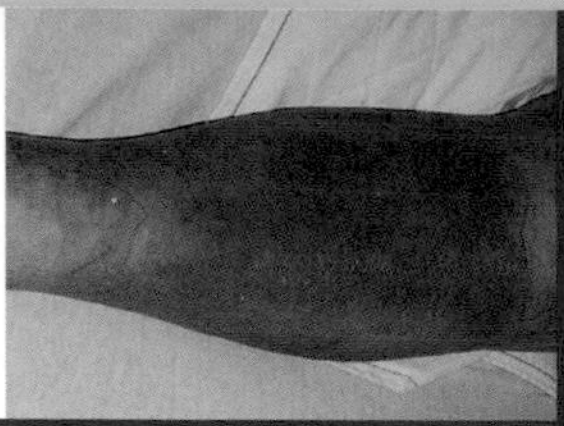

CAREER STATISTICS

➤ More than 20 million cases each year
➤ Common infection in athletes
➤ Can occur on any area of the body

CAREER HIGHLIGHTS

➤ Causes redness and pain
➤ No pus
➤ Serious infections may be accompanied by fever and other symptoms
➤ Most commonly caused by *Streptococci* and *Staphylococci*
➤ Skin injuries and chronic skin conditions (eg, eczema or athlete's foot) are risk factors for this common infection

Figure A3A.1 Bacterial infection of the upper skin layers. (Reproduced with permission from: Berg D, Worzala K. *Atlas of Adult Physical Diagnosis*. Philadelphia: Lippincott Williams & Wilkins; 2006. Copyright © 2006 Lippincott Williams & Wilkins.)

Appendix 3B

MRSA

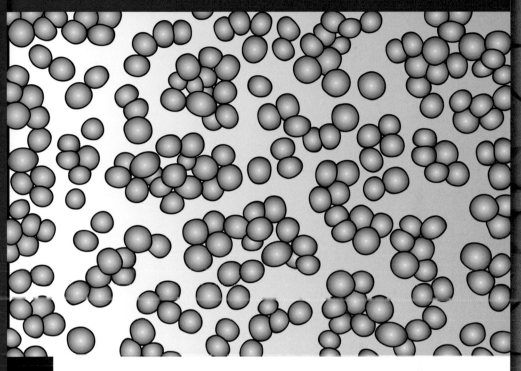

Methicillin-resistant *Staphylococcus aureus*

© Wolters Kluwer. All Rights Reserved.

Activate your eBook

Deverick J. Anderson

Infection
Prevention
in Athletes

Wolters Kluwer

Wolters Kluwer

MRSA

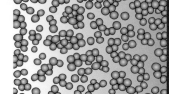

CAREER STATISTICS

- ➤ #1 antibiotic-resistant bacteria
- ➤ 4–22% of athletes are colonized with MRSA
- ➤ Increasingly common in community settings

CAREER HIGHLIGHTS

- ➤ Leading cause of pus
- ➤ Common cause of skin infections in athletes but can cause many other types of infection
- ➤ Can cause mild or very serious infections
- ➤ Transmissible between players, typically by skin-to-skin contact

Figure A3B.1 Methicillin-resistant *Staphylococcus aureus*.

ABSCESS

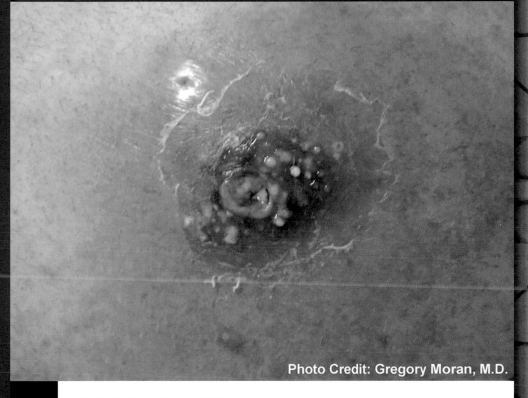

Photo Credit: Gregory Moran, M.D.

Skin infection with pus

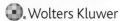

© Wolters Kluwer. All Rights Reserved.

ABSCESS

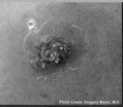

Photo Credit: Gregory Moran, M.D.

CAREER STATISTICS

- ➤ 60% to 70% caused by MRSA
- ➤ Most common in young men between 18 and 40 years
- ➤ More than 1.5 million abscesses occur each year in the United States

CAREER HIGHLIGHTS

- ➤ Pus accompanied by pain and redness
- ➤ Typically requires drainage of pus and antibiotic treatment
- ➤ Many names and varieties, including folliculitis, furunculosis, and carbuncle
- ➤ Cover skin lesion until healed

Figure A3C.1 Skin infection with pus. (Photo credit: Gregory Moran, MD.)

HERPES GLADIATORUM

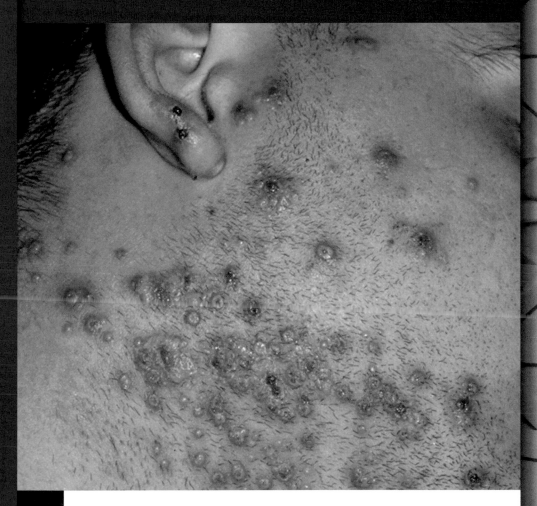

Herpes infection of the skin

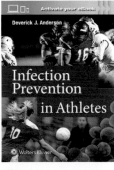

© Wolters Kluwer. All Rights Reserved.

Wolters Kluwer

HERPES GLADIATORUM

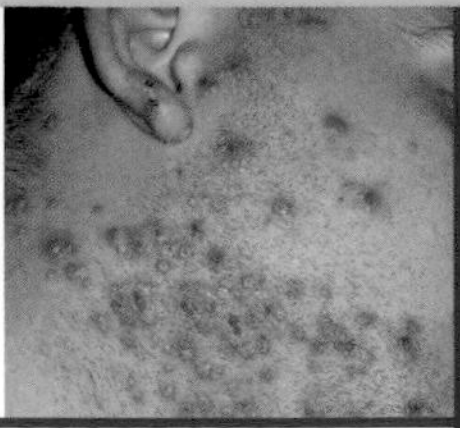

CAREER STATISTICS

- More than 50% of people have herpes simplex virus (HSV)
- Unique infection in athletes
- Incubation period is 4 to 11 days

CAREER HIGHLIGHTS

- Occurs when HSV enters scratches or breaks in skin (typically from saliva)
- Often mistaken for bacterial skin infection
- Most common in wrestlers but can occur in any contact-sport athlete

Figure A3D.1 Herpes infection of the skin. (Reprinted with permission from Craft N, Fox LP, Goldsmith LA, et al. *VisualDx: Essential Adult Dermatology*. Philadelphia, PA: Wolters Kluwer Health; 2010.)

HAND, FOOT, AND MOUTH DISEASE

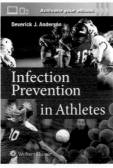

Typical lesions of HFMD are red and some have central clearing

© Wolters Kluwer. All Rights Reserved.

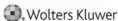

Wolters Kluwer

HAND, FOOT, AND MOUTH DISEASE

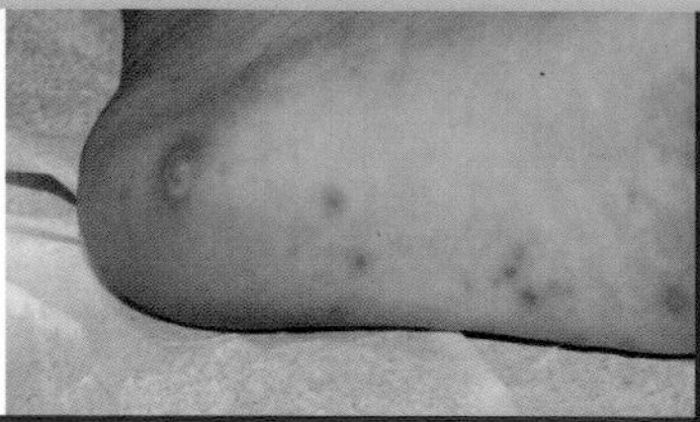

CAREER STATISTICS

➤ Increasingly common
➤ Symptoms last 2 to 7 days

CAREER HIGHLIGHTS

➤ Typically mild illness
➤ Most common in summer and fall
➤ Children may have lesions in mouth; adults probably won't
➤ Spread by fecal-oral route
➤ Highly transmissible

Figure A3E.1 Hand, foot, and mouth disease. (Reprinted with permission from Goodheart HP, Gonzalez ME. *Goodheart's Photoguide to Common Pediatric and Adult Skin Disorders*. 4th ed. Philadelphia, PA: Wolters Kluwer; 2015.)

TINEA

Fungal infection of the skin

© Wolters Kluwer. All Rights Reserved.

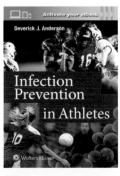

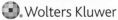

TINEA

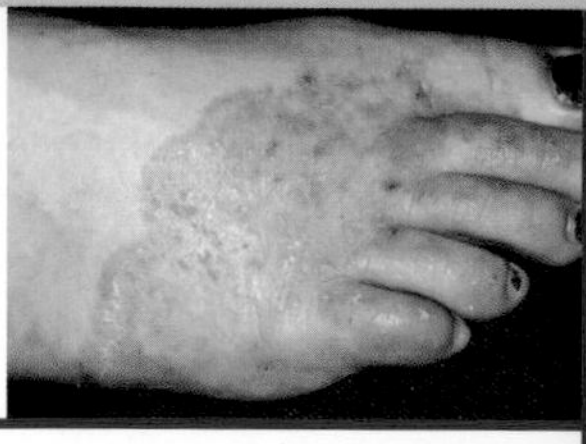

CAREER STATISTICS

➤ Causes more than 25% of skin infections in athletes
➤ Symptoms are persistent; treatment can be prolonged

CAREER HIGHLIGHTS

➤ Leads to localized scaly, red rash
➤ Often itchy and painful
➤ Can occur in multiple locations, most common is on foot (tinea pedis)
➤ Predisposes to bacterial skin infection
➤ Wear sandals in the locker room shower to avoid the infection

Figure A3F.1 Fungal infection of the skin. (Reprinted with permission from Chung EK, Atkinson-McEvoy LR, Lai NL, Terry M. *Visual Diagnosis and Treatment in Pediatrics*. 3rd ed. Philadelphia, PA: Wolters Kluwer Health; 2014.)

HEPATITIS A AND B

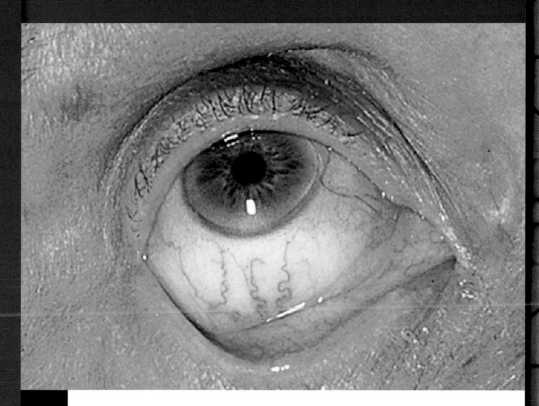

Viral infections of the liver

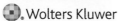

Infection
Prevention
in Athletes

Deverick J. Anderson

Wolters Kluwer

© Wolters Kluwer. All Rights Reserved.

HEPATITIS A AND B

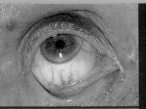

CAREER STATISTICS

- ➤ Vaccination has led to a big decrease in incidence
- ➤ Many outbreaks of hepatitis A have occurred in the last several years
  - More than 27,000 cases have occurred since 2016, leading to 16,000 hospitalizations and almost 300 deaths
- ➤ Hepatitis B infection is common throughout the world but much less common in the United States

CAREER HIGHLIGHTS

- ➤ Both viruses are vaccine preventable
- ➤ Hepatitis A is typically acquired through contaminated food via fecal-oral route
  - Hepatitis A is shed in stool for weeks
- ➤ Hepatitis B is typically acquired through blood or body fluid exposure
- ➤ Hepatitis B can lead to chronic infection of the liver
- ➤ Accompanied by fever, jaundice, decreased energy, and abdominal pain

Figure A3G.1 Viral infections of the liver. (Used with permission from Bickley LS, Szilagyi P. *Bates' Guide to Physical Examination and History Taking*. 8th ed. Philadelphia, PA: Lippincott Williams & Wilkins; 2003:147.)

NOROVIRUS

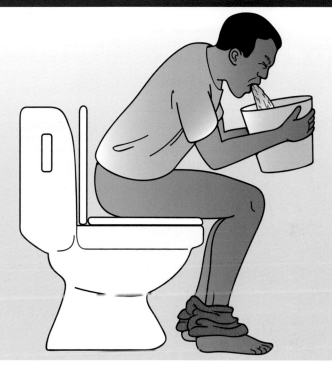

Leading cause of vomiting and diarrhea

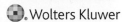

© Wolters Kluwer. All Rights Reserved.

. Wolters Kluwer

NOROVIRUS

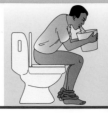

CAREER STATISTICS

➤ Highly infectious; exposure to 100 viral particles can lead to infection
➤ Peaks in the winter but can occur sporadically throughout the year
➤ Symptoms typically last less than 72 hours
➤ Quick incubation period (<48 hours)

CAREER HIGHLIGHTS

➤ Infection leads to nausea, vomiting, diarrhea, abdominal pain and cramping, and sometimes fever
➤ Children are key source of transmission
➤ Outbreaks often occur through contaminated food or among people in close proximity via the fecal-oral route
➤ Not eliminated by standard disinfectants. Need to use bleach- or hydrogen peroxide–based disinfectants to eliminate from environmental surfaces

Figure A3H.1 Leading cause of vomiting and diarrhea.

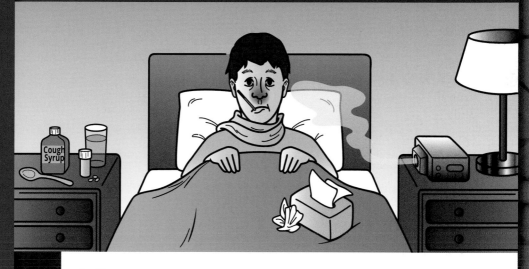

Influenza

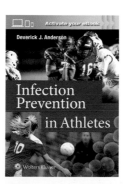

© Wolters Kluwer. All Rights Reserved.

Wolters Kluwer

THE FLU

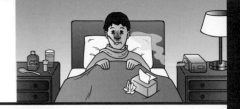

CAREER STATISTICS

➤ Veteran player—has caused human infections for centuries
➤ Causes 10 to 50 million infections each year in the United States
➤ "Flu season" typically lasts from November to March and typically peaks in January
➤ Symptoms can last for more than a week

CAREER HIGHLIGHTS

➤ Flu transmission typically occurs through exposure to respiratory droplets when infected people cough, sneeze, or talk. Less often, flu can be transmitted on contaminated surfaces
➤ Vaccines are imperfect but remain the best prevention strategy
➤ Classic "flu" symptoms include fevers, chills, muscle aches, joint pain, headache, fatigue, nonproductive cough, sore throat, and runny nose
➤ Influenza infection will decrease respiratory and overall performance

Figure A31.1 Influenza.

MONO

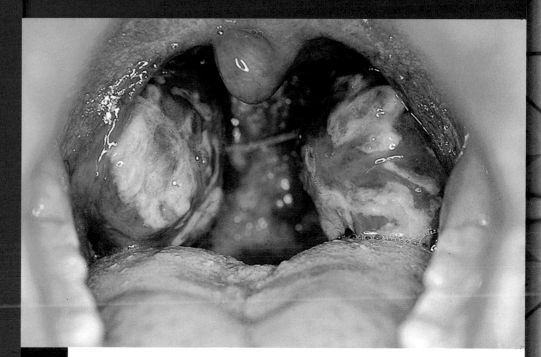

Infectious mononucleosis or "the kissing disease" is caused by Epstein-Barr virus (EBV)

© Wolters Kluwer. All Rights Reserved.

Activate your eBook

Deverick J. Anderson

Infection Prevention in Athletes

Wolters Kluwer

Wolters Kluwer

MONO

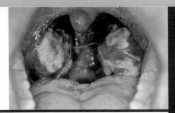

CAREER STATISTICS

➤ More than 3 million cases in the United States each year
➤ Frequently in the game—90% of the world's population has been infected with Epstein-Barr virus (EBV) during childhood
➤ Highest risk occurs from late teens to early 20s
➤ Source of exposure can be difficult to determine, as the incubation period can be up to 4 to 7 weeks

CAREER HIGHLIGHTS

➤ Transmitted through body fluids such as saliva
➤ Leads to fatigue, fever, rash, swollen lymph nodes, enlarged tonsils, and an enlarged spleen
➤ Athletes are typically held out of competition until the spleen is no longer enlarged

Figure A3J.1 Infectious mononucleosis or "the kissing disease" is caused by Epstein-Barr virus (EBV). (Reprinted with permission from Hatfield NT. *Introductory Maternity and Pediatric Nursing*. 3rd ed. Philadelphia, PA: Wolters Kluwer Health; 2013.)

WHOOPING COUGH

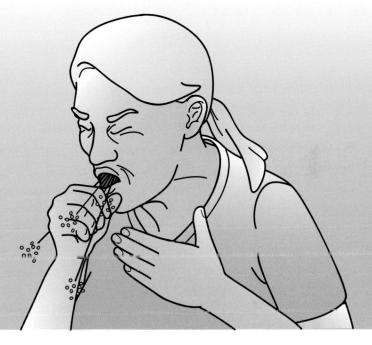

Coughing spell that leads to vomiting? Think pertussis (*Bordetella pertussis*)

© Wolters Kluwer. All Rights Reserved.

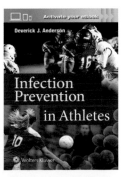

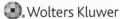

WHOOPING COUGH

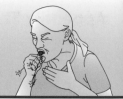

CAREER STATISTICS

➤ More common than people think; 2 million cases occur each year in the United States
➤ Once labeled as a "childhood disease," more than 60% of cases now occur in adults
➤ Incubation period is typically 5 to 10 days
➤ Symptoms can be prolonged (weeks) without treatment

CAREER HIGHLIGHTS

➤ Immunization is the leading prevention strategy but immunity from the vaccine wanes over time
➤ Recent guidelines recommend a vaccine booster (Tdap) after childhood
➤ Infection typically progresses from mild (fatigue, mild cough, runny nose, sometimes fever) to more severe (severe coughing paroxysms that often lead to vomiting)
➤ Athletes with pertussis may miss more than a week of playing time

Figure A3K.1 Coughing spell that leads to vomiting? Think pertussis (*Bordetella pertussis*).

TUBERCULOSIS

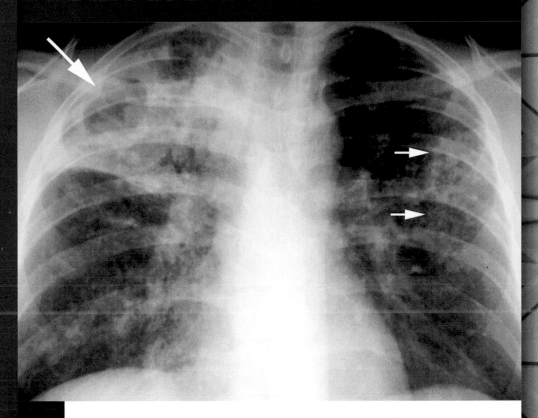

Tuberculosis (*Mycobacterium tuberculosis*) leads to cavitary lung lesions (arrows)

© Wolters Kluwer. All Rights Reserved.

Activate your eBook

Deverick J. Anderson

Infection Prevention in Athletes

Wolters Kluwer

Wolters Kluwer

TUBERCULOSIS

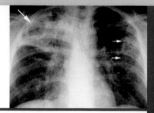

CAREER STATISTICS

➤ Fights for the #1 infection ranking in the world
➤ Nearly one of every three people in the world has been infected with tuberculosis (TB)
➤ Rare in the United States (<200,000 cases each year)

CAREER HIGHLIGHTS

➤ Most cases occur in people who have lived in countries where the infection is more common
➤ TB can persist quietly in the lungs for years after exposure ("latent TB")
➤ Latent TB is not contagious but can convert to active TB
➤ Active TB is contagious, as TB can spread to others via aerosols from coughing
➤ Active TB infection is typically in the lungs but can cause infection in just about any part of the body
➤ Treatment of TB is complicated and often overseen by the Health Department

Figure A3L.1 Tuberculosis (*Mycobacterium tuberculosis*). (Reprinted with permission from Webb RW, Higgins CB. *Thoracic Imaging*. 3rd ed. Philadelphia, PA: Wolters Kluwer Health; 2016.)

CHICKEN POX

Varicella zoster virus (VZV)

© Wolters Kluwer. All Rights Reserved.

Wolters Kluwer

CHICKEN POX

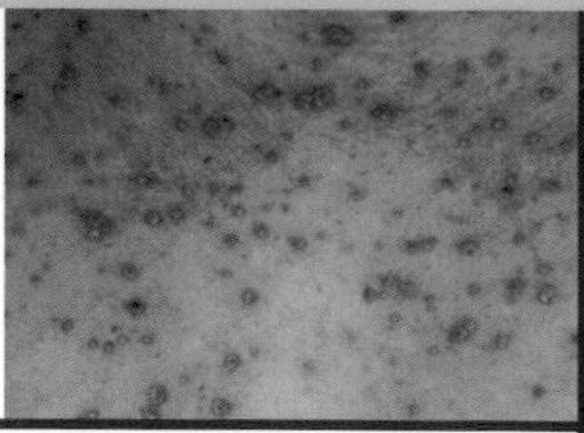

CAREER STATISTICS

➤ Previously ubiquitous during childhood, now fewer than 200,000 cases occur each year in the United States
➤ Great reduction in cases since vaccine introduced in the 1990s
➤ Two doses of vaccination lead to >90% immunity
➤ Incubation period is 1 to 2 weeks
➤ Symptoms last up to a week

CAREER HIGHLIGHTS

➤ Infection leads to fever, fatigue, headache, and rash
➤ Tell-tale rash typically includes between 250 and 500 itchy, blister-like lesions
➤ Highly contagious
➤ No longer contagious once pox have dried up or "crusted over"
➤ Can occasionally cause severe infections of the lungs, particularly in adults who become infected

Figure A3M.1 Varicella zoster virus (VZV). (Reprinted with permission from DeLong L, Burkhart NW. *General and Oral Pathology for the Dental Hygienist*. 3rd ed. Philadelphia, PA: Wolters Kluwer Health; 2018.)

MEASLES

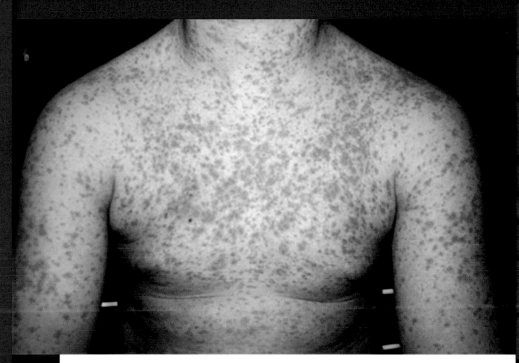

Comeback player of the year

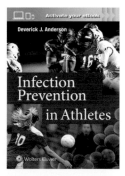

© Wolters Kluwer. All Rights Reserved.

. Wolters Kluwer

MEASLES

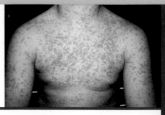

CAREER STATISTICS

➤ Declared to be eradicated from the United States in 2000, the number of measles cases in the United States in 2019 is the highest of the last 2 decades
➤ One of the top ranked players for contagiousness; 9 of 10 unvaccinated people exposed to a sick individual will become infected
➤ The incubation period lasts 7 to 21 days

CAREER HIGHLIGHTS

➤ Early infection includes fever and the 3Cs (cough, coryza [runny nose], and conjunctivitis)
  • Infection can be severe or life-threatening
➤ The tell-tale rash occurs 3 to 7 days after onset of symptoms
➤ Vaccination remains the #1 strategy for prevention
➤ Two doses of vaccination are 97% effective
➤ Requires "herd immunity" for complete protection. Unfortunately, herd immunity is decreasing as people refuse vaccination

Figure A3N.1 Characteristic measles rash. (Courtesy of Kathleen Cronan, MD. Reprinted with permission from Chung E. *Visual Diagnosis in Pediatrics.* 3rd ed. Philadelphia, PA: Wolters Kluwer; 2014.)

MUMPS

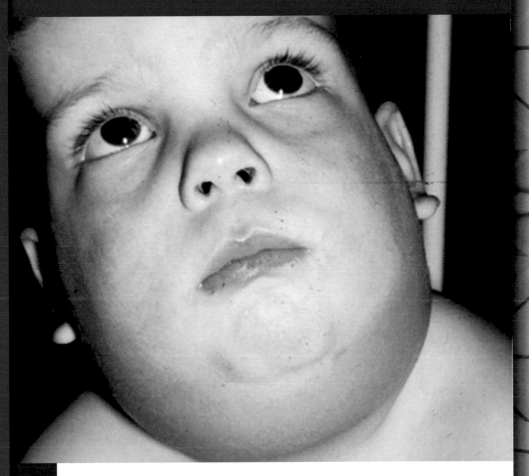

Swollen tender cheeks or parotid glands? Think mumps

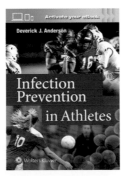

Activate your eBook

Deverick J. Anderson

Infection
Prevention
in Athletes

Wolters Kluwer

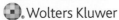. Wolters Kluwer

© Wolters Kluwer. All Rights Reserved.

MUMPS

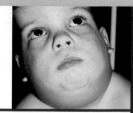

CAREER STATISTICS

➤ Vaccination led to a 99% decrease in incidence
➤ Increasing number of cases and outbreaks in the last 15 years due to declining vaccination rates and declining herd immunity
➤ Incubation period is approximately 17 days
➤ Symptoms persist 4 to 10 days

CAREER HIGHLIGHTS

➤ Highly infectious through saliva or respiratory secretions
➤ Infection typically causes fever, headache, fatigue, and muscle aches; the characteristic parotid gland swelling begins 1 to 2 days after symptom onset
➤ Vaccination is #1 prevention strategy
➤ Two doses of vaccination are 88% effective
➤ Requires "herd immunity" for complete protection

Figure A30.1 Swollen tender cheeks or parotid glands? Think mumps. (Reprinted with permission from Kyle T, Carman S. *Essentials of Pediatric Nursing*. 3rd ed. Philadelphia, PA: Wolters Kluwer; 2016.)

HIV

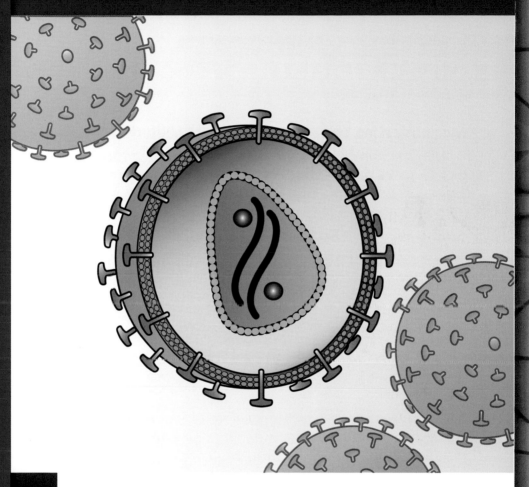

Human immunodeficiency virus

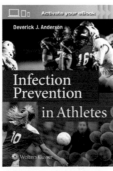

© Wolters Kluwer. All Rights Reserved.

. Wolters Kluwer

HIV

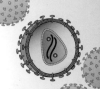

CAREER STATISTICS

➤ Approximately 1 million people in the United States have human immunodeficiency virus (HIV) infection
➤ 14% of people with HIV infection don't know they have the virus
➤ African Americans have the highest number of new HIV infections of any race or ethnic group tracked by the CDC

CAREER HIGHLIGHTS

➤ Acute HIV leads to a influenza-like illness including fevers, chills, rash, night sweats, muscle aches, sore throat, fatigue, swollen lymph nodes, or mouth ulcers
➤ Spreads through contact with infected body fluids (blood, semen, vaginal fluid, rectal fluids, breast milk)
➤ Does NOT spread through saliva
➤ If untreated, HIV destroys part of the immune system and can lead to AIDS and death

Figure A3P.1 Human immunodeficiency virus.